Improving
the Quality of
Long-Term Care

Gooloo S. Wunderlich and Peter O. Kohler, *Editors*

Committee on Improving Quality in Long-Term Care

Division of Health Care Services

INSTITUTE OF MEDICINE

NATIONAL ACADEMY PRESS
Washington, D.C.

NATIONAL ACADEMY PRESS • 2101 Constitution Avenue, N.W. • Washington, DC 20418

NOTICE: The project that is the subject of this report was approved by the Governing Board of the National Research Council, whose members are drawn from the councils of the National Academy of Sciences, the National Academy of Engineering, and the Institute of Medicine. The members of the committee responsible for the report were chosen for their special competences and with regard for appropriate balance.

Support for this project was provided by the Robert Wood Johnson Foundation, the Archstone Fund, Irvine Health Foundation, Department of Veterans Affairs, and Health Care Financing Administration. The views presented in this report are those of the Institute of Medicine Committee on Improving Quality in Long-Term Care and are not necessarily those of the funding agencies.

Library of Congress Cataloging-in-Publication Data

Institute of Medicine (U.S.). Committee on Improving Quality in Long-Term Care,
    Improving the quality of long-term care / Gooloo S. Wunderlich and Peter Kohler,
    editors ; Committee on Improving Quality in Long-Term Care, Division of Health Care
    Services, Institute of Medicine.
        p. ; cm.
    Includes bibliographical references and index.
    ISBN 0-309-06498-8
        1. Long-term care facilites—Quality control. 2. Long-term care of the sick—Quality
    control. 3. Quality assurance. 4. Nursing homes—Quality control. I. Wunderlich, Gooloo
    S. II. Kohler, Peter O., 1938- III. Title
        [DNLM: 1. Long-Term Care—United States. 2. Outcome and Process Assessment
    (Health Care)—United States. 3. Quality Assurance, Health Care—United States. W 84.7
    I587 20001]
    RA997 .I57 2001
    362.1′6′0685—dc21
                                                        00-067864

Additional copies of this report are available for sale from the National Academy Press, 2101 Constitution Avenue, N.W., Box 285, Washington, D.C. 20055. Call (800) 624-6242 or (202) 334-3313 (in the Washington metropolitan area), or visit the NAP's home page at **www.nap.edu.**

For more information about the Institute of Medicine, visit the IOM home page at **www.iom.edu.**

The serpent has been a symbol of long life, healing, and knowledge among almost all cultures and religions since the beginning of recorded history. The serpent adopted as a logotype by the Institute of Medicine is a relief carving from ancient Greece, now held by the Staatliche Museen in Berlin.

*"Knowing is not enough; we must apply.
Willing is not enough; we must do."*
—Goethe

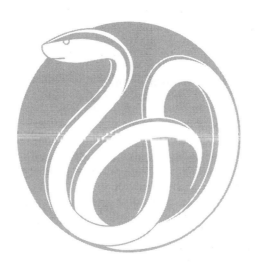

INSTITUTE OF MEDICINE

Shaping the Future for Health

THE NATIONAL ACADEMIES

National Academy of Sciences
National Academy of Engineering
Institute of Medicine
National Research Council

The **National Academy of Sciences** is a private, nonprofit, self-perpetuating society of distinguished scholars engaged in scientific and engineering research, dedicated to the furtherance of science and technology and to their use for the general welfare. Upon the authority of the charter granted to it by the Congress in 1863, the Academy has a mandate that requires it to advise the federal government on scientific and technical matters. Dr. Bruce M. Alberts is president of the National Academy of Sciences.

The **National Academy of Engineering** was established in 1964, under the charter of the National Academy of Sciences, as a parallel organization of outstanding engineers. It is autonomous in its administration and in the selection of its members, sharing with the National Academy of Sciences the responsibility for advising the federal government. The National Academy of Engineering also sponsors engineering programs aimed at meeting national needs, encourages education and research, and recognizes the superior achievements of engineers. Dr. William A. Wulf is president of the National Academy of Engineering.

The **Institute of Medicine** was established in 1970 by the National Academy of Sciences to secure the services of eminent members of appropriate professions in the examination of policy matters pertaining to the health of the public. The Institute acts under the responsibility given to the National Academy of Sciences by its congressional charter to be an adviser to the federal government and, upon its own initiative, to identify issues of medical care, research, and education. Dr. Kenneth I. Shine is president of the Institute of Medicine.

The **National Research Council** was organized by the National Academy of Sciences in 1916 to associate the broad community of science and technology with the Academy's purposes of furthering knowledge and advising the federal government. Functioning in accordance with general policies determined by the Academy, the Council has become the principal operating agency of both the National Academy of Sciences and the National Academy of Engineering in providing services to the government, the public, and the scientific and engineering communities. The Council is administered jointly by both Academies and the Institute of Medicine. Dr. Bruce M. Alberts and Dr. William A. Wulf are chairman and vice chairman, respectively, of the National Research Council.

COMMITTEE ON IMPROVING QUALITY IN LONG-TERM CARE

PETER O. KOHLER (*Chair*), President, Oregon Health Sciences University

RICHARD DELLA PENNA, Regional Elder Care Coordinator, Southern California Permanente Group, Kaiser Permanente

PENNY HOLLANDER FELDMAN, Director, Center for Home Care Policy and Research, Vice President, Research and Evaluation, Visiting Nurse Service of New York

JANET GEORGE, Former Vice President, Quality Improvement, Manor Care, Inc., Gaithersburg, Maryland

CHARLENE A. HARRINGTON, Department of Social and Behavior Sciences, University of California

ROSALIE A. KANE, Director, National LTC Resource Center, University of Minnesota

VINCE MOR, Director, Center for Gerontology and Health Care Research, Brown University

VIVIAN OMAGBEMI, Program Manager, Health and Human Services, Aging and Disability Services, Montgomery County, Maryland

JAMES PERRIN, Associate Professor of Pediatrics, Harvard Medical School, Director, Division of General Pediatrics, and Director, MGH Center for Child and Adolescent Health Policy, Massachusetts General Hospital for Children, Boston

LAURIE E. POWERS, Associate Professor and Co-Director of the Center on Self-Determination, Oregon Health Sciences University

ELLEN REAP, Vice President, Senior Living Services, Adventist Health Care, Rockville, Maryland

JOHN F. SCHNELLE, UCLA/Jewish Home Borun Center, Sepulvada VA Hospital, Reseda, California

PAUL M. SCHYVE, Senior Vice President, Joint Commission on Accreditation of Healthcare Organizations, Oakbrook Terrace, Illinois

ERIC TANGALOS, Professor of Medicine and Chair, Division of Community Internal Medicine, Mayo Clinic, Rochester, Minnesota

ARTHUR Y. WEBB, President and CEO, Village Care of New York/Village Center for Care, Inc.

JOSHUA M. WIENER, Principle Research Associate, The Urban Institute, Washington, D.C.

KEREN BROWN WILSON, Former President and CEO, Assisted Living Concepts, Inc., Portland, Oregon

Acknowledgments

The Institute of Medicine (IOM) Committee on Improving Quality in Long-Term Care acknowledges with appreciation the many persons and organizations, not all of whom can be individually listed, who contributed to the success of the study.

The primary support for this study was provided by the Robert Wood Johnson Foundation. Generous support was also provided by the Archstone Foundation, Irvine Health Foundation, Department of Veterans Affairs, and Health Care Financing Administration.

Many individuals shared unselfishly with the committee the results of their work and background information from their organizations. The committee appreciates the organizations and individuals that presented testimony at a public hearing. These individuals are listed in Appendix A.

During the course of the study the committee held meetings at which experts made thoughtful presentations on various aspects of the committee's mandate. The presenters are listed in Appendix A; their contribution of time and knowledge is appreciated.

We are grateful to the authors of the commissioned papers prepared for the study. Their names and the subjects of their papers are listed in Chapter 1. The papers were used by staff and committee to guide them in drafting the report.

A number of people within IOM provided support and assistance to the study committee. The committee acknowledges with gratitude their contributions. Marilyn Field served as study director until May 1999. Many other staff assisted her and the committee at various times and in various capacities. Kay Harris and later Jennifer Cangco (since March 2000) helped keep our budget in order. Claudia Carl managed the logistics of the report review process, and Mike Edington shepherded the report through the editing and production process. Sally Stanfield at the National Academy Press was supportive as always.

We also acknowledge Janet Corrigan, Director, Division of Health Care Services, for her support in a difficult time by providing staff from her division to complete the study. We are grateful to Nicole Amado and Kathleen Nolan for their enormous efforts in staffing the study through its completion. They cheerfully labored over 30 pages of references correcting them and making the citations and references consistent and the text accurate, developing the charts and tables in the report, and reviewing and editing the report drafts for accuracy and style under very tight deadlines. We appreciate Nicole's meticulous work formatting the manuscript for prepublication release.

Finally we would like to thank Gooloo Wunderlich for the enormous contribution she made to this study. Gooloo's professionalism, knowledge, and extraordinary commitment were critical to resolving many policy and technical issues and completing the study.

Reviewers

The report was reviewed by individuals chosen for their diverse perspectives and technical expertise in accordance with procedures approved by the National Research Council's Report Review Committee. The purpose of this independent review is to provide candid and critical comments to assist the authors and the Institute of Medicine in making the published report as sound as possible and to ensure that the report meets institutional standards for objectivity, evidence, and responsiveness to the study charge. The content of the review comments and the draft manuscript remain confidential to protect the integrity of the deliberative process. The committee wishes to thank the following individuals for their participation in the report review process:

Floyd Bloom, Chairman, Department of Neuropharmacology, The
Scripps Research Institute, La Jolla, California
Robert Butler, President and Chief Executive Officer, International
Longevity Center-USA, Ltd., New York City
Karen Davis, President, The Commonwealth Fund, New York City
Toby Edelman, Attorney, National Senior Citizens Law Center,
Washington, D.C.
Catherine Hawes, Senior Research Scientist, Myers Research Institute,
Menorah Park Center for the Aging, Beachwood, Ohio
Susan Hughes, Professor, Health Research and Policy Centers,
University of Illinois at Chicago

Mathey Mezey, Director, The John A. Hartford Foundation Institute for
the Advancement of Geriatric Nursing Practice, New York University

Robert J. Newcomer, Professor and Chair, Department of Social and
Behavioral Sciences, University of California at San Francisco

Joe Ouslander, Co-Director, The Southeast Center for Excellence in
Geriatric Medicine, Emory Clinic at Wesley Woods, Atlanta, Georgia

David R. Zimmerman, Director, Center for Health Systems Research
and Analysis, University of Wisconsin

Although the reviewers listed above have provided many constructive comments and suggestions, they were not asked to endorse the conclusions or recommendations nor did they see the final draft of the report before its release. The review of this report was overseen by Frank Sloan, Professor, Duke University, appointed by the Institute of Medicine, and Mary Jane Osborn, Professor and Head, Department of Microbiology, University of Connecticut Health Center, appointed by the NRC's Report Review committee, who were responsible for making certain that an independent examination of this report was carried out in accordance with institutional procedures and that all review comments were carefully considered. Responsibility for the final content of this report rests entirely with the authoring committee and the institution.

Contents

EXECUTIVE SUMMARY   1

1 INTRODUCTION   21
Long-Term Care Needs, 22
The IOM Study, 25
Basic Concepts and Definitions, 27
Scope and Limitations, 34

2 PROFILE OF LONG-TERM CARE   36
Characteristics of Long-Term Care Users, 38
Providers of Long-Term Care, 41
Financing Long-Term Care, 62
Coordination of Long-Term Care Services, 69
Conclusion, 72

3 STATE OF QUALITY OF LONG-TERM CARE   73
Measurement of Quality of Care, 74
Current State of Quality of Care, 76
Conclusion, 108

**4 INFORMATION SYSTEMS FOR MONITORING
QUALITY**   110
On-Line Survey and Certification Assessment Reporting
System, 112

The Resident Assessment Instrument and the Minimum Data
Set for Nursing Homes, 115
Outcome and Assessment Information Set for Home Health
Care, 120
Challenges in Using Assessment Data, 122
Assessment and Quality Monitoring Instruments for Other
Settings, 124
Incorporating Consumer Perspectives in Measurement of
Quality, 127
Measurement Considerations for Children and
Young Adults, 132
Conclusion, 134

5 **IMPROVING QUALITY THROUGH EXTERNAL
OVERSIGHT**   135
Central Role of Government, 136
Basic Standards of Quality, 140
Residential Care Facilities, 163
Home Health Agencies, 169
Home Care and Related Services, 173
The Role of Advocacy, 174
Accreditation, 178
Conclusion, 179

6 **STRENGTHENING THE CAREGIVING WORK FORCE**   180
Nursing Homes, 182
Education and Training of Staff in Nursing Homes, 196
Residential Care Settings, 202
Home Health Agency Staff, 205
Home Care, 209
Education and Training Recommendations, 210
Labor Force Issues, 211
Conclusion, 218

7 **BUILDING ORGANIZATIONAL CAPACITY**   220
Recent Initiatives to Improve Caregiving Capacity in
Long-Term Care, 220
From Rules, Data, and Guidelines to Effective Practice, 221
Quality Management Systems, 222
Organizational Capacity to Translate Knowledge into Practice, 223
Identifying Effective Interventions, 227
Care Process Implementation and Improvement, 228

Measurement Issues, 231
Improving Organizational Capacity, 233
Conclusion, 234

8 **REIMBURSING TO IMPROVE QUALITY OF CARE**   235
Reimbursement and Quality, 236
Limited Nursing Home Bed Supply and Quality of Care, 244
Conclusion, 246

9 **CLOSING REMARKS**   248

REFERENCES   253

APPENDIXES
A Committee Meetings and Presenters of Testimony, 283
B Separate Dissenting Opinions, 287

ACRONYMS   295

BIOGRAPHICAL SKETCHES OF COMMITTEE MEMBERS   299

INDEX   307

Tables and Figures

TABLES

2.1 Demographic Characteristics of Long-Term Care Users Aged 18–64 and Aged 65 and Older Living in the Community and in Nursing Homes: United States, 1994 and 1996, 39

2.2 Number of Long-Term Care Facilities and Beds: United States, 1992 and 1998, 43

2.3 Number and Percent Distribution of Nursing Homes, Beds, and Residents, by Facility Characteristics: United States, 1997, 44

2.4 Number and Percent Distribution of Certified Home Health Agencies and People Served, by Agency Characteristics: United States, 1996, 52

2.5 Total Medicaid Personal Care Services and 1915(c) Home and Community-Based Services Waivers: United States, 1997–1998, 56

2.6 Number and Percent of Selected Categories of Occupations Employed in Selected Long-Term Care Settings and in Hospitals: United States, 1998, 61

2.7 Expenditures and Source of Funds for Nursing Home and Home Health Care: United States, 1997, 64

2.8 Medicaid Payments, by Type of Service and Category of Beneficiary: United States, 1997, 66

xvi

5.1 Average Number of Deficiencies per Certified Facility and Percent of Facilities with No Deficiencies, by State: United States, 1992–1998, 146

5.2 Level of Deficiencies, Based on Scope and Severity of Substandard Care, and the Remedy Categories Available to States for Each Level of Deficiency, 155

6.1 Nursing Staff Levels per Resident Day, by Facility Type and Region for Nursing Homes: United States, 1998, 185

6.2 Distribution of Combined Nursing Hours per Resident Day in All Certified Nursing Facilities: United States, 1998, 186

6.3 Comparison of Average Nursing Hours per Resident Day for OSCAR Data, HCFA Time Studies, and Time Proposed by Experts, 187

FIGURES

2.1 Distribution of assisted living facilities by bed size: United States, 1998, 48

2.2 Percent distribution of ownership of home health and hospice agencies: United States, 1996, 53

2.3 Percent of patients receiving home health care services by type of service: United States, 1996, 53

2.4 Percent of patients receiving home health care services by service provider: United States, 1996, 54

3.1 Top 10 deficiencies of nursing facilities and percent of facilities with the deficiency cited: United States, 1998, 78

4.1 Proposed classification scheme for measuring a person's perspective about his/her quality of medical care, 129

5.1 Average number of deficiencies and percent of facilities without deficiencies: United States, 1991–1998, 145

5.2 Surveyor evaluations of the scope and severity of deficiencies, as a percentage of total deficiencies, cited in all nursing facilities: United States, 1996, 1997, and 1998, 157

6.1 Mean staffing hours per resident day for nursing facilities in the United States surveyed in calendar year 1998, 184

6.2 Average nursing hours per resident day in all certified nursing facilities: United States, 1991–1998, 188

Executive Summary

The quality of long-term care has raised concerns over the years among local, state, and national policy makers and the public, including the users of services and their families. The nursing home sector in particular remains the focus of continuing concern about the quality, cost, and accessibility of care and the adequacy of oversight and enforcement mechanisms. These concerns about problems in the quality of long-term care persist despite some improvements in recent years, and are reflected in, and spurred by, recent government reports, congressional hearings, newspaper stories, and criminal and civil court cases. Debate also continues over the effectiveness and appropriate scope of state and national polices to regulate long-term care, reduce poor performance of providers, and improve the health and well being of those receiving care. These questions and debates extend beyond nursing homes to home and community-based services and residential care facilities.

Long-term care covers a diverse array of services provided over a sustained period of time to people of all ages with chronic conditions and functional limitations. Their needs range from minimal personal assistance with basic activities of everyday life to virtually total care. Those needs are met in a variety of care settings such as nursing homes, residential care facilities, or people's homes. Of the 190 million people aged 18 years of age and older in 1994, nearly 9 million were using formal (paid) and informal (unpaid) long-term care. Of these, 6.5 million were over 65 years and older. The proportion of long-term care users who reported using only informal care dropped from 51 percent in 1984 to 40 percent in 1994, while the proportion who reported using institutional care increased from approximately 26 percent to 30 percent during the same period. Elderly people using long-term care in 1994 were older than in 1984 (mean age up from 79.2 to 80.5 years) and more likely to be women, to be cognitively impaired, and to have a greater number of limitations with activities of daily living than those using long-term care in 1984.

The aging of the U.S. population and the projected growth of the oldest age bracket (85 years and older) will have a major effect on the demand for and supply of long-term care services and on the resources needed to provide those services. The implications of these changes are enormous as evidenced by the widespread public and policy focus on the elderly population in discussions of such care. The population aged 85 years and older is the fastest-growing age group in the United States, and it is the most rapidly growing age group among the elderly population (65 years and older). Most of the increase in demand for long-term care services is expected to occur when the "baby boom" generation enters the elderly ages. The first of this generation will reach age 65 in the year 2011 and the last will do so around 2030.

The older population today, on average, is in better health than its counterpart of a few decades back. Recent studies have reported declines in the prevalence of chronic disability among elderly people. Although their overall health has improved, many elderly persons are dependent and frail with one or more chronic conditions and the consequent disabling conditions that increase with age. Also, with life expectancies continuing to rise for most groups, a larger proportion of people lives to age 90 and beyond. Hence the absolute number of years that people with disabling conditions require long-term care is likely to grow substantially, even if significant declines in disability rates are assumed.

Although long-term care creates the image of an elderly person in a nursing home, it is not limited to the needs of older persons or to care provided in nursing homes. Needs can occur at any age. The number of children and adolescents with severe long-term health conditions, although small in comparison to the elderly, has grown substantially over the past two decades and will continue to do so. Advances in medicine and surgical technologies now allow many children who would have died in previous eras to survive to adulthood, although often with psychological and physical impairments. Continuing improvements in medical care that allow more children and non-elderly adults with serious congenital or chronic disorders and injuries to survive for longer periods also are likely to contribute to a growing demand for long-term care services.

Most formal long-term care service is provided through organized service providers ranging from home and community-based services such as those provided by home health agencies, nonmedical personal care and supportive services in individuals' homes; to community-based residential care facilities; to institutional facilities such as nursing homes. Definitions of many of these long-term care service providers vary; states may label similar services differently or apply similar labels to services that differ. Although discussions of long-term care policy appropriately emphasize the role of paid professionals, paraprofessionals, and other workers, much long-term care is provided by unpaid, informal caregivers, including family members, neighbors, friends, volunteers from religious and community organizations, and others. Nearly 65 percent of caregivers are either the spouses or the children of the long-term care recipients.

In 1986, the Institute of Medicine (IOM) Committee on Nursing Home Regulations issued its report *Improving the Quality of Care in Nursing Homes.* Its recommendations provided the basis for Congress to enact a major reform of nursing home regulations embedded in the Omnibus Budget Reconciliation Act of 1987 (OBRA 87). Since the IOM issued its 1986 report, many changes have occurred. Long-term care is no longer synonymous with nursing home care. The use of alternative non-institutional settings for long-term care has increased to include home health care, personal care, residential care, care management, and other services.

In the context of these evolving long-term care options and needs and persistent concerns about the quality of long-term care, especially care in nursing homes, the Robert Wood Johnson Foundation requested that the Institute of Medicine undertake another examination of the quality of long-term care provided in nursing homes and other long-term care settings. The Archstone Foundation, Irvine Health Foundation, Department of Veterans Affairs, and Health Care Financing Administration provided additional support. The IOM was asked to examine the following:

- the demographic, health, and other characteristics of individuals requiring long-term care;
- the roles of different long-term care settings in community health care systems, and the movement of people among long-term care and other settings (their relationship to other components of community care systems);
- the current quality of long-term care settings and the extent to which this has improved or deteriorated in the past 10 to 15 years;
- the impact of regulations, especially the Nursing Home Reforms in OBRA 87, on such matters as the use of physical and chemical restraints, advance care planning, provision of adequate nutrition, identification of substandard facilities or programs, and public access to information on quality of care; and

- the strengths and limitations of existing approaches to measure, oversee, and improve quality of care and outcomes in nursing homes and
  other long-term care settings and ways of improving them to promote better quality of care and other outcomes, regardless of setting.

The IOM appointed a committee of experts to examine the above
issues. This report responds to that request. To address its charge in a
systematic manner, the committee conducted a number of activities. It
reviewed and analyzed an extensive body of research, both published
and unpublished, and other relevant reports; analyzed data from various
sources; conducted site visits; heard from a large number of experts and
interest groups at public hearings and a workshop; and commissioned
several background papers.

The scope of the study is broad and complex, covering a wide range
of settings for providing long-term care and the broad range of issues that
affect long-term care. Although the committee recognizes their growing
importance, lack of available data as well as resource and time constraints
prevented the committee from addressing every possible long-term care
service and service setting, population group, and issue. Thus, a fuller
consideration of the quality of long-term care for children, adolescents,
and younger adults with developmental disabilities; personal attendant
services; services for people with severe cognitive impairment; severe
and persistent mental illness; AIDS; and other conditions can and should
be the subjects of separate studies. Likewise, settings such as intermediate
care facilities for the mentally retarded and long-term psychiatric hospitals also are not covered in this report.

In responding to its charge, the committee decided to devote most of
its attention to older adults, both because they are the major users of long-
term care, with prospects for further growth in their numbers, and because
the long-term care literature and policy agendas focus primarily on aged
adults and adults with disabilities. The committee also examined nursing
homes in more depth than other service settings, because of the long-
standing problems of quality of care in these settings, and because of the
paucity of literature on the quality of care in other settings.

Three complementary approaches are generally used for ensuring
quality of care and life in long-term care. They are: (1) standards set and
enforced by government and accrediting agencies, and incentives for
quality improvement through Medicare and Medicaid, and other payers;
(2) consumer information, choice, and market competition; and (3) organizational and professional commitment to quality improvement.

The committee believes that all three must be pursued effectively to
promote and improve quality in the provision of long-term care. These
approaches to assure and improve quality of care and life in long-term

care should not be considered as alternatives; they are interdependent. The regulatory approach does not preclude consumer choice, and both these external approaches require internal organizational mechanisms to ensure quality.

The committee's major findings and conclusions based on this review and its deliberations are summarized below, followed by the text of the recommendations.

FINDINGS AND CONCLUSIONS

Assessment of Quality of Long-Term Care

Defining or evaluating quality of long-term care is fraught with problems, made more difficult by the unevenness of the available empirical evidence. Although information to evaluate quality of care in nursing homes is extensive and systematic, for most other settings it is nonexistent or very limited and lacking in uniformity. Moreover, opinions about what constitutes excellent, good, or poor quality also are changing and sometimes conflicting. Some of the available information is open to interpretation, and conclusions are sometimes based on personal and clinical experience rather than on empirical evidence.

Standards for evaluating whether quality is good or bad are shaped by several considerations and circumstances. The committee identified three specific aspects of long-term care that are relevant for assessing quality. First, long-term care is both a health program and a social program. For the health services component, judgments about quality emphasize medical and technical aspects of care, and such judgments are generally based on achieving desired health and functional outcomes and on adherence to correct processes of care. For the social services aspect, judgments about quality place more emphasis on the opinions and satisfaction of consumers (or their surrogate agents). Second, the potential and actual role of consumers is an essential element in long-term care. Although a relatively new concept, long-term care, and therefore the basis for evaluating the quality of such care is being redefined. At least in some care settings, consumers have assumed a larger role in choosing, directing, and evaluating many features of their care. Third, for nursing homes and residential care facilities, the physical environment of the facility can contribute to the physical safety and functional mobility of residents and, more broadly, to their quality of life. Privacy is an important aspect of the physical environment, and is intimately tied to the consumer-centered principles that the committee endorses.

In nursing homes, the committee found that since the implementation of the Omnibus Budget Reconciliation Act of 1987 (OBRA 87), the quality of care has generally improved over the past decade, even though nursing homes are serving a more seriously ill population. For example, many facilities have successfully reduced the inappropriate use of physical and chemical restraints. The focus of increased regulatory scrutiny on these two areas of care was a major contributing factor in reductions in both of these. Yet in many nursing homes quality of care continues to be problematic. Despite these improvements, serious quality-of-care problems persist in some nursing homes. Pain, pressure sores, malnutrition, and urinary incontinence have all been shown to be serious problems in recent studies of nursing home residents. The committee recognizes, however, that change in eliminating or reducing persistent and serious problems is a long process requiring diligent monitoring and enforced adherence to standards.

The quality of life for nursing home residents also has shown some improvements, but to a lesser extent. As a result of OBRA 87 and in response to market competition, the quality of life and the physical environment in nursing homes have improved somewhat, but concerns remain. Outside of nursing homes, little is known about the quality of care or outcomes of services provided by medically oriented home health agencies, and even less about the quality of social service oriented home- and community-based services. Residential care facilities, including assisted living, present a mixed picture in terms of both quality of care and quality of life. Some offer individualized, high-quality care in facilities that afford privacy, dignity, and individualization. However, others appear to lack adequately trained staff, and offer neither sufficient amount of care nor privacy and "homelike" settings. Also, there are indications that consumers may receive too little information to make informed choices regarding these facilities and the services provided.

Evidence regarding the quality of home care is more limited than that for nursing home care, but also points to a mixed experience. Moreover, most of the research in this area measures satisfaction and unmet need and not quality of care. Medicare-funded home health care generally appears to be of adequate quality in terms of the transactions between caregivers and care users. However, the program has suffered from problems of overuse and inappropriate use, leading to new constraints on payments that may adversely affect the availability of services for those with the most severe care needs. Access to home and community-based services and especially personal care services for people with disabilities is not uniformly available across states and appears to be largely unmet. The committee believes that access to, and choice of appropriate services, is essential to the quality of care and quality of life for individuals with disabilities. It concluded that research is needed towards developing an appropriate array of community-based long-term care services to meet the needs of consumers and assess the quality of the services and outcomes.

Problems with the quality of care being provided in some situations across all types of long-term care settings remain. Better mechanisms are needed to more adequately assess quality in these settings. More attention should be given to these issues including safety, consumer choice in quality improvement, and broadened participation in decision making.

Assessment Tools for Monitoring Quality

Information based on valid, reliable, and timely data about the care provided, the recipients, the facilities, and the caregivers is fundamental to all strategies for monitoring and improving the quality of long-term care. Such information is of interest to many constituencies, including consumers, caregivers, provider organizations, managers, regulators, purchasers, and researchers. The committee reviewed the current state of the major data systems in long-term care and their application for clinical assessment, quality monitoring, and reimbursement.

At the federal level, three data systems provide basic information on monitoring compliance with regulations and on the quality of long-term care offered by nursing homes and home health agencies: (1) the On-line Survey Certification and Reporting (OSCAR) System for nursing homes and home health care is a computerized national database for long-term care facilities used for maintaining and retrieving survey and certification data for providers that are approved to participate in the Medicare or Medicaid programs. It provides information on how well a nursing home has met the regulatory standards in the past and provides on-site surveyors with background information on past performance. It also has compiled nationwide data on resident characteristics and conditions, facility characteristics, staffing, survey deficiencies including scope and severity, and complaints. As such, it serves as a quality assessment tool. OSCAR data also are used to provide information to consumers through a HCFA-supported web site on the Internet that contains data on every nursing home in the United States. The data are collected and updated on a regular basis by state licensing and certification agencies under contract with HCFA to conduct Medicare and Medicaid certification surveys.

(2) OBRA 87 reforms require nursing homes to develop a uniform Resident Assessment Instrument (RAI) for all nursing home residents. The RAI provides a structured approach to assessment of a nursing home resident's need for care and treatment in preparing a plan of care. Its primary use is clinical, to assess the functional, cognitive, and affective levels of residents on admission to the nursing home and at least annually thereafter and when any significant change in status occurs. Individual-

ιʑeu, restorative care plans are developed at this time. The RAI includes a set of core assessment items, known as the Minimum Data Set (MDS) for assessment and care screening and more detailed Resident Assessment Protocols (RAP) in 18 areas that represent common problem areas or risk factors for nursing home residents. The reliability, validity, and sensitivity of individual MDS data elements, and composite scales constructed from these data elements, have been tested and analyzed extensively.

(3) The Outcome and Assessment Information Set (OASIS) for home health care is a group of data elements that represent core items of a comprehensive assessment of an adult home care patient, and that form the basis for measuring patient outcomes for purposes of outcome-based quality improvement. OASIS is a key component of Medicare's partnership with the home care industry to foster and monitor improved home health care outcomes and is proposed to be an integral part of the revised conditions of participation for Medicare certified home health agencies.

The committee identified a number of technical and methodological challenges involved in using the data collected in these systems for quality assessment and other policy related purposes. Despite such problems, the committee believes that continued use and evaluation of these data systems is essential.

Other types of long-term care settings, such as assisted living facilities and non-Medicare-certified home health care providers, have introduced various consumer-based information systems that include data on the individual recipients of care. Because a variety of residential care facilities offer room, board, and supervision to frail individuals without certification by the Medicaid or Medicare programs, several states have developed assessment systems for use in such residential care environments, based on the RAI and MDS for nursing homes.

States have also designed assessment instruments to determine an applicant's eligibility for services under Medicaid waiver programs for home and community-based services and then to guide the development of a plan of care and referrals to service agencies for those who are eligible. Many states use these instruments only for Medicaid reimbursed clients. The nature of the information collected by states varies enormously both across and within states, and although all states use assessments to develop a care plan, the comprehensiveness of the assessment varies and most states do not have standardized terms. Also, most states do not require training in the administration of the instrument despite its importance.

Interest is increasing in the possibility of identifying an instrument or set of core assessment elements that is applicable to all users of long-term care regardless of the setting. This interest stems in part from a growing recognition of the overlap among the characteristics of long-term care populations served in different settings and from a desire to compare the quality of care across settings. The availability of such assessment tools also might help in monitoring individuals as they move from one care level or setting to another. Uniform definitions of various community-based services and programs, common measures, and common sets of codes for categorizing care users' physical, cognitive, and emotional functioning would facilitate a common language for assessing long-term care needs and the outcomes of care. However, much work is needed first to examine the diversity across states of the services provided, service settings and service arrangements, and the infrastructure for monitoring quality and then to develop agreements on common core data elements and uniform definitions of various community-based arrangements across states.

Quality Assurance Through External Oversight

Organizations providing long-term care are staffed with professional, paraprofessional, and support staff, and often volunteers. In the final analysis, the quality and safety of long-term care depends on the actions of these individuals. External forces, however, can and do influence their actions by providing guidance and setting expectations for outcomes. They also can provide incentives, financial or otherwise, for specific actions that will affect access to and safety of care, and the quality of care and of life in long-term care settings. These external forces include formal quality oversight mechanisms, purchasers of long-term care, and families. The committee recognizes that other forces—including the mass media, care management and monitoring programs, and contractor standards set by purchasers—also influence provider behavior.

Federal and state governments share regulatory responsibilities for long-term care. Overall, the federal government has a dominant presence in nursing home and home health regulation through certification for Medicare and Medicaid participation. States, however, play the major role in regulating other kinds of long-term care. For example, they set licensure and other standards for various kinds of residential care arrangements. States also perform many of the certification procedures under contract with HCFA.

The major goals of long-term care regulation have been described as consumer protection (specifically, ensuring safety, the quality of the care received, and the legal rights of consumers) and accountability for public funds used for care. The central elements of long-term care regulation at the federal or state level are: establishing quality and related standards for service providers; designing survey processes and procedures to measure and monitor actual conditions of residents or clients and to assess compliance with the standards; and specifying and imposing remedies or sanctions for noncompliance.

To assess compliance by nursing homes with Medicare and Medicaid requirements for participation, HCFA relies on a survey and certification process administered under contract by state agencies. In recent years, HCFA has taken several steps or has proposed needed steps to improve specific areas of weakness, but the committee believes that more should be done to ensure adequate enforcement of standards. Although the basic standards for nursing homes are sound, the survey and enforcement of the standards has been weak with widespread variability across states. The committee identified a number of ways in which the regulatory system can be improved. HCFA can revise some aspects of the survey and enforcement processes it uses to monitor nursing homes. Some of the suggested changes include targeting chronically poor performing providers, paying more attention to chain facilities, focusing on resident problems, improving sampling techniques and sample sizes, reducing the predictability of the surveys, strengthening consistency of survey determinations, improving complaint investigations, and certifying the accuracy of nursing home data.

Residential care programs such as board and care homes have been around for a long time. The regulation of residential care facilities including assisted living occurs primarily at the state level. In general, the states have broad discretion in carrying out this oversight. The state role includes licensing and monitoring compliance with health and safety regulations covering such matters as building safety, food handling, medication storage and distribution, and staffing. State standards are highly variable for these care arrangements including assisted living facilities, a relatively recent subset of residential care. This variability begins with the very definition of the kinds of settings subject to particular regulation and extends to eligibility for service, services provided, staff requirements, and configuration of personnel and social living spaces.

Unresolved questions remain about the appropriate role of state regulatory standards in meeting the needs and preferences of the diverse population using long-term care. Research studies have raised serious questions about the effectiveness of state regulation and licensure promoting quality in residential care. The committee pointed to a range of actions that might help improve state-level regulation, beginning with research to examine the effectiveness of state survey and enforcement activities, especially in terms of quality of care, quality of life, staffing, and other measures related to residential care. Although not all committee members agree on the specifics of how state regulatory systems should be modified, there was consensus in the committee that, at this time, these mechanisms need not mirror the extensive federal regulatory system that is in place for nursing homes.

Outside of government, advocacy by consumers, family members, and committed community members historically has played a critical role in shaping long-term care policy and services. Perhaps the best-known advocacy effort is the Long-Term Care Ombudsman Program, which was mandated under the Older Americans Act in 1978. Program staff investigate and resolve problems made on behalf of residents living in long-term care facilities, and they also help educate the public and facility staff on complaint filing, new laws governing facilities, and best practices used in improving quality of care and evaluating care options. Other advocacy efforts involve resident representatives; resident councils; and family councils that participate in a variety of activities in nursing homes, assisted living facilities, and other residential settings; as well as independent state and national organizations devoted to long-term care issues. Such efforts are essential to consumer protection and, with adequate funding, will remain an important part in the overall effort to improve the quality of long-term care.

Strengthening the Caregiving Work Force

Provision of formal long-term care requires an adequate, skilled, and diverse work force. Registered nurses, licensed practical nurses, nursing assistants or aides, and home health aides represent the largest component of personnel in long-term care. Other professionals—such as physicians, social workers, therapists (physical, occupational, and speech), mental health providers, pharmacists, dietitians, and dentists—provide many different kinds of essential services to at least some of those using long-term care. Nonprofessionals, who provide the majority of personal care services, such as assistance with eating or bathing, have a major impact on both the health status and the quality of life of those receiving care. In addition to the direct caregivers, administrative, food service workers, housekeeping staff, and other personnel play essential roles in long-term care.

Long-term care services are labor intensive, and therefore the quality of care depends largely on the performance of the caregiving personnel. Personnel standards vary considerably across long-term care settings. Federal standards have been set for some personnel in nursing homes and home health agencies, but not for personnel providing care in other types of long-term care settings. Some states also have their own requirements for personnel in the facilities and programs that they regulate, particularly regarding health professionals and long-term care administrators, but these requirements vary widely across states.

Most of the research on the relationship between staffing and quality of long-term care has focused on nursing homes. Some studies have examined home health care workers, but few of these studies have examined the relationship between work force characteristics and quality of care. Little is known about the relationship of staffing to quality of care in other long-term care settings.

The committee reviewed the research literature, OSCAR data and HCFA's time studies to determine if staffing as a measure of quality in nursing homes has increased since implementation of the 1987 nursing home reforms embedded in OBRA 87. A slight but noticeable increase in staffing level has occurred in recent years. This increase may be attributed in part to the requirements of OBRA 87 and in part to the increased acuity of residents and the consequent staffing required to provide specialized services. The committee found a wide range of staffing levels[1] in nursing facilities. Many facilities have adequate staffing levels and provide high quality of care to residents. However, current staffing levels in some facilities are not sufficient to meet the minimum needs of residents for provision of quality of care, quality of life, and rehabilitation. Research provides abundant evidence of quality-of-care problems in some nursing homes and such problems are related in part to inadequate staffing levels.

The importance of having adequate staffing is highlighted by a number of studies, focused on nurses in particular, that point to a positive association between staffing levels and the processes and outcomes of nursing home care. Abundant research evidence indicates that both nursing-to-resident staffing levels and the ratio of professional nurses to other nursing personnel are important indicators of high quality of care, and that the participation of registered nurses in direct caregiving and in the provision of hands-on guidance to nurse assistants is positively associated with quality of care. Several studies have shown the importance of nursing management by professional nursing staff and gerontology specialists in making improvements in quality of care. A limited number of studies of other types of non-nursing services, such as physical therapy, also have found positive benefits in terms of residents' functional status and the costs of care. The research literature, however, does not answer the question of what particular skill mix is optimal. Nor does it take into account possible substitutions for nursing staff and ways to best organize all staff.

Moreover, nurse staffing levels alone are a necessary, but not a sufficient, condition for positively affecting care in nursing homes. Many factors influence the quality of care provided by staff to consumers of

---

[1]In this report "staffing levels" includes numbers of staff, ratios of staff to residents, and the mix of different types of staff in nursing homes and residential care facilities.

long-term care and their quality of life. In addition to staffing levels, education and training of staff, supervision, environmental conditions, leadership and management, attitudes and values, job satisfaction and turnover of staff, salaries and benefits, and management and organizational capacity of the facility are all essential elements in the provision of quality care to residents.

Reflecting on the role of each of these factors, the committee proposes recommendations for the development of training, education, and competency standards that prepare staff to care competently for all long-term care users with different needs and characteristics, including participation in consumer-directed service programs. Furthermore, the committee recommends that staff not be retained if they have been convicted of a felony or any crime involving the abuse, neglect, or exploitation of others. The committee therefore proposes federal legislation requiring timely background checks before hiring for all personnel in all long-term care settings.

The committee recognizes that the recommended enhancements would entail additional costs for care providers. Substantial improvements in the long-term care work force are not possible without increased resources for care providers. Government policies of reimbursing for long-term care have an important influence in improving quality of care. At the same time, there is evidence that some staffing changes, such as increased professional nurse staffing, might in some cases produce cost savings. For example, savings could accrue if an increased presence of professional nurses reduced the incidence of medical problems requiring hospitalization. Or, higher worker productivity might result if better staffing improved staff morale, lowered turnover, and reduced on-the-job injuries, which now are common in nursing homes.

Meeting current and emerging work force needs in long-term care may be challenged by the nation's booming economy, which is worsening the shortage of nurses, home health aides, personal care workers, and other workers in the health community. The Bureau of Labor Statistics has projected, for example, that jobs in the long-term care sector will increase by 1.64 million, or 53 percent, between 1996 and 2006. Considering the growing emphasis on the provision of care at home or in alternative residential care settings rather than in nursing homes, total employment in nursing facilities is projected to grow less quickly, but still substantially. Many of these new jobs will be in what today are relatively low-paid, low-benefit positions. As recruitment efforts build, it may be more important than ever to expand training and education and to develop and implement additional competency standards to ensure that all staff—new and in place—are able to perform their jobs well and in a manner that is respectful of those receiving the care. Wages, benefits, and working conditions need to be improved in order to recruit, retain, and stabilize the long-term care work force in a competitive market.

Building Organizational Capacity

Measurement tools, quality standards, and external oversight mechanisms all are important for providing quality long-term care, but they do not ensure that all providers will have the capacity to use the measures correctly, implement the standards effectively, or respond to oversight as intended. The committee examined the organizational capacity of providers to manage information and personnel, the technology and resources needed to translate knowledge into improved long-term care, and the management needed for meeting policy makers' demands for accountability. Although the committee focused mostly on nursing homes, many issues are applicable, directly or with some adaptation, to providers in other long-term settings and home health care.

The committee found major challenges in all of the areas examined. For example, a large gap exists between the current state of scientific knowledge and the capacity of most long-term care providers to implement that knowledge. In many cases, the missing components are the number and competence of staff and the amount and type of resources.

In recent years, a number of initiatives have been put in place to facilitate the ability of nursing homes to produce better outcomes for people using long-term care. The committee examined four initiatives. These are: (1) Regulatory standards articulated in OBRA 87 provide nursing homes with a specific definition of quality; (2) standardized clinical information systems have been developed in the form of the MDS (this data set is designed to help nursing homes organize their clinical activities to meet regulatory expectations for quality of care); (3) evidence-based practice guidelines, providing the best scientific advice available on how to treat common health problems, have been developed for some long-term care settings and common geriatric conditions; and (4) Quality Improvement Systems that have been successful in settings outside of health care have been embraced by some nursing homes.

Taken together, these four initiatives logically begin with policies to define goals for better nursing home care and help providers meet these goals. However, there is no strong evidence that these approaches have solved major quality problems in nursing home care. The guidelines appear neither routinely nor effectively implemented by nursing home providers nor known by direct care nursing home staff. At least part of the problem is that practice guidelines are developed rarely with an eye toward also getting providers to understand what personnel would most appropriately implement them and what costs are associated with them.

The committee reviewed several intervention studies and found that simple (i.e., not technically complicated) interventions can improve nursing home resident outcomes, but it is doubtful that there is enough staff to implement these simple but time-intensive interventions. Furthermore, improvement management models for implementing validated care processes require a significant expenditure of time for measurement and analysis. These expenses increase the total cost. Multiple studies indicate that staffing in nursing homes is inadequate to provide care that meets consumer expectations or maximizes residents' independence, leaving little time for data collection and evaluation.

The committee concluded that OBRA 87 regulations, information systems for MDS, practice guidelines, and quality management systems fail to emphasize the critical capacity issues, perhaps because the technical expertise of long-term care providers and the necessary tangible resources are assumed. Practice guidelines, for example, provide specific recommendations about how to treat nursing home residents based on the best knowledge available in the clinical research literature. None of the guidelines, however, includes a description either of the personnel necessary to implement the recommended treatment steps or of the implementation costs. Clearly, research is needed to test the feasibility and cost effectiveness of implementing clinical practice guidelines and proven care interventions in long-term care settings.

Most nursing homes, even highly motivated ones, may lack the technical expertise and resources—including but not limited to staffing levels—necessary to translate OBRA 87 regulations, practice guidelines, and quality improvement systems into practice. This report emphasizes the inadequacy of nursing home staffing levels and the consequent deficiency in long-term care services. However, increasing staffing without simultaneously improving management systems will most certainly result in less-than-expected improvement. The management problems related to accurate measurement described in this chapter, as well as numerous other management issues, will have to be addressed to realize fully the benefit of increased staffing. These problems should not be used by any stakeholders to justify abandoning efforts to improve care.

Reimbursing to Improve Quality of Care

Quality improvement initiatives are unavoidably intertwined with issues of costs and reimbursement. Yet, few efforts have highlighted the role that reimbursement can play in promoting or inhibiting the quality of long-term care. Contributing to the lack of emphasis on reimbursement is the paucity of conclusive data on the subject. Some studies have linked diminished quality of care in nursing homes to low Medicaid payment it others have posited that quality-of-care deficiencies should be ?d to factors such as excess demand. Although relatively little is known about the effect of reimbursement on quality of care in nursing homes, virtually nothing is known about its impact on home and community-based services.

The impact of changes in reimbursement on the quality of long-term care is difficult to assess. Almost all of the research literature on the relationship between financing and quality is limited to nursing homes, is based on very old data, and does not reflect the regulatory changes required by the OBRA 87. Moreover, several studies are focused on data from one or a few states, making it hard to generalize to the nation as a whole.

Two recent developments have directed new attention to the relationship between reimbursement and the quality of long-term care. The federal Balanced Budget Act of 1997 (the Act) repealed federal standards for reimbursing nursing home care under the Medicaid program, giving states virtually unlimited freedom in setting payment rates. For Medicaid home and community-based waiver services, states have always had complete freedom in determining reimbursement levels.

Second, the Act also dramatically altered Medicare reimbursement methods for nursing homes and home health care agencies and combined these changes with large budget savings. In some cases, the changes have been major. Many observers maintain that both federal actions have led to payment reductions that far exceed those intended by policy makers.

As states gain new freedom to set Medicaid nursing home reimbursement levels and the federal government reduces Medicare payments, it becomes increasingly important for states to understand and to be able to evaluate the possible impact of these changes for access to, and quality in, long-term care. Recent changes in payment policies are creating great turmoil in the long-term care sector. The withdrawal of substantial resources from long-term care providers is troubling, especially because many of the recommendations in this report require more, not less, funding.

Research on reimbursement and its potential impact on the quality of care generally focuses on two broad areas of concern: (1) what is the relationship between the costs of long-term care and the quality of care and (2) does the method of payment (e.g., flat rate, prospective payment, use or type of case-mix adjustment), independent of its level, affect the quality of care? The first policy question is important because as in most areas of Medicaid policy, nursing home reimbursement levels and methods vary dramatically by state. The second question is potentially very important because government policy makers have considerable control over these policy levers.

Measuring cost and payment levels is comparatively straightforward, but measuring the quality of care is not, and the way quality is assessed can significantly affect the results of studies that examine the relationship between the two. All of the studies examined by the committee focused on nursing homes.

Most studies have analyzed the relationship between cost or payment levels and quality by using some form of input (e.g., staffing levels) or process indicator as a measure of quality. This analysis found a small but positive relationship between Medicaid reimbursement and nurse staffing levels (except for nurse assistants) and reported fewer certification deficiencies in facilities with higher staffing levels. The complexity of the relationship among costs, inputs, and outcomes and the dilemma for states in trying to establish payment rates that are adequate to produce quality care is illustrated in other studies that found a relationship between cost or reimbursement level and staffing intensity. All these analyses found that professional staffing had a positive and significant relationship to quality of care in terms of outcomes. However, the effects of higher cost or reimbursement levels on staffing, and of staffing on outcomes, were not large enough for cost or reimbursement to have a significant impact on quality as measured by outcomes. Research is lacking in understanding the effect of changes in payment policies on providers, on accessibility of services, and on the quality of care.

Although there does not appear to be a simple relationship between cost and quality, logic suggests that there is some minimal level of reimbursement below which it will be either difficult or impossible for nursing homes to provide an adequate level of care. Moreover, continuing quality-of-care problems in long-term care should make policy makers alert to the possible negative impact of reducing the resources available to providers.

RECOMMENDATIONS

On the basis of its findings and conclusions, the committee has developed five categories of recommendations: (1) access to appropriate services, (2) quality assurance through external oversight, (3) strengthening the work force, (4) building organizational capacity, and (5) reimbursement issues. The committee's recommendations, grouped according to these categories, follow. They are keyed to the chapters in which they appear in the body of the report. The sequence in which the recommendations are presented does not reflect a priority order.

RECOMMENDATIONS ON ACCESS
TO APPROPRIATE SERVICES

Recommendation 3.1: The committee recommends that the Department of Health and Human Services, with input from states and private organizations, develop and fund a research agenda to investigate the potential quality impact associated with access to, and limitations of, different models of consumer-centered long-term care services, including consumer-directed services.

RECOMMENDATIONS ON QUALITY ASSURANCE
THROUGH EXTERNAL OVERSIGHT

Recommendation 4.1: The committee recommends that the Department of Health and Human Services and other appropriate organizations fund scientifically sound research toward further development of quality assessment instruments that can be used appropriately across the different long-term care settings and with different population groups.

Recommendation 5.1: The committee recommends that:

- Federal and state survey efforts focus more on providers that are chronically poor performers by surveying them more frequently than required for other facilities, increasing penalties for repeated violations of standards, and decertifying persistently substandard providers;
- HCFA's monitoring in all areas of state survey and sanction activities be improved by ensuring greater uniformity in state surveyor interpretation and application of survey regulations, and be reinforced by assistance and sanctions as necessary to improve performance; and
- An analysis to examine if increased funding is needed to allow HCFA to improve the state survey and certification processes for nursing homes should be commissioned.

Recommendation 5.2: The committee recommends that state agencies working with the private sector develop programs to disseminate information to consumers on (a) the various types of long-term care settings available to them, and (b) where applicable, the compliance of individual long-term care providers with relevant state standards.

Recommendation 5.3: The committee recommends that all states have appropriate standard-setting and oversight mechanisms for all types of settings where people receive personal care and nursing services. The committee recognizes that before this recommendation can be implemented, research examining the effectiveness of state survey and enforcement activities for residential care must be undertaken.

Recommendation 5.4: The committee recommends that the federal and state governments encourage the development of effective consumer advocacy and protection programs by providing funding and support for the following types of activities:

- consumer education and information dissemination initiatives; and
- complaint resolution programs and processes targeted at consumers of community-based long-term care.

RECOMMENDATIONS ON STRENGTHENING THE WORK FORCE

Staffing in Nursing Homes

Recommendation 6.1: The committee recommends that HCFA implement the IOM 1996 recommendation to require RN presence 24 hours per day. It further recommends that HCFA develop minimum staffing levels (number and skill mix) for direct care based on casemix-adjusted standards.

Recommendation 6.2: The committee recommends that Congress and state Medicaid agencies adjust their Medicaid reimbursement formulas for nursing homes to take into account any increases in the requirements of nursing time to meet the casemix-adjusted needs of residents.

Education and Training

Recommendation 6.3: The committee recommends that for all long-term care settings, federal and state governments, and providers, in consultation with consumers develop training, education, and competency standards and training programs for staff based on better knowledge of the time, skills, education, and competency levels needed to provide acceptable consumer-centered long-term care.

Labor Force Issues

Recommendation 6.4: For all long-term care service workers and settings, the committee recommends that federal and state governments, as appropriate, undertake measures to improve work environments including competitive wages, career development opportunities, work rules, job design, and supervision that will attract and retain a capable, committed work force.

Recommendation 6.5: The committee recommends federal legislation requiring timely performance of criminal background checks before hiring for all personnel in all long-term care settings.

RECOMMENDATIONS ON BUILDING ORGANIZATIONAL CAPACITY

Recommendation 7.1: The committee recommends that the Department of Health and Human Services fund research to examine the actual time and staff mix required in different long-term care settings to provide adequate processes and outcomes of care consistent with the needs and variability of consumers in these settings, and the fit between these needs and other existing staffing patterns. The Committee further recommends that the Department of Health and Human Services, by establishing Centers for the Advancement of Quality in Long-Term Care, initiate research, demonstration, and training programs for long-term care providers to redesign care processes consistent with best practices and improvements in quality of life.

RECOMMENDATIONS ON REIMBURSEMENT ISSUES

Recommendation 8.1: The committee recommends that, before making decisions to reduce reimbursements, state officials carefully assess the impact on access to services and on quality of care of any proposed reductions in Medicaid reimbursements for nursing home, home health and other home and community-based services.

Recommendation 8.2: The committee recommends that the Department of Health and Human Services fund and support research to better understand the effects of payment policies on accessibility and quality of long-term care services, including the following:

- the effects of low reimbursement rates or changes in Medicare and Medicaid reimbursement policies on providers of nursing home, home health, or other long-term care services;
- the effects of current payment systems, such as prospective payment for nursing facilities and interim payment systems for home health agencies, on the accessibility and quality of services; and
- whether states with low Medicaid reimbursement rates (adjusted for geographic variation in prices and other state-specific requirements) have lower quality of nursing home care.

1

Introduction

The quality of care in nursing homes and other long-term care settings is a major concern for local, state, and national policy makers and is becoming an ever-pressing issue. Recent reports of poor conditions in nursing homes[1] have captured national attention and raise questions not only for providers but also for the state and federal agencies responsible for ensuring quality of care in these settings. In 1986, the Institute of Medicine (IOM) Committee on Nursing Home Regulations issued its report *Improving the Quality of Care in Nursing Homes*. Its recommendations provided the basis for Congress to enact a major reform of nursing home regulations embedded in the Omnibus Budget Reconciliation Act of 1987 (OBRA 87). The legislation was refined through subsequent enactments in 1988, 1989, and 1990. The Health Care Financing Administration (HCFA) issued the enabling regulations in 1990, which were implemented in 1990 and 1991. The enforcement regulations were issued in 1994 and became effective in July 1995. OBRA 87, and its implementing regulations, substantially extended and reshaped the regulation of nursing homes aimed at improving the quality of care provided in these facilities.

Since the IOM issued its 1986 report, many changes have occurred. Long-term care is no longer synonymous with nursing home care. The

---

[1]Throughout the report, the terms "nursing home" and "nursing facility" are used interchangeably.

use of alternative noninstitutional settings for long-term care has increased to include home health care, personal care, residential care, and care management and other services. Within institutional settings such as nursing homes, specialized units often termed "special care" units and "subacute care" units have emerged in an effort to meet the needs of subgroups of residents such as those with Alzheimer's disease or with relatively short-term post-acute care needs, respectively. Over the past decade, federal Medicare policies dramatically expanded and then more recently contracted coverage for home health care. Moreover, the increased use of preadmission screening for nursing homes, the expanded role of Medicaid home and community-based waivers, the introduction of Medicare and Medicaid managed care programs, the general trend toward prospective payment and more rapid discharges from hospitals, and the emergence of various long-term care provider industries, all have altered the patterns of long-term care. These arrangements also offer more alternatives for long-term care users and their family members.

This expanding range of services and service settings reflects, among other things, better understanding of the preferences and values of people needing long-term care; medical and technological advances that allow more care to be provided outside hospitals and other institutions; and pressures to cut costs by shifting more care from hospitals to other settings that are thought to be less costly. Managed care organizations have not been major participants in long-term care delivery, but their decisions about hospitalization, home care, rehabilitation, and similar matters have spillover effects to the long-term care sector.

Changing cultural perspectives about people with long-term care needs also are influencing the nature of long-term care. These individuals are being viewed as people not only with needs and vulnerabilities but also with preferences to retain some control over major elements of the care they receive. As encouraged by the 1986 IOM report and by others, assessment of the quality of long-term care increasingly includes attention to the quality of life, including satisfaction with care, experienced by those receiving such care.

LONG-TERM CARE NEEDS

The implications of the aging of the population for the demand for long-term care and for the widespread public and policy focus on the elderly population in discussions of such care are a long-standing concern. The U.S. population is aging and the elderly population is growing older. The population aged 85 years and older is the fastest-growing age group in the United States, and it is the most rapidly growing age group among the elderly population. Most of the increase in demand for long-term care services is expected to occur when the "baby boom" generation enters the elderly ages. The first of this generation will reach age 65 in the year 2011 and the last will do so around 2030. The proportion of the population aged 65 or older is expected to increase from 13 percent in 1996 to 20 percent in 2030, and the number of people in this age group is projected to more than double, from 33.9 million to 69.4 million (Census, 1996). During this same period, the number of people 85 years of age and older is expected to more than triple, increasing from about 2.3 million to about 8.8 million, and will continue to grow as the baby boomers reach these oldest ages. This rapid growth in the oldest-old population (85 years and older) will have a major effect on the demand for and supply of long-term care services and the resources needed to provide these services. Friedland and Summer (1999) project that by 2030, between 10.8 million and 14 million older Americans will need long-term care, and between 4.3 million and 5.3 million of these will need nursing home care.

An important question for long-term care planning is whether people will experience disabling conditions and need long-term care for a smaller fraction of their years in old age compared to their predecessors. The older population today, on average, is in better health than its counterpart of a few decades back. Recent analyses have reported declines in the prevalence of chronic disability among elderly people, with declines greater in recent (1989–1994) than in earlier (1982–1989) years (Manton et al., 1993, 1997; Singer and Manton, 1998). These findings have led some to suggest that the increasing number of older people may not bring a corresponding magnitude of increase in the number requiring long-term care. Although their overall health has improved, many elderly persons are dependent and frail with one or more chronic conditions and the consequent disabling conditions that increase with age. Some of these conditions may be life threatening; others affect quality of life. Also, with life expectancies continuing to rise for most groups, a larger proportion of people lives to age 90 and beyond. Hence the absolute number of years that people with disabilities require long-term care is likely to grow substantially, even if significant declines in disability rates are assumed.

Although long-term care conjures up the image of the elderly person in a nursing home, it is not limited to the needs of older persons. This need can arise for any age group—children, adolescents, and younger adults. Nearly 58 percent of people with limitation of activity caused by a chronic condition or impairment are of working age; about 32 percent are elderly, and approximately 10 percent are children (Trupin and Rice, 1995). The number of children and adolescents with severe long-term health conditions, although small in comparison to the elderly, has grown substantially over the past two decades and will continue to do so. They include children with chronic conditions and those who are dependent on technology. Advances in medicine and surgical technologies now allow many children who would have died in previous eras to survive to adulthood, although often with psychological and physical impairments. Continuing improvements in medical care that allow more children and nonelderly adults with serious congenital or chronic disorders and injuries to survive for longer periods also are likely to contribute to a growing demand for long-term care services. Such care for children requires more than a scaled-down version of care for adults; it requires provision of social support services and coordination with the educational system.

Others with long-term care needs that differ from those of the elderly include a growing population of physically and developmentally disabled[2] adults, some of whom have outlived the ability of their aging parents to care for them. This group includes both individuals who have always lived in the community and those who formerly lived in institutions, sometimes until legal action prompted states to support noninstitutional alternatives for their care. People with severe and persistent mental and cognitive problems also have distinctive long-term care needs (Kuntz, 1995; Levin and Petrila, 1996). Over time, they may cycle through alternating periods of needing long-term care services and being able to function without them.

Continuing Concerns About Quality

Concerns about problems in the quality of long-term care, especially care in nursing homes, persist despite some improvements in recent years. The nursing home sector in particular remains the focus of continuing concern about the quality, cost, and accessibility of care and the adequacy of oversight and enforcement mechanisms. These concerns are reflected in, and spurred by, recent government reports, congressional hearings, newspaper stories, and criminal and civil court cases (GAO, 1998a, 1999a–e; HCFA, 1998a; OIG, 1998). Consumers often dread the loss of control signaled by admission to a nursing home and express anxiety about quality of life. Debate also continues over the effectiveness and appropriate scope of state and national polices to regulate long-term care, reduce

---

[2]For purposes of determining eligibility for government programs, developmental disabilities, originally defined on a condition-by-condition basis (e.g., mental retardation, cerebral palsy), are now defined as severe, chronic functional limitations that are due to mental or physical impairments, manifested before age 22, and likely to continue indefinitely (Braddock et al., 1998). The limitations must affect three of seven areas of major life activities: receptive and expressive language, learning, mobility, self-care, self-direction, capacity for independent living, and economic self-sufficiency. The majority of those with developmental disabilities are mentally retarded.

poor performance of providers, and improve the health and well-being of those receiving care. These questions and debates extend beyond nursing homes to home and community-based services and residential care facilities, with emphasis on contracting and disclosure practices, consumer education, and staff training.

THE IOM STUDY

Committee Charge

Now, more than a decade since the 1986 IOM report, it is timely to take another look at the state of quality in long-term care and to consider quality assessment and improvement strategies. In the context of evolving long-term care options and needs and persistent concerns about the quality of nursing home care, the Robert Wood Johnson Foundation requested the Institute of Medicine to undertake another examination of the quality of long-term care provided in nursing homes and other long-term care settings. Additional support was provided by the Archstone Foundation, Irvine Health Foundation, Department of Veterans Affairs, and Health Care Financing Administration. The IOM was asked to examine the following:

- the demographic, health, and other characteristics of individuals requiring long-term care;
- the roles of different long-term care settings in community health care systems, and the movement of people among long-term care and other settings (their relationship to other components of community care systems);
- the current quality of long-term care settings and the extent to which this has improved or deteriorated in the past 10 to 15 years;
- the impact of regulations, especially the Nursing Home Reform Act of 1987 (OBRA 87), on such matters as the use of physical and chemical restraints, advance care planning, provision of adequate nutrition, identification of substandard facilities or programs, and public access to information on quality of care; and
- the strengths and limitations of existing approaches to measure, oversee, and improve quality of care and outcomes in nursing homes and other long-term care settings and ways of improving them to promote better quality of care and other outcomes, regardless of setting.

The broad mandate of this study reflects the evolution of long-term care since the 1986 committee report was issued.

The IOM appointed a committee of 17 members representing a range of expertise related to the scope of this study. The members of the committee consisted of academic health professionals, researchers, health providers, and long-term care advocates. This report presents the results of the examination by the committee, which began its work in early 1997.

Study Method

The committee examined the statutory requirements for long-term care services; conducted extensive reviews of research literature and empirical evidence; and gathered information during site visits, a public hearing, and two workshops. It relied mainly on existing information from a variety of sources, reviewing and analyzing research literature on the varied topics covered in this report.

From early 1997 to April 2000, the committee met on eight separate occasions to discuss long-term care dynamics with a focus on quality. Some of these meetings consisted of workshops that were open to the public. They provided an opportunity for the committee to expand its perspective and views by obtaining a wide range of opinions from interested and concerned groups—such as health care associations and advocacy groups from skilled nursing facilities, home health agencies, and assisted living agencies—on matters under consideration, especially ideas and concepts of how the presenters perceive, measure, and evaluate quality within the different long-term care settings. A listing of the meetings and the presenters can be found in Appendix A.

The committee commissioned five background papers in order to obtain expert and detailed analysis of some of the key issues.

1. "Issues in the Quality of Long-Term Care for Children," by Ruth E.K. Stein, M.D.
2. "The Characteristics of Long-Term Care Users," by William D. Spector, Ph.D., John A. Fleishman, Ph.D., Liliana E. Pezzin, Ph.D., and Brenda Spillman, Ph.D.
3. "Quality of Care Problems Persist in Nursing Homes Despite Improvements Since the Nursing Home Reform Act," by Marie F. Johnson, M.D., and Andrew M. Kramer, M.D.
4. "Work Force Issues and Quality of Long-Term Care," by Penny Hollander Feldman, Ph.D.
5. "Long-Term Care Financing and Quality of Care," by Joshua M. Wiener, Ph.D., and David G. Stevenson.

The committee appreciates and values their contributions.

BASIC CONCEPTS AND DEFINITIONS

Long-Term Care

For purposes of this report, *long-term care* is broadly defined as an array of health care, personal care, and social services generally provided over a sustained period of time to persons with chronic conditions and with functional limitations.

Functional limitations are typically assessed as limitations in *activities of daily living (ADLs)* or *instrumental activities of daily living (IADLs)*. ADLs reflect an individual's capacity for self-care. They usually refer to the five basic functions: bathing, dressing, eating, transferring in and out of bed or chair, and using the toilet. Mobility assistance is often included. IADLs involve more complex tasks that enable an individual to live independently in the community. These include doing light housework, managing money, shopping for groceries or clothes, using the telephone, preparing meals, taking medications, and communicating verbally or in writing. For children, especially very young ones, ADLs and IADLs become very difficult to measure. Given the basic dependence of young children on adults around them, developmental milestones may form more reliable comparisons.

Health care includes medical, nursing, and other care provided by nurses, nursing aides, therapists, physicians, and other health workers serving people who need long-term care. *Personal care* services include assisting people of all ages with chronic conditions and limitations with ADLs. These services are "provided by an individual qualified to provide such services" (42 C.F.R. 440.167). (Skilled services that may be performed only by a licensed health professional are not considered personal care services.) *Social services* are diverse and include linking people to a range of community resources and services, assisting in the resolution of family or financial problems, and arranging social and educational activities. A *sustained period of time* has no official definition but is often considered to be three months or more.

Formal long-term care refers to a range of health care and supportive services provided by individuals and organizations paid to provide such services. Much long-term care, however, is *informal*—provided on an unpaid basis by family members and friends. Most discussions of quality assessment and improvement focus on formal care, but support for and assessments of informal services are also relevant to a comprehensive understanding of the experiences of those receiving long-term care.

Long-term care is generally distinguished from acute and primary care both by its duration and by its greater emphasis on personal care and social services, but the boundaries can blur, especially for people with serious chronic illness. Moreover, people receiving long-term care also require a variety of preventive, primary, and acute care services, some of which (e.g., immunizations) may be delivered by long-term care providers.

Long-term care goals and strategies may vary for different populations. For children, the definition and goals of long-term care have to take developmental status into account. Many of the services (e.g., assistance with dressing and financial matters) that might meet the definition of long-term care for adults would be provided as a matter of routine to developmentally normal children, especially younger children.

Consumer-Centered Care

Consumer-centered care, or patient-centered care, is health care that is closely congruent with and responsive to patients' wants, needs, and preferences (Gerteis et al., 1993). The term is used to refer to a shift from a more professional-driven health care system to one that recognizes and incorporates an individual patient's perspectives (Laine and Davidoff, 1996). Elements of consumer-centered care include individualized care planning and delivery of services; participation of a consumer or a consumer's family and other intimate caregivers in care planning and delivery; consideration of consumer values, culture, traditions, experiences, and preferences in the definition and evaluation of the quality of care; and recognition and support of consumer self-care capabilities, including integration of formal services with informal supports.

The notion of consumer-centered care is not a new one, but it has accelerated rapidly in recent years and there is now tangible evidence, at least in the acute and primary care encounters, of consumer-centered care in many facets of health care delivery and financing, medical law, and quality assessment (Laine and Davidoff, 1996).

Historically much health care, particularly institutional care, has operated in a health care environment managed by professionals whose training and medical ethics standards have traditionally emphasized expertise, responsibility, and benevolence more than patient autonomy and informed decision making (see Cassell, 1991; Gerteis et al., 1993; Goodwin, 1999). Over the last three decades, however, there has been a shift in health care decision-making approaches from the more paternalistic patient-physician relationships to deliberative models that engage the patient in active discourse in order to incorporate the patient's perspective when determining the optimal course of action (Slack, 1977; Kassirer, 1983; Quill, 1983; Emanuel and Emanuel, 1992; Laine and Davidoff, 1996).

Legislative developments lend support to various aspects of consumer-centered care, specifically, greater recognition of consumer preferences in health care decision making and expansion of health care delivery options.

The Americans with Disabilities Act of 1990 (ADA) has set the standard for various legal and policy efforts. The Patient Self-Determination Act (PSDA) of 1990 requires every health care facility that participates in Medicare and Medicaid to inform adult patients about advance directives (P.L. 101-508). Although the actual impact of the PSDA is debatable, the intent is to empower patients to take part in health care decisions that affect the duration and condition of their lives (Emanuel et al., 1993; Laine and Davidoff, 1996).

The term *consumer-directed services* goes beyond the concept of consumer-centered care to address the capacity of individuals to "assess their own needs, determine how and by whom these needs should be met, and monitor the quality of services they receive" (National Institute on Consumer-Directed Long-Term Services, 1996, p. 1). To date, consumer-directed services for long-term care are most often considered within the context of home and community-based personal attendant services (Litvak et al., 1987; Doty et al., 1996; Scala and Mayberry, 1997). Much of the foundation for the development of consumer-directed services for long-term care can be traced to the Housebound and Aid and Attendance Allowance Program operated by the Veterans Administration (Cameron, 1993), and to the models of personal assistance services for persons with physical disabilities developed through the independent living movement (DeJong et al., 1992). Consumer-directed models of long-term care services for these populations include: (1) consumer selection, training, and supervision of caregivers and providers of service; (2) individualized supports essential to maintaining the consumer's health and quality of life in the community (e.g., personal assistance, assistive devices, environmental modifications, consumer education, service coordination, and family and social supports); (3) consumer involvement in the development and approval of support plans and the authorization of payment; and (4) consumer monitoring of the quality of care (DeJong et al., 1992; Fenton et al., 1997; Scala and Mayberry, 1997). Such models have been applicable mostly to people with physical and developmental disabilities using personal attendant services, although some approaches to consumer-directed services are beginning to emerge for the elderly population with chronic illness and functional limitations.

Quality of Care

Assessments of the quality of the health, personal, and social services that make up long-term care draw not only on concepts used in assessing the quality of health care but also on concepts of quality of life. Broadly defined, *quality of life* reflects "subjective or objective judgment concerning all aspects of an individual's existence, including health, economic, political, cultural, environmental, aesthetic, and spiritual aspects" (Gold et al., 1996, p. 405). *Health-related quality of life* refers to those aspects of a person's overall well-being that are affected by health status or health care (Gold et al., 1996). The *quality of health care* has been defined as "the degree to which health services for individuals and populations increase the likelihood of desired health outcomes and are consistent with current professional knowledge" (IOM, 1990, p. 21).

The reference to desired health outcomes and quality of life emphasizes health and well-being as viewed and valued by people for themselves, not just as defined by health professionals or others. The importance that people using long-term care assign to various dimensions of health and well-being will vary depending on their circumstances (e.g., nature of health problems, age, family situation), expectations, and values. In some cases, efforts to improve one desired outcome (e.g., independence) may compromise another (e.g., avoidance of injury to self or others), and different people may value and balance these and other outcomes differently. In some cases, people may reject health care that would improve certain health outcomes at the expense of their quality of life. A commonly cited example is a person who rejects difficult therapies that might extend life for a few days or weeks and opts, instead, for palliative care that emphasizes physical and emotional comfort.

Another consideration in assessing the quality of long-term care is the nature of desired and expected outcomes and the appropriate care to achieve those outcomes, all of which may vary for different populations. Unlike acute care, which is usually expected to restore people to good health, the desired outcome of long-term care (and chronic care generally) will often be preventing or slowing further declines in health status and functional capacity for people with disabling conditions. After initial periods of more intensive service including habilitative or rehabilitative service,[3] many people adapt to their chronic conditions and disabilities and can sustain themselves for long periods with limited medical, personal, or social assistance. In particular, the long-term needs of children and adolescents may change drastically over several years. They may require long-term care services for lengthy periods, but the goal—often but not always achieved—is eventual independence from long-term care services and integration into the community as participating members of society.

---

[3]Rehabilitative services aim to restore function that once existed, whereas habilitative services are aimed at initially developing a function that had not existed (e.g., helping children with congenital disabilities achieve more than they would without special assistance).

A consumer-centered approach to long-term care would necessitate a fundamental shift in the approach to determining and evaluating the quality of that care. The locus for defining quality of care and desired outcomes would need to be extended from the care provider to the alliance of provider and consumer. The *definition* of quality of care would need to be expanded beyond health and safety outcomes to include outcomes such as quality of life and autonomy. The *measurement* of consumer-centered care would be incorporated as a complement to those of patient health and safety, and effectiveness and efficiency of care. Outcomes and other indicators of the quality of care likewise would need to be extended from traditional clinical health assessment to include consumer-reported experiences of care, processes of care, satisfaction with care, as well as consumer self-report of the achievement of health outcomes and quality of life goals specified in a care plan. Finally, the *collection* of data to assess the quality of care would need to be accomplished by providers and consumers jointly seeking to identify processes of care and environments that achieve desired outcomes, to target areas for care improvement, and to assign responsibilities for implementing these improvements. These approaches to evaluation of consumer-centered quality of care, although understood at a conceptual level, are just beginning to be translated into a valid and reliable technology for quality of care assessment and improvement (see, for example, the Picker Institute, 1995).

General Principles

The committee was guided in its deliberations by several working principles including a mix of value statements and empirically based assumptions. These principles are not absolutes, and in some situations they may conflict with one another or with other important principles that guide health care or public policy. For example, accommodating the desire to live at home or in other settings that offer more independence than a nursing home may, because of the higher risk of injury, conflict with society's commitment to establishing basic safety standards for certain products and services. Despite the potential for such conflicts, the committee believes that these principles should help shape efforts to protect and improve the quality of long-term care.

1. *Long-term care should be consumer-centered* rather than solely provider-centered. Consumer-centered care focuses on the needs, circumstances, and preferences of people using care and their families, and involves them, to the extent possible, in planning, delivering, and evaluating long-term care. Provider needs and circumstances (e.g., the need for cost efficiency and to react to short staffing) are important

but secondary. Although the principle may seem clear and simple, caregivers, providers, policy makers, and others can find it difficult to remain consumer-centered when confronted with the practical, day-to-day realities of organizing, delivering, financing, and regulating care across the array of long-term care settings and services. Moreover, given resource constraints and the frail condition of many of those using long-term care services, especially residents in nursing homes, often it may be impractical to ask people about how they experience and value the care they receive. Inadequate staffing in terms of numbers as well as education and training, combined with high turnover rates, also tends to lead to care that is provider-centered rather than consumer-centered.

2. *A system of consumer-centered long-term care should be structured to serve people with diverse characteristics and preferences.* The system should provide for people of all ages, race and ethnicity, income, family support, and all kinds and levels of physical, mental, and cognitive illnesses and functional limitations.

3. *Reliable and current information about the options available and the quality of care provided should be easily accessible to allow people to make informed choices about long-term care.* The growth and variability of options in long-term care service, the diversity of state programs to license or monitor them, and even the inconsistent language used in talking about long-term care needs and services make the development of coherent information and its communication particularly important.

4. *Access to appropriate long-term care services is both a quality of care and a quality of life issue.* Historically, long-term care has been nearly synonymous with institutional long-term care. Individuals with severe disabling conditions may need an array of services ranging from institutional services, residential care, and home care, to a variety of home and community-based personal assistance services. The ability to choose the type of services and the setting of services that are most appropriate to the needs and wants of the individual is an important consideration. Access to such services can make an important difference in the quality of life and quality of care for individuals with chronic conditions and functional limitations who want to remain at home or in the community.

5. *Measures of the quality of long-term care should incorporate its many dimensions, especially quality of life.* Such measures should reflect the broad range of social, psychological, physical, and medical needs of consumers of long-term care service. Quality of life was emphasized in the 1987 nursing home reforms, and assessment of quality of life is especially relevant for evaluating care for people with chronic dis-

abling conditions that substantially limit their control over their life and environment.

6. *Providers should be held accountable for their performance in providing high-quality long-term care, including the outcomes of care that they could affect.* A system of accountability requires (1) identification of standards of acceptable performance, (2) measurement tools and information systems that allow informed measurements and assessments of performance, and (3) dissemination of these assessments to the parties to whom accountability is owed.

7. *A motivated, capable, and sufficient work force is critical to quality long-term care.* Although the physical environment and other factors are important, the final common pathway for providing high-quality long-term care is the individual caregiver. If staff are poorly educated, trained or supervised, mismatched in skills to the needs of those requiring care, demoralized by their working conditions, or overwhelmed by their workload, it is virtually impossible to achieve acceptable quality care, especially care that is consumer-centered.

8. *Improving the quality of long-term care requires sustained government commitment to develop and implement fair, effective regulatory and financing policies.* Policy makers and payers have a fiduciary responsibility to see that public funds for long-term care are used well. They also have a broader responsibility to protect public health and safety. In setting forth the basic standards for providers of care, federal and state policies provide a foundation and safeguard for the other principles enumerated here. Although consumer choice and market forces have roles to play in the evolution of more consumer-centered long-term care, neither can operate effectively without a basic regulatory framework that covers contracting, information provision, complaint handling, and similar matters.

9. *Improving quality of care must be an ongoing objective. Building the capacity for high-quality long-term care depends on improved knowledge of the practices and policies that contribute to the well-being of people using that care.* Improvement in quality of care should be informed by scientific evidence linking alternative modes of care to desired outcomes and be guided by structured procedures to evaluate processes and outcomes of care, to identify areas of improvement, and to design and test actions that improve care.

Although not stated as a formal principle, the committee also urges consideration of the value of two principles for guiding and improving individual behavior that are grounded in centuries' worth of social evolution. One rests on the ideal of *high personal ethics*. This ideal applies to informal and formal caregivers alike, as well as to managers, policy makers, and all those making decisions about long-term care for others. Building on and going beyond this ideal is the principle of *professionalism*. External regulations, internal management structures, and impersonal market forces cannot compensate for caregivers, managers, and others involved in long-term care who lack an engaged conscience informed by personal and professional standards and values.

SCOPE AND LIMITATIONS

The scope of the study is very broad and complex, covering a wide range of settings for providing long-term care. Although the committee recognizes their growing importance, for reasons of lack of available data as well as resource and time constraints, the committee was unable to address every possible long-term care service and setting, population group, and issue that might be considered relevant or related to its charge. For instance, a fuller consideration of the quality of long-term care for children, adolescents, and younger adults with developmental disabilities; personal attendant services for people with severe cognitive impairment, severe and persistent mental illness, AIDS, and other conditions; and some settings such as intermediate care facilities for the mentally retarded, long-term psychiatric hospitals, and others can and should be the subjects of separate studies. The committee discussed the issues surrounding the movement of people among long-term care settings and providers, but time and resource constraints, as well as lack of sufficient information, prevented the committee from fully addressing this issue.

This report addresses the current status of long-term care quality and proposes ways to build a better policy environment in long-term care. Three criteria guided the committee in the content of the report and its recommendations. First, the subjects examined should be within the purview of the committee, and the topics should be relevant to and within the scope of the study. Second, the evidence must be sufficient to support and justify its findings, and recommendations must be adequately supported by evidence and analysis. Third, a recommendation should be attainable at reasonable cost. The committee deliberated long and hard on the various issues, findings and conclusions. Not all agreed on all recommendations, but most agreed with the overall report. Some disagreed with the wording of recommendation 3.1 and some expressed dissatisfaction with the report's discussion of regulatory issues. Their separate dissenting opinions are included in Appendix B.

Organization of the Report

The various services and settings for the provision of long-term care represent related but separate sectors of care often facing different issues with regard to topics studied by the committee. As stated earlier, the nature and extent of systematic empirical information also vary by providers and settings. In fact, a major problem in developing a balanced examination of the issues across settings is the paucity of reliable and systematic data and research for most of the care settings with the exception of nursing homes. Therefore, for the most part they are discussed separately within each chapter.

Chapter 2 summarizes the profile of long-term care in terms of who uses it, who provides it, and how it is currently financed.

Chapter 3 provides a framework for assessing the quality of long-term care and summarizes what is known about the current state of quality in different settings of long-term care. Chapter 4 discusses the current information systems for monitoring performance that could be used to assess, monitor, and improve quality of care.

Chapters 5 through 9 examine a range of issues and needed changes leading toward building a better policy environment in long-term care. These efforts include improvements in defining and enforcing basic standards of care, maintaining an adequate and qualified work force, building organizational capacity to improve care, and finally, designing reimbursement methods that encourage both quality and efficiency in care.

Although the committee has made every effort to obtain data and objective evidence based on research, some of its conclusions are necessarily derived from professional judgment based on the expertise and experience of committee members and on testimony and information provided by constituencies. In such cases, the committee has so indicated.

The report considers similarities and differences in the circumstances and concerns of various users of long-term care, including children, but it devotes more attention to older adults, both because they are the major users of long-term care, with prospects for further growth in their numbers, and because the long-term care literature and policy agendas also focus on aged adults and adults with disabilities. The report reviews nursing homes in more depth than other service settings because of long-standing problems of quality of care in these settings and because the literature on the quality of care in other settings is very limited.

2

Profile of Long-Term Care

L ong-term care covers a diverse array of services provided over a sustained period of time to people of all ages with chronic conditions and functional limitations. Their needs for care range from minimal personal assistance with basic activities of everyday life to virtually total care. Those needs are met in a variety of care settings such as nursing homes, residential care facilities or people's homes. People follow various paths in long-term care, reflecting differences in their health and functional status, variations in individual and family preferences and values, economic circumstances, and geographic location. In combination, these factors shape both the options and resources available to people needing long-term care and the ways in which they understand and evaluate their choices. Transitions in care occur not only because of changing care needs, but also because of changing family or financial circumstances and changing options or preferences for care. In some cases, regulatory policies, funding strategies, and provider capabilities, can require a person to move from one setting to another. Such transitions in care—voluntary or involuntary—can lead to difficulties that range from emotional to social, physical, and logistical.

This chapter presents a brief overview of the characteristics of the people using long-term care, the settings in which such care is provided, financing of the care, and coordination of care. As indicated in Chapter 1, learning about people who use long-term care and the various providers of care is complicated by the lack of comprehensive and systematic data across all long-term care settings and uniform definitions within settings.

Although an effort has been made in this report to touch on all aspects of the long-term care landscape, not all possible users and providers of long-term care are addressed. The discussion often emphasizes the elderly and care in nursing homes. The information on providers and users of long-term care services in this chapter is based mostly on the periodic national surveys of nursing homes and home health and hospice care conducted by the National Center for Health Statistics (NCHS) and a few ad hoc studies of other providers such as board and care homes and assisted living facilities. It also draws heavily from the analysis of the characteristics of long-term care users by Spector and colleagues (1998) using data drawn from four principal data sources, with varying reference dates and sometimes varying definitions of terms such as disability.[1] The data in their analysis rely on household surveys or surveys specifically of the elderly or of nursing home residents. Only one survey provides data on children using home and community-based services, and none includes people in state mental hospitals or in intermediate care facilities for people with mental retardation.

Adler (1995) estimated that in 1990, approximately 12.7 million people living in the community including certain institutional settings (about 5 percent of the total population) had long-term care needs. Nearly 58 percent of those with long-term care needs were aged 65 or over, and almost 81 percent were living in the community rather than in institutions such as nursing homes. The population with long-term care needs represented about 30 percent of a larger population of 42.7 million people (17 percent of the total population) who had disabilities.

Use of long-term care services may not always equate with need for such services. Some people who, by their own assessment or according to expert criteria, need long-term care services may be unable or unwilling to obtain care, even informal care from family members. Others who use formal long-term care services may not have functional limitations. For example, one national survey reported about 3 percent of nursing home residents needed no assistance with activities of daily living (ADLs) (Krauss and Altman, 1998). These residents, however, may have clinically complex conditions that require daily nursing care and monitoring.

Even though different long-term care settings tend to emphasize different types of care, they commonly serve mixed populations with

---

[1]Much of the analysis was taken from the background paper commissioned from Spector, Fleishman, Pezzin, and Spillman for use by the Institute of Medicine committee. The principal data sources for this analysis are the 1994 Disability Supplement to the National Health Interview Survey, the National Long-Term Care Survey, the Assets and Health Dynamics of the Elderly Survey, and the nursing home component of the Medical Expenditure Panel Survey.

overlapping characteristics. Moreover, states differ in their regulations regarding "appropriate" residential care settings for people with specific characteristics and care needs. For example, some state policies allow assisted living facilities to serve people who meet the criteria for nursing home admission, whereas other states explicitly prohibit the admission or retention of such individuals in these settings (Mollica, 1996, 1998). Thus, the characteristics of the assisted living populations may vary across states, depending on such admissions policies. Unfortunately, no single comprehensive source of data exists on the various settings and the users of long-term care.

CHARACTERISTICS OF LONG-TERM CARE USERS

Adults

Of the approximately 190 million people aged 18 or over in 1994, nearly 9 million were using formal and informal long-term care (Spector et al., 1998). Of these, 6.5 million were over age 65. Between 1984 and 1994, the number of persons 65 years and older using formal and informal long-term care remained about the same, but the percentage of this age group using long-term care dropped from 19.7 to 16.7 (Spector et al., 1998). The proportion of long-term care users who reported using only informal care dropped from 51 percent in 1984 to 40 percent in 1994, while the proportion who reported using institutional care increased from approximately 26 percent to 30 percent during the same period. Elderly people using long-term care in 1994 were older than in 1984 (mean age up from 79.2 to 80.5 years) and more likely to be women, to be cognitively impaired, and to have a greater number of ADL limitations.

Table 2.1 summarizes the demographic characteristics and levels of functional limitations of elderly and nonelderly users of long-term care in nursing homes and community-based settings, broadly defined to include both formal and informal services. Ninety-one percent of those using nursing home services are elderly; the vast majority of long-term care users are women, but among the small number of nonelderly nursing home residents, the proportion of men and women is nearly equal. In both age groups, nursing home residents are, on average, older than those using community-based services and also more disabled, as reflected in the substantially higher proportion needing assistance with three or more ADLs. Even among the older population, almost half of those using community-based long-term care services required assistance only with instrumental activities of daily living (IADLs).

For persons living in the community, the types of conditions that create a need for long-term care are different for younger and for older

TABLE 2.1 Demographic Characteristics of Long-Term Care Users Aged 18–64 and Aged 65 and Older Living in the Community and in Nursing Homes: United States, 1994 and 1996

Characteristics of Users	Community-Based Users (1994)		Nursing Home Users (1996)	
	18–64	65 and Older	18–64	65 and Older
	Number (000)			
Population (thousands)	3,363	3,823	138	1,425
	Years			
Mean age (years)	44.5	79.1	51.0	84.6
	Percent			
Gender				
Female	57.6	67.3	51.0	73.9
Male	42.4	32.7	49.0	26.1
Race				
White	77.0	86.4	76.1	89.9
Black	19.0	11.6	19.2	7.9
Other	4.0	2.0	4.7	2.2
Marital status				
Married	47.3	37.2	16.4	16.7
Never married	29.2	4.2	27.0	11.3
Divorced	18.4	6.6	46.3	7.5
Widowed or separated	4.8	51.8	10.3	64.5
Education				
Less than 12 years	34.3	51.5	42.9	43.6
12 years	39.4	27.5	23.8	18.9
Greater than 12 years	23.5	17.4	16.9	15.6
Missing	2.7	3.7	16.4	21.9
Level of IADL and ADL Disability[a]				
IADL Only	55.9	49.4	7.7	2.1
1–2 ADLs	26.7	29.0	14.5	13.9
3–6 ADLs	17.4	21.7	75.5	83.2

NOTE: Data from the 1994 Disability Supplement to the National Health Interview Survey (community-based users) and from the 1996 Medical Expenditures Panel Survey—Nursing Home Components (nursing home users). Except as indicated, entries are percentages. Missing data are indicated only if they represent more than 2% of cases.

[a]ADLs are defined as activities necessary for personal care, including eating, dressing, bathing, transferring (e.g., from bed to chair), and using the toilet. IADLs describe activities necessary to live independently in the community, such as doing light housework, managing money, shopping for groceries, using the telephone, preparing meals, and taking medications. SOURCE: Adapted from Spector et al., 1998.

adults. Among those aged 18 to 64, the most common conditions cited in one analysis were back problems, mental retardation, mental illness, coronary heart disease, and respiratory conditions; among those aged 65 and over, the leading conditions were arthritis, coronary heart disease, visual impairments, stroke, and respiratory conditions (Adler, 1995). For nursing home residents, dementia was the most common health condition (Krauss and Altman, 1998).

Children and Adolescents

Among the small number of children with severe disabilities requiring long-term care, about 45 percent have major developmental problems (primarily mental retardation), 35 percent have severe physical limitations, and 20 percent have primarily mental health problems (SSA, 1999). The physical conditions include major lung diseases such as cystic fibrosis and severe asthma, severe arthritis, and childhood cancers; major development problems include mental retardation and other developmental disorders, and mental illness (Hobbs et al., 1985). Some conditions necessitate lifelong care, but others may require special care only during childhood. For example, children born prematurely who survive their experience in newborn intensive care units may have long-term central nervous system or lung disease that often requires home and community-based services for a few years, but with time and good growth, these needs may largely disappear for some children.

Reports based on national long-term care surveys typically do not include data on long-term care users under age 18 because the numbers are so small and because definitions of disability for children differ from those for adults. The definitions for children reflect their developmental status and usually focus on limitations in play and school activities. Depending on the assumptions made about existing data from surveys and other sources, estimates of children potentially needing long-term care vary greatly. On the conservative side, the 1990 census reported that about 0.1 percent of children in the United States (approximately 92,000) were in long-term care institutions (Newacheck et al., 1998). Data from other sources produced estimates of another 170,000 children with long-term care needs who were living in the community in 1990 (Adler, 1995). On the high side, the 1994 National Health Interview Survey—Disability Supplement (NHIS-D) estimated that 18 percent of children (more than 12.6 million) had "a chronic physical, developmental, behavioral, or emotional condition and required health and related services of a type or amount beyond that required by children generally" (Newacheck et al., 1998, p. 117).

PROVIDERS OF LONG-TERM CARE

The question, Who provides long-term care? can be addressed in several ways, for example, by distinguishing between formal and informal caregivers, professional and paraprofessional workers, employees and independent contractors, and organized providers and individual workers. Organized providers include residential institutions and long-term care facilities (such as nursing homes and residential care facilities), as well as nonresidential service providers (such as agencies that manage home health and hospice care services). Individual caregivers include those providing professional, paraprofessional, and other services on a formal paid basis and those providing informal, generally unpaid services (often family members or friends).

Organized Providers of Long-Term Care Services

Most formal long-term care is provided through organized service providers that operate in specific settings ranging from an individual's home to residential facilities within a community to institutional facilities such as nursing homes. Definitions of these long-term care service providers vary. States may label similar services differently or apply similar labels to services that differ.

1. *Institutional providers* include nursing homes (used here to include what some regulations differentiate as skilled nursing facilities), rehabilitation hospitals, intermediate care facilities for those with mental retardation, long-term psychiatric hospitals, and long-term care units of acute care hospitals.
2. *Community-based residential care facilities* include a broad and diverse category of facilities that provide supervision and assistance in settings ranging from apartments (private rooms, kitchens, baths, and door locks), ward-like settings with multiple beds; licensed or unlicensed personal care homes providing nonprofessional supervision and assistance to one or more residents; and licensed group homes with trained staff to supervise and assist people with mental retardation or mental illness to live as independently as possible.
3. *Home and community-based services* include nonresidential community-based services provided by home health care agencies; nonmedical personal care services in individual homes and congregate residential settings; a variety of supportive services, such as adult day care or night care (e.g., when a family member works the night shift) in a protective setting; agencies that supply durable medical equipment

to home users; and agencies that assist people in directing their own arrangements for such services.

Within these general categories, considerable variation exists, which may affect the quality of life and quality of care for people using such services and the ability of those monitoring quality to detect problems or prompt improvements.

Other providers and settings are sometimes included in discussions of long-term care. For example, hospice care organizations provide services over a period of weeks or months for those approaching death.[2] Such services are also provided by many home health agencies, and some hospitals and nursing homes have hospice units or teams. Continuing Care Retirement Communities are another type of setting that might be included in discussions of long-term care. They have been developed to provide a geographically adjacent, commonly managed spectrum of care options primarily for older adults who hope, insofar as possible, to age in place and minimize disruptive moves. The options offered may include a skilled nursing facility and assisted living units, in addition to independent housing units. They serve primarily the upper- and middle-class elderly population. Table 2.2 shows the distribution of selected long-term care facilities by size for 1992 and 1998.

Nursing Homes

According to the Health Care Financing Administration (HCFA) survey and certification reporting, the number of nursing home beds and facilities has grown substantially in recent decades. Between 1978 and 1998, the number of facilities increased from about 14,200 to 17,800 (a 25 percent increase), and the number of beds increased from about 1.31 million to 1.81 million (a 39 percent increase) (Harrington et al., 1998b).

According to the National Nursing Home Survey conducted by NCHS there were about 17,000 nursing homes in the United States with a total of 1.8 million beds and caring for 1.6 million residents in 1997 (NCHS, 2000).[3]

---

[2]These and other providers such as psychiatric hospitals and intermediate care facilities for the mentally retarded are not addressed at any length in this report.

[3]Nursing homes are defined by NCHS as facilities with three or more beds that routinely provide nursing care services. Facilities may be certified by Medicare or Medicaid, or not certified but licensed by the state as a nursing home. These facilities may be freestanding or a separate unit of a larger facility. Other surveys, such as the nursing home component of the Medical Expenditures Panel Survey (MEPS) conducted by the Agency for Healthcare Research and Quality (AHRQ), use a narrower definition of nursing home that requires the home to be certified and to provide 24-hour skilled nursing care.

TABLE 2.2 Number of Long-Term Care Facilities and Beds: United States, 1992 and 1998

Type of Facility	Facilities		Beds	
	1992	1998	1992	1998
		Number		
Nursing facilities—certified	16,804	17,458	1,714,756	1,806,944
Home care agencies				
State licensed	8,116	13,537	N/A	N/A
Medicare/Medicaid certified	6,240	9,726	N/A	N/A
Residential care facilities	37,770	51,227	614,804	878,804
Intermediate care facilities				
for the mentally retarded	5,888	6,553	137,114	125,909
Adult day care	1,847	3,590	N/A	N/A

SOURCE: Harrington et al., 2000c.

As shown in Table 2.3, proprietary nursing homes accounted for 67 percent of all facilities. Fifty-six percent of the facilities were part of a "chain" (multi-facility organizations). More than three-fourths (77.7 percent) were certified by both Medicare and Medicaid, and nearly all nursing homes had some form of certification in 1997. The average-size nursing homes had 107 beds, with an occupancy rate of 88 percent. Half of the total facilities had 100 or more beds occupied by 71 percent of the residents (NCHS, 2000). The majority of nursing home residents were elderly people, white, and female. About 91 percent were 65 years and older, and 46 percent were 85 years and older. The average age of all residents at the time of the survey was 81 years.

In addition to increases over the years in the number of nursing homes and nursing home beds, the types of services offered by facilities have expanded. Some facilities have created special units to serve people with specific conditions such as Alzheimer's disease. Other such units referred to as "post-acute" or "subacute" care units serve the relatively short-term needs of people discharged from acute care hospitals to recuperate from surgery. Nursing homes also provide a considerable amount of long-term care for people with severe mental or cognitive problems, especially older people with dementia or people with other disabling health problems (Mechanic, 1998).

Over the past two decades, nursing homes in the United States have been transformed. First, rather than merely being permanent settings for frail elders to live out their remaining years of infirmity, many nursing homes now serve multiple populations, and nursing homes in general

TABLE 2.3 Number and Percent Distribution of Nursing Homes, Beds, and Residents, by Facility Characteristics: United States, 1997

Facility Characteristics	Facilities	Beds	Residents
		Number	
Total	17,000	1,820,800	1,608,700
Ownership			
Proprietary	11,400	1,213,900	1,054,200
Voluntary nonprofit	4,400	465,400	422,700
Government and other	1,200	141,500	131,700
Certification			
Medicare only	800[a]	61,000	47,400
Medicaid only	2,300	184,700	156,300
Both	13,200	1,526,000	1,365,500
Not certified	700[a]	49,000	39,400[b]
Affiliation[c]			
Chain	9,600	1,035,700	909,400
Independent	7,400	772,800	690,200
		Percent	
Ownership			
Proprietary	67.1	66.7	65.5
Voluntary nonprofit	26.1	25.6	26.3
Government and other	6.8	7.8	8.2
Certification			
Medicare only	4.7[a]	3.4	3.0
Medicaid only	13.6	10.1	9.7
Both	77.7	83.8	84.9
Not certified	4.1[a]	2.7	2.5
Affiliation[c]			
Chain	56.3	56.9	56.5
Independent	43.2	42.4	42.9

[a]Figures should not be assumed reliable because the sample size is between 30 and 59, or the sample size is greater than 59 but has a relative standard error greater than 30 percent.
[b]Facilities need not certify all their beds for Medicare or Medicaid residents.
[c]Excludes a small number of homes and residents with unknown affiliations.
SOURCE: NCHS, 2000.

have become more heterogeneous (Banaszak-Holl et al., 1996). More than 2,500 Medicare- or Medicaid-certified nursing facilities in the country today are hospital based, and another 10 percent of the remaining free-standing facilities concentrate on serving relatively short-stay Medicare patients. The entry of nursing homes into the post-acute and recuperative market began in the early 1980s but accelerated in the late 1980s with the introduction of the short-lived Medicare Catastrophic Coverage Act. This trend continued throughout the 1990s with the emergence of managed care and its focus on reducing hospital use by contracting with alternate providers (Laliberte et al., 1997). Comparison of the level of functional impairment of nursing home residents in 1987 and 1996 in the two national nursing home surveys reveals that the proportion of all residents with impairment in three or more ADLs increased from 72 to 83 percent. Furthermore, there has been a substantial drop in the proportion of residents in nursing homes that manifest serious behavioral problems. This reported decline could be a product of several factors. For example, the implementation of the Pre-admission and Assessment Screening and Annual Resident Review (PSSRR) regulations restricting the use of nursing homes for persons with psychiatric diagnoses could contribute to this decline. Improved behavior management interventions in the period following the Omnibus Budget Reconciliation Act of 1987 (OBRA 87) is another possible explanation.

Community-Based Residential Care

Community-based residential care has been the mainstay of long-term care services for many years. Some residential care arrangements, such as board and care homes, adult foster homes for older persons and small group homes for those with mental retardation, are intended to be like family homes; and others, such as assisted living facilities, are intended to be more like apartments and sometimes like hotel rooms. Depending on the state and the services provided, residential care settings may or may not be licensed. Even when they are licensed, labels and definitions for residential services and facilities differ markedly between, as well as within, states (Mollica, 1996, 1998) and they are often unclear to consumers (GAO, 1999a). National comprehensive and systematic trend data are almost nonexistent.

Board and Care Homes. Residential care facilities, known colloquially as board and care homes but rarely licensed under that name, for decades have been major providers of shelter and light levels of service. They are non-medical community-based facilities that provide at least two meals a day and routine protective oversight to one or more residents with functional limitations. Board and care homes are licensed and regulated under more than 25 different names (Hawes et al., 1993). Terms commonly used for these settings are group homes, domiciliary care homes, and personal care homes. Data from the 1991 National Health Provider Inventory indicate that there were about 30,000–34,000 licensed board and care homes in the United States serving over half a million persons (Clark, et al., 1994).

In addition there are an unknown number of unlicensed homes. Historically they provided care especially to people with mental illnesses or developmental disabilities. A quarter of the people with chronic mental illness live in some kind of sheltered care facility. Nearly three-quarters of them lived in licensed homes of this sort (Barnes, 1993).[4] The label board and care home today is widely applied to settings that provide care to mostly older people who need some supervision and assistance with activities of daily living and cannot live, or choose not to live, in an independent household. In 1991, only about 32 percent of the homes primarily served a mental health population (Clark, et al., 1994). These homes increasingly are serving people with physical impairments. State regulations allow increasing levels of impairment to be admitted to and retained in residential care facilities (Mollica, 1998).

These homes vary greatly in size, resident characteristics, services, and cost both within and across states. The majority of residents were elderly and two thirds were women. They also vary greatly in the amount, type and extent of regulations across states, and little systematic information is available about the quality of care provided or the quality of life in these settings.

In order to fill the need for systematic information on what are known as board and care homes and the quality of care provided, a major probability 10-state study of board and care homes and their residents was conducted in late 1993 by Hawes and colleagues under contract with the Department of Health and Human Services. The 1993 study found that 92 percent of licensed homes and 62 percent of unlicensed homes provided personal care, such as assistance with ADLs (Hawes et al., 1995a).[5] Most homes provided three meals a day and assistance with storage and supervision of medication. Many homes provided organized activities, recreation, and transportation, and some reported providing money management. About 25 percent of licensed facilities and 27 percent of unlicensed facilities provided professional nursing care, but many of these services were arranged through home health care agencies (Hawes et al., 1995a). Most of the 3,257 residents studied were elderly white women, who were widowed, divorced, or never married. Compared to nursing homes, residents in board and care homes are on the average less impaired. Yet 40

---

[4]The committee did not address care that may be needed by or provided to people with serious mental illness in other "sheltered settings" such as jails, prison, and homeless shelters.

[5]Hawes and colleagues (1995a) have pointed out that the term "personal care" also has varied meanings in state regulations for board and care facilities. In some states, it refers to hands-on care, whereas in others, some types of hands-on care (e.g., assistance with transfers or toileting) are explicitly excluded.

percent were moderately or severely cognitively impaired, 23 percent had urinary incontinence, 15 percent used a wheelchair, and 7 percent were bedfast or chair-fast.

The cost of board and care homes varied widely. Many states offer a small variety of income transfers; 40 states and the District of Columbia offer State Supplemental Payments to the federal Supplemental Security Income. Interviews with local agencies revealed that for various reasons many community-based services are available to none or only a limited number of board care residents, although they may be eligible for most services. Staff in many areas were unable to provide estimates of services available.

Assisted Living Facilities. Although no single definition of assisted living exists, the term tends to be used to connote a residential setting that is similar to a board and care home or residential care facility (and is often licensed as a subset of that category rather than separately), but that undertakes to provide or arrange for personal care and routine nursing services to address ADL needs. When the term was developed in Oregon, assisted living was envisioned to be a setting that combined much of the high level of care provided in a nursing home with desirable features of apartment life. In practice, the name has spread widely, but many facilities known as assisted living facilities have neither the service capability nor the privacy and homelike accommodations envisaged by advocates of these settings (Hawes et al., 1999).

Some states use licensing criteria to limit assisted living to people with lower levels of disabling conditions than nursing home residents. Other states treat assisted living as an alternative to nursing home care. In terms of physical environments, some states reserve the term for facilities that offer apartments containing full baths and kitchenettes; other states allow for varying physical arrangements; and still others have no criteria for the physical settings. Lack of a uniform definition of assisted living hinders efforts to understand this subset of residential care facilities and its role in providing long-term care to the frail elderly, the quality of life and care provided, or to obtain uniform trend data across states on various measures including the characteristics of the facilities, staffing, quality of care, and other relevant issues.

Hawes and colleagues (1999), reporting on the 1998 national probability sample survey of administrators of 2,945 assisted living facilities, found significant variations within the industry. In 1998, there were an estimated 11,459 assisted living facilities in the United States, with approximately 611,300 beds and 521,500 residents. They differ widely in ownership, auspices, size, and philosophy. These facilities are relatively new; they have been in operation an average of 15 years—more than half

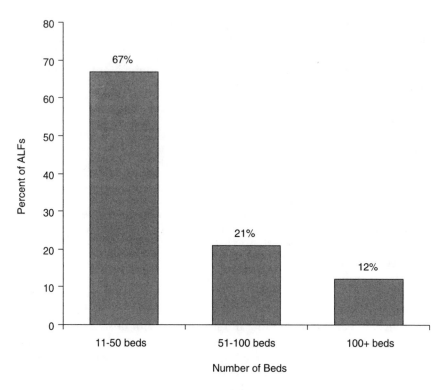

FIGURE 2.1 Distribution of assisted living facilities by bed size: United States, 1998. SOURCE: Hawes et al., 1999.

(58 percent) for 10 years, and 32 percent for no more than 5 years (Hawes et al., 1999).[6] Figure 2.1 shows the distribution of assisted living facilities by number of beds. The average facility had 53 beds, with the majority of facilities having 50 beds or fewer. Although most facilities had less than 50 beds, the majority of residents lived in the larger facilities.

---

[6]Unless otherwise noted, the data on assisted living facilities (ALFs) discussed in this chapter are based on the National Study of Assisted Living for the Frail Elderly. The survey was conducted under contract with the Department of Health and Human Services. A probability telephone sample survey of administrators of 2,945 facilities was conducted. Facilities included in the survey met the three eligibility criteria: the facility has more than 10 beds, serves a primarily elderly population, and represents itself as an ALF or offers at least basic level of services such as 24-hour staff oversight, housekeeping, at least two meals a day, and personal assistance in two out of the following three services: medication, bathing, or dressing.

The facilities varied in terms of accommodations, privacy, and bathroom facilities. Of the accommodations surveyed, 57 percent were rooms and 43 percent were apartments. Despite a distinct preference by consumers for private accommodations to maintain privacy and dignity, the majority of facilities reported some shared units. Only 27 percent of the facilities had all private accommodations, and slightly more than a quarter (28 percent) reported at least one bedroom shared by three or more residents. Although a majority of facilities reported having shared units, 73 percent of units across all facilities were private, 25 percent were shared, and only 2 percent were ward-type rooms. There appeared to be less privacy in the use of bathrooms. Although nearly three-quarters of the accommodations were private, only 62 percent of the units surveyed offered a private full bathroom and an additional 5 percent had a private half-bath. Thus more than a third of the units required the residents to share a bathroom.

With respect to admission and retention policies, most administrators of the facilities in the survey reported willingness to admit residents with moderate physical limitations such as needing a wheelchair, but fewer than half were willing to admit residents who needed assistance with transfers or residents with moderate to severe cognitive impairments. In terms of retention of residents, nearly one-third of the ALFs stated that they would not retain a resident who used a wheelchair and 38 percent would discharge a resident who needed assistance with locomotion. Fewer than half would retain a resident with moderate to severe cognitive impairment, and 76 percent would not retain residents with behavioral symptoms such as wandering. Further, 76 percent would not retain a resident who needed nursing care for more than 14 days, and 72 percent had discharged a resident within the last six months because the resident needed skilled nursing care. An estimated 24 percent of the residents received help with three or more activities of daily living, and about 34 percent had moderate to severe cognitive impairments.

Adult Foster Care and Small Group Homes. Variously known as adult foster care, small group homes, family homes, domiciliary homes, and other titles, these settings are private homes that house and provide care for small numbers of people, typically ranging from one to six. State licensing often sets the maximum number of residents somewhere between three and six. In a 1996 study of foster care programs in 26 states, Folkemer and colleagues (1996) found that 24-hour supervision is the key feature of adult foster care and that often one or more care providers live in these settings. In 19 of the states, the adult foster care program was largely supported by public funds, including Supplemental Security Income (SSI), state SSI supplements, and Medicaid home and community-based services

(HCBS) waivers. However, in five states studied (Michigan, Montana, Ohio, Oregon, and Washington) the majority of residents were private paying and in two (Kentucky and Nevada) there was an even division between private-pay and public-pay consumers. Expansive definitions of services permitted in adult foster care in Oregon, Washington, Minnesota, and Wisconsin allow adult foster care to be a lifetime setting if the consumer and provider so choose, whereas in other states, it is seen as a strategy for light care (Folkemer et al., 1996). The authors also noted a trend towards corporate or multiple ownership of foster homes by a single provider who staffs the homes with live-in or shift personnel. Such consolidation may offer some economies of scale and bring greater resources to adult foster homes, though the model also changes to a less personalized one.

Home Health and Hospice Care Agencies

Home health and hospice care agencies are usually defined in terms of the type of care they provide. *Home health care* is provided to individuals and families in their place of residence for the purpose of promoting, maintaining, or restoring health or for maximizing the level of independence while minimizing the effects of disabilities and illness, including terminal illness. Home health care as embodied in Medicare and Medicaid was conceived by Congress as a post-acute care benefit. Although the average length of service use was 334.0 days in 1996, most Medicare home health beneficiaries have relatively short episodes of care; only 42.4 percent of users have episodes longer than 180 days, and 33.8 percent of recipients use services for 60 days or less (NCHS, 1999b).

Hospice care is defined as a program of palliative and supportive care services providing physical, psychological, social, and spiritual care for dying persons, their families, and other loved ones. Hospice services are available in both home and inpatient settings and may be provided by home health care agencies or hospices (NCHS, 1998).

In 1996, an estimated 2.5 million individuals received care from 13,500 home health and hospice care agencies in the United States (NCHS, 1998). An estimated 10,600 of the 13,500 agencies had only home health care patients, 1,300 had only hospice care patients, and 1,600 had both types. Medicare's prospective payment system for hospital services combined with Medicare's coverage of home health care has contributed to the rapid growth of home health care agencies and to more frequent and intense use of post-acute services, including home health care, nursing homes, or both (Neu and Harrison, 1988; Shaughnessey and Kramer, 1990). The number of agencies rose from 8,000 in 1992 to 13,500 in 1996—a 68 percent increase. During the same period, the number of people receiving care increased by 92 percent, from 1.3 million in 1992 to 2.0 million in 1994 and 2.5 million in 1996 (NCHS, 1998, 1999a). However, since the implementation of the Balanced Budget Act of 1997, the use of, and Medicare expenditures for, home health care have decreased significantly. The number of Medicare-certified home health agencies dropped from 10,444 in 1997 to 7,747 in 1999, a figure that is still far above the number of agencies in the early 1990s (NAHC, 2000).

Nearly 62 percent of home health agencies were proprietary and 66 percent were part of a group or chain. More than 90 percent of these agencies were certified by either Medicare or Medicaid to provide home health or hospice care; 88 percent were certified for home health under Medicare and 85 percent were certified under Medicaid (NCHS, 1999a).

In looking at the distribution of users of home health care, in 1996, home health agencies provided care to 2.4 million patients receiving home health care and 59,400 receiving hospice care. As in previous years, most home health care patients were elderly women. Two-thirds of the home health care patients were women; 72 percent (1.75 million) were 65 years and older when they were admitted for care. Of these, nearly 70 percent were 75 years and older. About two-thirds were female, more than 60 percent were white, and 47 percent were widowed. Over 90 percent of patients were living in a private residence (NCHS, 1999b). More than 95 percent of the patients were served by agencies certified by Medicare or Medicaid to provide home health. About 50 percent of the patients were served by voluntary nonprofit agencies, and about 42 percent were served by proprietary agencies (Table 2.4). The majority of home health care patients received services from agencies that were certified by Medicare, Medicaid, or both. Forty-two percent were served by an agency that was part of a chain of agencies, and about one-third were served by a hospital-affiliated agency.

The ownership of agencies serving home health care patients differed significantly from those serving hospice patients (see Figure 2.2). About half of the home health care patients were served by voluntary nonprofit agencies and about 42 percent were served by proprietary agencies, compared to 85 percent of hospice care patients who were served by voluntary nonprofit agencies and only 11 percent who received care from proprietary agencies.

Figures 2.3 and 2.4 summarize the distribution of the types of services received by patients from home health care agencies and the types of caregivers providing services. Most frequently received services were nursing services, homemaker and household services, and physical therapy (Figure 2.3). Frequently seen caregivers were registered nurses, home health aides, physical therapists, and licensed practical nurses (Figure 2.4).

TABLE 2.4 Number and Percent Distribution of Certified Home Health Agencies and People Served, by Agency Characteristics: United States, 1996

Agency Characteristic	Agencies	People Served
	Number	
Total	10,600	2,427,500
Ownership		
Proprietary	6,600	1,010,900
Voluntary nonprofit	2,600	1,190,000
Government and other	1,200	226,600
Certification		
Certified	9,700	2,324,600
Medicare	9,300	2,242,300
Medicaid	9,000	2,271,000
Not certified	1,000	102,900
Affiliation		
Affiliated	7,000	1,540,300
Independent	3,600	887,200
	Percent	
Ownership		
Proprietary	61.7	41.6
Voluntary nonprofit	24.3	49.0
Government and other	11.4	9.3
Certification		
Certified	90.9	95.8
Medicare	87.8	93.1
Medicaid	85.0	93.6
Not certified	9.1	4.2
Affiliation		
Affiliated	65.8	63.5
Independent	34.2	36.5

SOURCE: NCHS, 1999b.

Home and Community-Based Services (HCBS) Organizations

All 50 states and the District of Columbia now have one or more HCBS waivers to provide long-term care to various populations[7] (see Table 2.5). For example, waivers have been granted for elderly persons, persons with physical disabilities, persons with persistent and serious

---

[7] All 50 states offer HCBS services; however, Arizona's Medicaid program is administered differently and they do not specifically have separate waivers for their HCBS programs.

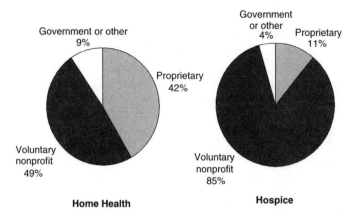

FIGURE 2.2 Percent distribution of ownership of home health and hospice agencies: United States, 1996.
SOURCE: NCHS, 1998.

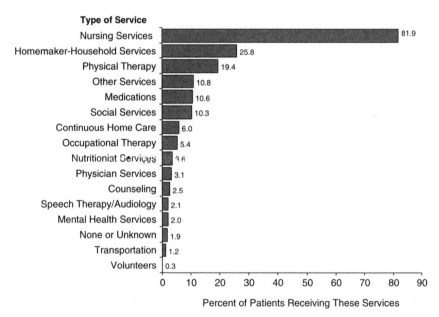

FIGURE 2.3 Percent of patients receiving home health care services by type of service: United States, 1996.
NOTES: Values for "transportation," "volunteers," and "none or unknown services" should not be assumed reliable because the sample size is between 30 and 59, or the sample size is greater than 59 but has a relative standard error greater than 30 percent.
SOURCE: NCHS, 1999b.

Type of Provider

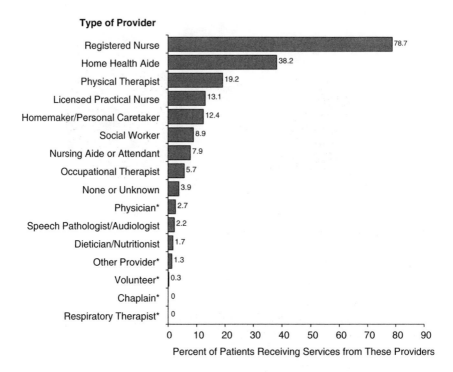

FIGURE 2.4 Percent of patients receiving home health care services by service provider: United States, 1996.
NOTES: Asterisk denotes values that should not be assumed reliable because the sample size is between 30 and 59, or the sample size is greater than 59 but has a relative standard error greater than 30 percent.
SOURCE: NCHS, 1999b.

mental illnesses, persons with developmental disability, persons with AIDS, and persons with brain injury. In turn, both direct service providers and care management agencies have emerged to deliver the services offered under the waivers. Care management typically is also used in state-funded HCBS programs and in long-term care funded under the Older Americans Act; quite often, the same care management agency manages all of the funding streams in an attempt to create "seamless care management" for the consumer.

Personal care. Many states provide personal care services under the Medicaid HCBS waivers, (See Table 2.5). In some states, personal care service agencies are licensed but not Medicaid-certified. In those cases home health care agencies provide these services. The agencies themselves may have less reliance on nurses and other professionals in direct care roles than do home health agencies. In some instances, the care managers doing the purchasing provide some of the professional oversight. Medicaid and Medicaid waiver programs also allow the individual to receive personal attendant services or other services from a self-employed, individual provider.

These personal attendant programs are not available uniformly across states to elderly persons. However, in some states many elderly and adults with disabilities receive services from independent workers. For example, Benjamin (1998) recently studied California's large In-Home Supportive Services Program, which cares for about 200,000 Californians under the regular Medicaid program; 65 percent of the beneficiaries are over 65 years of age. Oregon has about 10,000 state employees who serve as client-employed home care workers; although employed by the client and often related to the client, the state pays these individuals and offers them employment benefits (Kane et al., 1998c). A variety of concerns have arisen about the tax-status and protection of workers in client-directed programs (Sabatino and Litvak, 1992). Such problems are partly alleviated when fiscal intermediaries serve as the employer of record. A range of such intermediary agencies exist, including those that offer some supportive services to the consumers such as training consumers as employers, helping with recruitment, checking applicant references, and the like (Flanagan and Green, 1997).

Younger people with disabilities may sometimes use centers for independent living as a focal point for managing their long-term care. Such centers, funded federally under the Rehabilitation Act of 1973, have as their core services information dissemination and referrals, independent living skills training, and advocacy. But they also offer a wide range of other services including counseling, rehabilitation technology, interpreter and reader services, employment empowerment, and many others. Increasingly, they are beginning to serve some older people (Kane et al., 1998c).

Care management. Although originally conceived as a means of assisting individuals and families in obtaining information and access to social, housing, and other non-medical services, care management has recently become a prominent mechanism for controlling service use and costs (Applebaum and Austin, 1990; Vourlekis and Green, 1991; Evashwick, 1996). In part because users of such assistance have viewed the term as reinforcing the image of consumers as "subservient to a powerful case manager" (Perrin and Bloom, 1994, p. 711), the terms "care management"

TABLE 2.5 Total Medicaid Personal Care Services and 1915(c) Home and Community-Based Services Waivers: United States, 1997–1998

State	Total Participants			Participants per 1,000 Population of State			Rank Order of State
	Personal Care Services (PCS)	Home and Community Based Services (HCBS)	PCS and HCBS	HCBS	Total PCS and HCBS		
Missouri	33,167	23,823	56,990	4.41	10.54		1
Arkansas	18,198	8,355	26,553	3.31	10.52		2
Oregon	2,483	25,665	28,148	7.91	8.68		3
New York	87,496	51,986	139,482	2.86	7.69		4
Michigan	55,046	9,753	64,799	1.00	6.63		5
Kansas	—	15,392	15,392	5.92	5.92		6
Rhode Island	—	5,712	5,712	5.79	5.79		7
Wisconsin	10,926	19,006	29,932	3.65	5.75		8
California	134,694	46,718	181,412	1.45	5.64		9
Montana	2,672	2,120	4,792	2.41	5.45		10
West Virginia	4,500[a]	5,257	9,757	2.90	5.38		11
Washington	8,854	19,364	28,218	3.45	5.03		12
Minnesota	6,487	16,379	22,866	3.49	4.88		13
Texas	59,562	29,598	89,160	1.53	4.60		14
Vermont	—	2,264	2,264	3.84	3.84		15
Colorado	—	14,243	14,243	3.66	3.66		16
Wyoming	—	1,744	1,744	3.63	3.63		17
South Dakota	808	1,860	2,668	2.52	3.62		18
South Carolina	—	13,281	13,281	3.51	3.51		19
North Dakota	—	2,089	2,089	3.26	3.26		20
Oklahoma	6,000[a]	4,697	10,697	1.41	3.22		21
Alaska	980	915	1,895	1.50	3.11		22
Kentucky	—	12,125	12,125	3.10	3.10		23

State						Rank
New Hampshire	137	3,489	3,626	2.98	3.09	24
Illinois	—	36,743	36,743	3.06	3.06	25
New Jersey	12,810	11,703	24,513	1.45	3.04	26
Connecticut	—	9,629	9,629	2.95	2.95	27
Maine	1,133	2,527	3,660	2.03	2.95	28
North Carolina	8,884	12,898	21,782	1.74	2.93	29
Massachusetts	3,700[a]	12,242	15,942	2.00	2.61	30
Nebraska	1,234	3,069	4,303	1.85	2.60	31
Ohio	—	27,115	27,115	2.42	2.42	32
Alabama	—	10,396	10,396	2.41	2.41	33
Washington, D.C.	1,205	1,205	—	2.27	34
Iowa	—	6,022	6,022	2.11	2.11	35
Georgia	—	15,199	15,199	2.03	2.03	36
Virginia	—	13,449	13,449	2.00	2.00	37
Idaho	1,000[a]	1,305	2,305	1.08	1.91	38
Florida	—	27,124	27,124	1.85	1.85	39
New Mexico	—	3,014	3,014	1.75	1.75	40
Maryland	4,499	3,741	8,240	0.73	1.62	41
Utah	159	2,861	3,020	1.39	1.46	42
Nevada	853	1,515	2,368	0.90	1.41	43
Delaware	—	951	951	1.29	1.29	44
Hawaii	—	1,129	1,129	0.95	0.95	45
Pennsylvania	—	10,900	10,900	0.91	0.91	46
Mississippi	—	2,036	2,036	0.75	0.75	47
Tennessee	—	3,747	3,747	0.70	0.70	48
Louisiana	—	2,736	2,736	0.63	0.63	49
Indiana	—	3,624	3,624	0.62	0.62	50
Arizona	—	—	—	—	—	—
Total	467,487	561,510	1,028,997	2.10	3.84	

[a]Estimates.

NOTE: PCS data from telephone survey conducted in 1998–1999. HCBS data from telephone survey conducted in 1997.

SOURCE: Harrington et al., 2000a.

or "care coordination" are preferred. Care management can be a vital service for those using long-term care, and has been viewed as an essential feature for HCBS services. Although definitions and specifications vary across states, many programs are designed and implemented with the objectives to identify and assess needs, recertify eligibility for benefits, develop a care plan and monitor its implementation, help locate, arrange and coordinate services, and provide support in decisions and direction of services.

States vary in the design of their care management programs. Some states delegate the function to local area agencies on aging, some delegate it to county health departments or county human services departments, other states create regional offices of a state agency. Still others contract the function out to a variety of agencies within the state, including care providers, such as home care agencies, hospitals, and nursing homes. States differ on whether they permit the agency vested with care management responsibilities to also provide the care. For children, states often delegate the care management function to state Maternal and Child Health programs for Children with Special Health Care Needs.

Regardless of the model used, care management programs have proliferated since the 1980s with widely varying costs (Davidson et al., 1991; Kane et al., 1991c). Care managers are often persons with a bachelor's degree in social work or other degrees, though some programs also employ nurses as care managers, or at least have nurses available to assist care managers when needed.

Care management has been viewed as an essential feature for HCBS services; it is found in HCBS programs for all target populations including persons with mental problems. Some believe that care managers can themselves be a vehicle for quality assurance by assessing and monitoring at the individual level and by building quality standards into contracting at a programmatic level. In that regard, one study found that some, but not most, of 128 care management programs studied consciously tried to monitor and improve care through care management (Kane and Degenholtz, 1997). Research is limited, however, about the efficiency and efficacy of these programs and the ability of these programs to assure quality of care.

Despite the essential nature of this service, problems and conflicts do arise. The use of separate agencies to handle different aspects of care management—such as determining coverage eligibility, authorizing payments, and advocating for clients—has led to problems that some systems have tried to avoid by having a single agency perform all these functions. Ethical conflicts can arise for care managers in trying to meet both client needs and organizational responsibilities for managing public and organizational resources. Heavy case loads and limited care options may also lead some care managers to become insensitive to the preferences and values of those they serve. Care managers and direct home care providers at times come into conflict, especially when their roles seem to overlap (Kane and Frytak, 1994). Some disability advocacy groups representing younger persons with disabilities (particularly spinal cord injuries) have criticized care management as overly intrusive and interfering with the abilities of consumers to manage their own care. Some programs are developing care management efforts in proportion to the consumers' needs for oversight and to establish continuing eligibility, rather than a way of micromanaging care in all cases (Kane et al., 1998c).

Other HCBS Services. HCBS includes a wide range of other services, such as adult day care, home-delivered meals, emergency response systems, telephone reassurance programs, transportation programs, respite programs, caregiver support programs, home modification programs, and equipment programs. Some of these are offered under the Older Americans Act. Others are offered by freestanding providers of the particular service, but often meal programs or adult day care programs are sponsored by organizations such as nursing homes and home health care agencies.

Individual Caregivers

Informal Caregivers

Although discussions of long-term care policy appropriately emphasize the role of paid professionals, paraprofessionals, and other workers, most long-term care is provided by unpaid, informal caregivers, including family members, neighbors, friends, volunteers from religious and community organizations, and others.

According to data from the 1994 National Long-Term Care Informal Care Survey, informal care remains the most prevalent source of care for the elderly population in the community, with two in five elderly care recipients receiving all care informally and three in five receiving some informal care. In 1994, 5.9 million informal caregivers provided care to 3.6 million elderly people in the community. Nearly 29 percent of persons caring for elderly long-term care users were themselves aged 65 or older. Most (64.7 percent) were either the spouses or the children of the long-term care recipients (Spector et al., 1998). About one-quarter of the caregivers were spouses of care recipients, but the largest group of caregivers were daughters. Other relatives accounted for slightly more than a quarter of all persons providing informal care and nonrelatives for about 9 percent. By far, most caregivers were women (63 percent), and roughly three in five were married. Informal caregivers were more likely to be caring for those with only IADL problems, although about one-third cared for elderly persons having problems with three or more ADLs. Roughly half of all caregivers shared a household with a care recipient, but more than one in four were children who did not live with a recipient parent (Spector et al., 1998).

Most informal care is provided in private homes. Care from family and friends is usually unpaid, but informal caregivers may sometimes receive some payment from those using care or from another family member or friend. The demands on informal caregivers vary tremendously. Some, for example, assist an elderly parent with shopping, bill paying, and similar activities, mostly on a weekly basis and causing relatively little financial or social strain. Others—for example, a spouse or adult child of an older person with severe impairments or parents of a severely disabled child—may provide substantial amounts of low- and high-technology nursing and personal care on a daily basis, sometimes drastically curtailing their own work and social lives as a result. Such demands can seriously strain relationships between caregiver and care receiver, between spouses, and among siblings and members of extended families.

Formal Caregivers and Other Long-Term Care Workers

Formal long-term caregivers range from highly trained professionals including physicians, geriatric nurse practitioners, registered nurses, and therapists to paraprofessionals such as nurse assistants, home care aides, and personal care workers who may have limited formal education and varying amounts of on-the-job training. The long-term care work force also includes many who are not involved in direct caregiving, such as administrators, housekeeping staff, kitchen and maintenance workers, and clerical personnel.

In 1998, there were more than 3 million paid jobs in nursing homes, residential care settings, and home health organizations. More than half of these jobs were accounted for by registered nurses (RNs), licensed practical nurses,[8] physical therapists, social workers, and paraprofessionals, including nursing and home health aides, personal care attendants, and orderlies (BLS, 2000). As Table 2.6 shows, the mix of caregivers varies among long-term care settings. Nursing aides, home health and personal care aides, and orderlies make up about two thirds of the caregivers. The table also shows the contrast between hospitals, which have a caregiving work force dominated by RNs (64 percent compared to 16 percent in long-term care settings), and long-term care settings, which rely heavily

---

[8]In two states, California and Texas, these nurses are called licensed vocational nurses. In all other jurisdictions they are known as licensed practical nurses. In this report, licensed practical and vocational nurses are both referred to as licensed practical nurses.

TABLE 2.6 Number and Percent of Selected Categories of Occupations Employed in Selected Long-Term Care Settings and in Hospitals: United States, 1998

| | Long-Term Care Settings | | | | |
Occupation	All Long-Term Care Settings	Nursing and Personal Care Facilities	Home Health Care Services	Residential Care Facilities	Hospitals
			Number		
Total, key caregivers	1,825,512	1,054,997	518,640	251,875	1,921,676
Registered nurses	294,932	149,355	129,304	16,273	1,238,720
Licensed practical nurses	255,936	196,480	40,849	18,607	219,299
Personal care and home health aides	412,920	28,173	283,940	100,807	43,195
Nursing aides, orderlies, and attendants	772,011	652,471	42,693	76,847	313,641
Physical therapists	20,850	7,918	12,475	457	39,615
Social workers	68,863	20,600	9,379	38,884	67,206
			Percent		
Registered nurses	16.2	14.2	24.9	6.5	64.5
Licensed practical nurses	14.0	18.6	7.9	7.4	11.4
Personal care and home health aides	22.6	2.7	54.7	40.0	2.2
Nursing aides, orderlies, and attendants	42.3	61.8	8.2	30.5	16.3
Physical therapists	1.1	0.8	2.4	0.2	2.1
Social workers	3.8	2.0	1.8	15.4	3.5

SOURCE: BLS, 2000.

on nursing aides and similar paraprofessional workers. Similar labor force data for home and community-based services, such as are funded by Medicaid waivers and state-funded programs, are not available. The long-term care work force issues are discussed in detail in Chapter 6. Staffing shortages and the low reimbursement rates are receiving much attention among policy makers and in the media. These problems have serious implications for the quality of care provided.

Although physicians play a key role in overseeing the medical aspects of long-term care, they are a small segment of the long-term care work force, reflecting in part the significance of nursing care and nonmedical services for those needing long-term care. Other factors that contribute to limiting the role of physicians are insufficient training to care for people with serious functional impairments residing either in the community or in nursing homes, and unattractive reimbursement rates for visits to nursing homes and personal homes (Ouslander et al., 1997). For frail older people, the issue of physician competence has been addressed with modest success by the creation of a specialty in geriatric medicine, which has been one step to improve physician training in both the assessment of medical needs of older people and the direction of their medical care within the long-term care context. The American Society of Internal Medicine and the American Board of Family Practice provide a "certificate of added qualification" in geriatrics. but a relatively small number of physicians have qualified for this certificate.[9] In addition, the American Medical Directors Association offers educational programs as well as a certificate for physician medical directors of long-term care facilities (Ouslander et al., 1997).

For children needing long-term care, the role of physicians also raises special issues of training and skills involving accurate diagnosis, appropriate medical interventions, coordination of medical and nonmedical services, developmental assessment, and family counseling and guidance (Hobbs and Perrin, 1985; Perrin et al., 1993).

FINANCING LONG-TERM CARE

Payment sources are themselves an important influence on long-term care services. The mix varies depending on the characteristics of the person receiving care, the type of care provided, and the provider. The long-term care industry is heavily reliant on government funds and therefore constrained to a large extent by government policies. Comprehensive data are not readily available on sources and amounts of expenditures for the broad array of long-term care services discussed in this report. Most available data are for nursing home care and home health care services. More-

---

[9]Reflecting concern about fragmentation of the medical profession, the American Board of Medical Specialties (ABMS), which recognizes 24 specialties, has developed explicit criteria for specialty recognition. Individual specialty boards, such as the American Board of Internal Medicine, in turn, have criteria for recognizing subspecialties. In addition to full specialty or subspecialty recognition (the latter through certificates of special competence), boards may establish certificates for added qualifications subject to less stringent conditions for ABMS approval.

over, expenditure data do not reflect the value of unpaid care provided by family, friends, and volunteers (for more information, see Arnoet al., 1999). Although national surveys track private spending on health services, data on out-of-pocket (uninsured) spending for many nonmedical personal care services and supportive housing services are limited.

Care provided in freestanding (not hospital-based) nursing homes[10] accounted for 8.5 percent (nearly $83 billion) of the $969 billion that Americans spent for personal health care in 1997 (Braden et al., 1998). Care provided by freestanding home health agencies accounted for another 3.3 percent ($32.3 billion) of the total personal health care expenditures. In the aftermath of Medicare's move to a prospective payment system for hospital services that provided incentives to shorten hospital stays, hospitals increased their sponsorship of nursing home and home care services. In 1996, hospital-sponsored services accounted for about 10 percent of total nursing home expenditures (up from 7 percent in 1990) and about 20 percent of home health expenditures (up from 11 percent in 1990) (Levit et al., 1997).

Long-term care services are costly. For example, the average cost of nursing home care in 1998 was more than $50,000 per year, typically exceeding individual financial resources. Because of these costs, about two-thirds of nursing home residents rely on government assistance to pay for care, either from the outset or after they have exhausted their own resources (NCHS, 2000). Medicaid coverage provides a safety net; approximately one-third of the nursing home residents pay out of private funds when admitted and eventually spend down to Medicaid eligibility. As shown in Table 2.7, in 1997 the Medicaid program accounted for almost 48 percent of nursing home expenditures and Medicare accounted for 12 percent (Braden et al., 1998). For home health care services including short-term services,[11] Medicaid accounted for only 14.6 percent of spending but Medicare accounted for almost 40 percent. Private health insurance played a small role in nursing home care (4.9 percent) but accounted for 11.5 percent of funding for home health care. Out-of-pocket payments represented a substantial share of funds for both types of care: 31 percent

---

[10]"Nursing home care" covers services provided by skilled nursing facilities and intermediate care facilities including those administered by the Department of Veterans Affairs and those provided in Medicaid funded Intermediate Care Facilities for people with mental retardation. Hospital-based nursing facilities and home health expenditures are included under hospital expenditures (Braden et al., 1998).

[11]Home health care services cover medical services provided in the home by freestanding agencies excluding medical equipment costs not billed through these agencies, nursing services provided by nursing registries, and nonmedical services such as housekeeping assistance and supervision (Levit et al., 1997).

.7 Expenditures and Source of Funds for Nursing Home and
ealth Care: United States, 1997

Source of Funds	Nursing Home Care		Home Health Care	
	Expenditures (billion dollars)	Percent of total	Expenditures (billion dollars)	Percent of total
Personal health care expenditures[a]	$82.8	100.0	$32.3	100.0
Medicare	10.1	12.2	12.8	39.6
Medicaid (federal and state)	39.4	47.6	4.8	14.9
Private health insurance	4.0	4.8	3.7	11.5
Out-of-pocket payments	25.7	31.0	7.0	21.7
Other	3.6	4.3	4.0	12.4

[a]HCFA's count of health care expenditures uses a narrow definition of home health expenditures, excluding personal care services and many other HCBS expenditures.
SOURCE: Braden et al., 1998, pp. 124–125.

for nursing homes and 22 percent for home health services (Braden et al., 1998). Funding for residential care involves widespread use of personal resources. Much of the cost of assisted living is paid for by consumers from their personal resources (Hawes et al., 1999). Board and care homes are funded mostly through Supplemental Security Income, State Supplemental Payments, and Medicaid.

Programs Funding Long-Term Care

Medicare Program

Although many Americans believe that the federal Medicare program covers long-term care, it does not. From the outset, however, the program has covered some nursing home and home health services, in part because they were seen as potential alternatives to more expensive, hospital-based acute care services.

Medicare covers nursing home care only when a beneficiary requires daily skilled inpatient nursing or rehabilitation services and has had a 3-day hospital stay in the 30 days prior to nursing home admission. The first 20 days of such care are covered in full; a maximum of 80 additional days per benefit period are covered with a copayment ($96.00 per day in

2000).[12] Medicare's adoption of a prospective payment system for hospital care created incentives for shorter inpatient stays and has encouraged nursing homes to develop post-acute care units to handle surgical and other patients who require skilled nursing care that formerly would have been provided in a hospital. Medicare covers skilled nursing post-acute care (within 30 days following discharge from an acute care hospital) not only in nursing homes, but also in rehabilitation facilities and through home health agencies. Post-acute providers accounted for 24 percent of Medicare Part A expenditures in 1994 before falling in 1995 and 1996 (ProPAC, 1997).

Medicare also covers certain health services provided in personal residences or community-based residential settings without requiring a prior hospital stay. To qualify for this coverage, beneficiaries must be homebound and under the care of a physician who orders part-time or intermittent skilled nursing care or certain other services, such as physical therapy.[13]

Medicaid Program

Under the Medicaid program, states set payment levels, establish eligibility criteria, and define covered services subject to broad federal guidelines. These guidelines require that states cover nursing facility care for those over age 20 and home health care for those eligible for skilled nursing services. In addition, states may receive federal matching funds to cover certain optional services including nursing facility care for people under age 21, services in intermediate care facilities for those with mental retardation, and personal care services. Table 2.8 shows the distribution of Medicaid spending across major types of services for each beneficiary group. Medicaid, a federal–state entitlement program, covered medical and related services for more than 41 million people at a cost of $123 billion in 1997 (Health Care Financing Review, 1999). Personal attendant services, a major vehicle for flexible, consumer-directed long-term care, are available as a Medicaid plan service in some states, though many states do not make this option available to people over age 65.

Long-term care, particularly care provided in institutional settings, accounts for a substantial portion of Medicaid expenditures. Overall, long-

---

[12]A benefit period, which is roughly similar to an episode of serious illness, starts when a beneficiary enters a hospital and ends after a break of 60 days in the use of inpatient hospital or skilled nursing care.

[13]Federally qualified health maintenance organizations serving Medicare beneficiaries are not restricted to the part-time, intermittent definition for the home health services they provide.

TABLE 2.8 Medicaid Payments, by Type of Service and Category of Beneficiary: United States, 1997

	Children	Adults 18–64	Adults 65 and Older	Disabled	Total
			(in millions)		
Total	$15,666	$12,298	$37,721	$54,192	$123,551
Inpatient hospital	5,288	4,557	1,931	10,423	23,143
Intermediate care facility for the mentally retarded	22	6	637	8,988	9,798
Nursing facility	39	39	24,591	5,448	30,504
Physician	1,848	1,889	791	2,298	7,041
Outpatient hospital	1,327	1,299	605	2,721	6,169
Home health	413	85	3,351	8,113	12,237
Prescribed drugs	1,010	881	3,343	6,518	11,972
Other	5,719	3,542	2,372	9,620	22,687

SOURCE: Health Care Financing Review, 1999, pp. 304–312.

term care expenditures accounted for 40.5 percent of Medicaid expenditures, but the percentage varied among states from less than 30 percent to nearly 60 percent (Wiener and Stevenson, 1997).

Medicaid Waivers for Home and Community-Based Care. Since 1975, states have had the choice to offer personal care services (PCS) as an optional state plan benefit in their Medicaid benefit package (42 C.F.R. 440.167). These services include assistance with activities of daily living (e.g., bathing, dressing, and eating) and instrumental activities of daily living (e.g., shopping and cooking). When a state offers PCS as an optional state plan benefit, the services must be made available statewide to all individuals meeting financial and need-based criteria (LeBlanc et al., 2000a).

The Medicaid HCBS waivers program was established with the passage of OBRA 87. This resulted in Section 1915(c) of the Social Security Act, which authorized states to exercise the option of providing HCBS as an alternative to institutional care (Miller, 1992; Miller et al., 1999a). As indicated earlier, currently, there are 1915(c) HCBS waivers active in the District of Columbia and in every state except Arizona (LeBlanc et al., 2000b). States are allowed to target waivers to specific population groups rather than offering services to all categorically or medically needy groups. States, however, must apply for a specific number of slots for individuals for each waiver, subject to the approval of HCFA. Because states are permitted to determine the specific types and mixes of services covered under these waivers, such services are not uniformly available across states.

A number of studies have examined recent trends in PCS and HCBS participants and expenditures (Miller et al., 1999a; Harrington et al., 2000f; LeBlanc et al., 2000a,b). Other studies have examined the predictors of HCBS participants and expenditures (Miller et al., 1999b; Harrington et al., 2000i). Between 1988 and 1998, both the PCS state plan benefit and HCBS waiver programs were growing at a rate surpassing the growth of nursing facility placements (Burwell, 1999). Nonetheless, the amount states spend on institutional care continues to far outweigh, by a factor of three, what they spend on home and community-based alternatives (Burwell, 1999). It should be noted, however, that Medicaid pays for room and board for those individuals living in institutions but not for those living in the community, which in part explains the higher spending for institutional services. The vast majority of spending under HCBS waivers covers services for younger people with mental retardation or developmental disabilities (Wiener and Stevenson, 1998).

Disability advocates have expressed frustration over the smallness of the PCS and HCBS waiver programs, which they feel are not adequate to allow access for all Medicaid participants with disabilities (National Blue Ribbon Panel on Personal Assistance Services, 1999). In 1998–1999, 26 states had PCS state plan optional benefits (see Table 2.5). Across the states, there were a total of 467,487 participants in the PCS state plan option in 1998-1999. Table 2.5 shows there were 211 HCBS waiver programs and 561,510 participants in the states in 1997, the most recent year for which participant data were available for all states. When all participants in the PCS program were combined with the HCBS waiver program, there were about 1 million participants in personal care and waiver programs.

To be authorized for the waiver program, states must provide assurances that the waivers will be cost-effective. The average Medicaid cost with the waiver should not be more than the average Medicaid cost without it. Many states also have imposed per-person spending caps. As a reflection of policy makers' fears of creating a much expanded long-term care benefit, and thereby greatly increasing costs, the total number of people who can be covered by waivers is generally limited. Some states, such as Colorado, screen people to assess, first, whether they need nursing home care and second, whether they are likely to enter institutional care (Wiener and Stevenson, 1998). This targeted approach, although consistent with federal legislative intent, has been criticized as being too restrictive and unduly limiting access to home and community-based services.

Supplemental Security Income Program

The primary source of public financing for residential board and care programs is the federal Supplemental Security Income (SSI) program (Title XVI of the Social Security Act), which provides a guaranteed minimum income to low-income adults and children with relatively severe disabilities who may have long-term care needs. The SSI eligibility requirements and benefit levels are nationally established. States have the option to provide State Supplemental Payments (SSP) to supplement the SSI payments. Many states offer higher supplementation for individuals living in board and care, personal care homes, or foster care homes. Each state sets its own rates for SSP and these rates determine the amount that many residential care facilities receive as monthly payments for services. The SSI/SSP payment amount was $3.8 billion in 1998.

The number of children and adolescents covered by the SSI program has grown from approximately 265,000 in 1989 to almost 847,000 in 1999 (SSA, 1999). Much of this growth may reflect changes in public policies and the types of disabling impairments that are recognized and diagnosed for benefits. Some of the growth also reflects marked improvements in survival of young people with more severe chronic health conditions (Perrin et al., 1998, 1999).

State-Funded Programs

States vary enormously in the proportion of their state dollars that go to nursing homes compared to home and community-based services. According to both a General Accounting Office (GAO) study (GAO, 1994) and an AARP study (Alecxih et al., 1996), several states have made substantial inroads into shifting the balance of funds from nursing homes to HCBS services; these states are typically characterized by strong state and local organizations with effective local case management to target and allocate services.

In addition to the Medicaid and SSP funding, states also fund long-term care with earmarked dollars from the Older Americans Act, from allocations of the Social Services Block Grant (Title XX), and from their own general revenues raised through taxes and other means. Title III of the Older Americans Act funds care management, home delivered meals, respite programs, and various caregiver programs. Social Services Block Grants can be used for long-term care as well; however, since the amounts of these grants have not increased, states have tended to convert the programs to Medicaid to access federal match. Most notably, in the early 1990s, California converted a huge In-Home Supportive Services program from Title XX to Medicaid.

States still use substantial amounts of their own money for long-term care without federal matching dollars or federal grants. Typically these moneys are used for consumers who do not quite meet the financial or functional eligibility for Medicaid. Occasionally, state dollars are used to pay spouses for care since spousal payments are not allowed under Medicaid. Some states use state money as a cushion to pay for care when Medicaid eligibility is denied. Those who make that decision can use presumptive eligibility for HCBS services to make up the shortfall. Substantial local public money also goes into long-term care, especially when states require local matches for state programs. Some communities have raised local tax levies earmarked for long-term care.

Long-Term Care Insurance

Private insurance for long-term care covers limited numbers of people, types of services, and percentage of expenses. Although private insurance accounts for about 5 percent of nursing home and 12 percent of home health spending, most of this is ordinary health insurance that, like Medicare, provides limited benefits for extended care. Among elderly Americans—those most at risk—perhaps 7 percent have long-term care insurance (Wiener and Stevenson, 1998), and few people under age 65 purchase it. Some large employers offer such insurance at group rates, and Congress is considering offering federal employees and retirees long-term care insurance, but the employee typically pays the full premium.

A major barrier to the growth of private long-term care insurance is its cost (Wiener et al., 1994). Access to long-term care insurance is also restricted by insurers' underwriting criteria that limit initial purchase of individual policies to those in reasonably good health who can take care of themselves.

COORDINATION OF LONG-TERM CARE SERVICES

The concept of coordination of care is not defined in a precise manner. It can be more or less formal and can involve all or only a subset of services that an individual might need. Wide disparities in this process exist across states and across categorical eligible groups.

Integration of care through a managed care system implies the greatest degree of coordination, though typically long-term care services are not covered in the care that is capitated. Moreover, managed care does not imply vigorous care management at the level of the individual enrollee. A few capitated demonstration programs for people who are dually eligible for Medicare and Medicaid (such as the Minnesota Senior Health Organization, Commonwealth Fund supported demonstrations in New York

State, and the Wisconsin Partnerships) are indeed attempting to institute a care management capability that follows the consumer over time and across services including acute care and the full range of long-term care services. Often nurse practitioners are responsible for this coordination, attempting to follow the consumer whether they are in clinics, hospitals, home care, or nursing homes. The PACE (Program of All-Inclusive Care for the Elderly) programs are care organizations that tend to enroll about 300 people, all of whom are low income and all of whom are nursing home eligible. In this case, the enrollees are closely managed by a multi-disciplinary team (R.L. Kane, 1999).

Most long-term care is coordinated by some combination of the consumers themselves or their families, who by default are typically left to coordinate fragmented services. Some people, because of illness or cognitive limitations, cannot coordinate their care and lack family members willing or able to do so. A private-pay care management industry has arisen to meet this need. As already mentioned above, the home and community-based waiver program tends to have built-in case management, responsible for initial and ongoing assessment, identifying services, and coordinating and monitoring a care plan. Given that services in residential care settings are often covered for Medicaid-eligible people in HCBS waivers, care managers also coordinate those services for eligible people.

At the same time, provider agencies have their own coordination capabilities and claims, and complex agencies often have a need to coordinate their own services across disciplines, as well as to coordinate with other agencies concurrently serving the client. Home health agencies, for example, not only coordinate care for their clients, but also undertake "skilled evaluation and planning." When performed by a nurse or therapist, it is also a Medicare-covered skilled service. The Minimum Data Set for nursing homes, discussed in Chapter 4, is meant to be a vehicle for nursing homes to do care planning. Although most Medicaid money is expended in nursing homes, very few states have a system whereby the care managers for HCBS follow the individual after admission to a nursing home.

For children, a primary care physician caring for a child with serious chronic illness will typically be coordinating a range of inpatient and home-based medical services including sub-specialist services that may require negotiation of conflicting perspectives and treatment recommendations. For example, a child with hemophilia may need a hematologist, orthopedist, physical therapist, specialized dentist, blood bank specialist, and social worker, as well as specialized nurses or home health aides. The physician will work with families and care managers or care coordinators (often nurses or social workers) to assess the child's developmental progress and needs, develop appropriate care plans suited to changing medical and developmental status, and advise on choices related to education options. The care coordinator will typically help link the family with appropriate services to implement the care plan, monitor the plan and outcomes, and generally assist the family and child in moving toward greater control and management of services (see Jessop and Stein, 1994; Perrin and Bloom, 1994).

Consumer-Centered Care

Consumer-centered care that reflects the preferences and choices of the consumers of the service is desirable for almost all people across all health care settings, including long-term care settings, although the specific elements may vary. Moreover, not all consumers of long-term care are as well positioned to exercise their preferences and choices as in acute care markets. Generally, nursing homes with a consumer-centered focus may emphasize resident service in staff training, actively involve residents and or their families in care planning, provide a physical environment that supports, to the extent applicable, resident privacy and autonomy, and regularly solicit feedback from residents and families regarding their experiences and satisfaction with care. The philosophy of residential care settings such as assisted living emphasize autonomy and they may be expected to allow for individual preferences and privacy. Likewise, small group homes for people with developmental disabilities and, to a lesser extent, mental illness are intended to allow for increased independence, choice, and involvement in the community. Consumer-centered approaches are also applicable in home care delivery through collaborative care planning, an emphasis on educating and building the self care capacity of recipients of care and their families, and efforts to integrate professional services with informal community care resources.

The principles of consumer-centered care for children have been extended to encompass family-centered care and family-directed care. Family-centered long-term care for children with physical and developmental disabilities has been mandated and supported through federal legislation, specifically the Individuals with Disabilities Education Act (1997) and its subsequent amendments (IDEA, 1997, P.L. 105-17, originally named Education for All Handicapped Children Act, PL 94-142). This legislation provides for early intervention services and an individualized and appropriate public special education for children with disabilities in the least restrictive environment, at no cost to families. By law, families must be included as team participants through referral, evaluation, and yearly assessments of progress. Eligible children receive special education services, physical and occupational therapy, speech and language therapy, and other related medical and social services as identified through coordinated service plans. Plans for families with infants and toddlers include services to support and strengthen families through assistance with employment, obtaining health insurance, and linking them with support networks. Family involvement in the care of children with long-term health conditions has been supported by a variety of family assistance services, including those provided by volunteers (Trachtenberg and Batshaw, 1997; Perrin, 1998).

CONCLUSION

This profile of long-term care highlights the diversity that characterizes the population using these services and the settings in which care is provided. It depicts a "system" of long-term care that is highly variable across states and communities, fragmented, and unevenly coordinated. Different kinds of long-term care services have evolved, in part to meet the varying needs and, to an uncertain degree, the preferences of users. A combination of forces including the needs and preferences of long-term care users, federal and state regulatory requirements, professional doctrines, and financial incentives created by payment mechanisms and capital markets have sometimes worked together to increase the availability of needed forms of long-term care, such as increasing options for noninstitutional care.

3

State of Quality of Long-Term Care

This chapter addresses a specific task in the committee's mandate—to determine the current quality of long-term care in the various settings and the extent to which it has improved or deteriorated in the past several years. The chapter begins with a brief description of the committee's criteria for judging quality of care and the measurement of quality of care in long-term care settings. It summarizes available evidence about the current status of quality of care, focusing in particular on areas of improvement and on the nature and extent of continuing problems. The chapter then discusses whether the legislative and regulatory efforts to improve quality have achieved their objectives, namely improvement of quality in long-term care.

The committee's task was made difficult by the unevenness of available empirical evidence. Although information to judge quality of care in nursing homes is extensive and systematic, for most other settings it is nonexistent or very limited, and lacks uniformity. Moreover, opinions about what constitutes excellent, good, or poor quality care are changing and sometimes conflicting. Some of the available information is open to interpretation, and conclusions are sometimes based on personal and clinical experience rather than empirical evidence. The discussion in this chapter is based on data from national data systems and surveys, on published research and studies in progress, and on testimony received by the committee.

MEASUREMENT OF QUALITY OF CARE

uality of care in long-term care "is a complex concept confounded by regulations [and] debates about what should be measured to assess quality" (IOM, 1996b, p. 129). Defining quality in long-term care has been a difficult process; it is defined both as an input measure and as an outcome. Since the mid-1960s, quality assessment has been measured in terms of three concepts: structures of care, processes of care, and outcomes of care (Donabedian, 1966). Over the years, nursing home quality has been measured by *structural* variables such as level, mix, and education and training of staff; and characteristics of the facilities in relation to characteristics of the residents such as demographics, payer mix, and casemix. *Process* measures assess the services actually provided to the residents. Deficiencies in processes of care can be described as overuse of care, underuse of care, or poor technical performance (see, for example, IOM, 1990; Chassin and Galvin, 1998). Other process problems in long-term care have been characterized as neglect (e.g., inattention to weight loss) or even abuse (e.g., physical assault).

Outcomes of care include changes in health status and conditions attributable to the care provided or not provided. Unlike acute care, for which successful outcomes often mean restoring patients to their level of functioning before the onset of illness, successful outcomes in long-term care are likely to be based on criteria such as maximizing quality of life and physical function in the presence of permanent, and sometimes worsening, impairment. The occurrence of specific problems, such as pressure sores or inappropriate weight loss, is generally viewed as evidence of poor quality of care. Because care processes and structural factors are the means through which desired outcomes are achieved, they are key components in defining quality. In principle, health and quality-of-life *outcomes* are the end results of the structures and processes of care. Outcomes of interest might include overall health status, the presence or absence of specific conditions (e.g., pressure sores), social and psychological well-being, and satisfaction with care. However, using outcomes to assess quality of care is often difficult because of conceptual and practical (e.g., cost) considerations in collecting information on health status and quality of life. As a result, measures of structure and process (e.g., staffing levels or rates of sedative use) are frequently used as proxies for outcome measures of quality of care in various long-term settings. Opinions in the literature and in testimony given to the committee, and even among the committee, vary widely about the empirical evidence linking specific structural features or processes of care to the outcomes in question. At the same time, adequate availability of structural measures, such as staffing and facility characteristics, is essential to the provision of consumer-oriented long-term care.

In evaluating the quality of long-term care, multiple perspectives have to be considered. Application of the concept of consumer-oriented long-term care requires that the quality of long-term care be judged not only in terms of the structure, processes, and outcomes of clinical care, but also in terms of access to care, the nonmedical personal assistance services that are an important part of long-term care, and the long-term care user's quality of life. Because perspectives can differ among recipients of long-term care services and between care recipients and care providers, one of the challenges is establishing priorities reflecting different perspectives.

Standards for evaluating whether the quality of long-term care is good or bad, improving or deteriorating, are shaped by several considerations including views of the nature and scope of long-term care, the operational definitions of quality, and the ways quality-of-care data and research findings are interpreted. Different observers such as physicians, nurses, consumers, family members, and society also will have different perspectives. Different circumstances will require assessing the views of these and other participants. Long-term care can encompass a broad range of services affecting many aspects of daily life. It is easy to see how observers might differ in their views on the nature and scope of the field and therefore the basis on which the quality of long-term care should be judged. The following are three aspects of long-term care that are relevant to the assessment of its quality:

1. Long-term care is *both a health and a social program*. Although many long-term care programs are currently identified and judged primarily as either social models or medical models (R.A. Kane, 1999), users' needs do not divide so readily. Some aspects of long-term care are based on services that require knowledge of health conditions and their treatment. Other aspects are aimed at services to help people with functional limitations live in ways that maximize their capability and productivity. Long-term care funding comes partly from health programs, but also from social service and income support programs. For the health services components of long-term care, judgments about quality of care emphasize medical and technical aspects of care. For other aspects of long-term care, judgments about quality of care reflect the opinions and satisfaction of consumers (or their surrogate agents).

2. *The potential and actual role of consumers* is an essential element in long-term care. As indicated in Chapter 1, long-term care, and therefore the basis for evaluating the quality of such care, is being redefined (at least in some care settings) by the growing recognition of the role of

consumers and their involvement in choosing and directing many features of their care and in assessing the adequacy of care.

3. For nursing homes and residential care settings including assisted living, the *physical environment* of the facility can contribute to the physical safety and functional mobility of residents and, more broadly, to their quality of life. Privacy is an aspect of the physical environment and is intimately tied to the consumer-centered principles the committee endorses.

CURRENT STATE OF QUALITY OF CARE

No single or simple formula is available to guide those attempting to evaluate the quality of long-term care. Evaluators must determine how to interpret a variety of data on health outcomes and provider performance, on many different aspects of care for many individual consumers, and on many providers over a period of time.

Regulatory quality standards often focus on deficiencies in care, defined by the presence or absence of specified problems. When such standards are applied, the quality of care is considered lower if problems are found than if they are not found. At the present time, most measurable standards of quality do not recognize excellence in care with criteria based on positive outcomes, such as maximizing physical functioning or, in the psychological sphere, going beyond minimizing depression and anxiety to maximizing well-being. The following sections examine the state of quality of care in each of the specific long-term care settings addressed in this report.

Nursing Homes

The committee reviewed a large volume of research and investigative reports to examine the quality of nursing home care. In addition, two sources of data are available on nursing home care: (1) the On-Line Survey and Certification Assessment Reporting (OSCAR) System from the federal survey and certification system permits the analysis of longitudinal patterns of deficiencies identified in nursing home inspections; and (2) studies using resident-level data from the Minimum Data Set (MDS), which permits tracing quality indicators in nursing homes. (These information systems are discussed in Chapter 4.) Other research studies provide information on the state of quality, as do recent studies by the General Accounting Office (GAO). Some information also can be inferred from testimony presented to the committee.

Evidence indicates that the quality of nursing home care in general has improved over the past decade, even though nursing homes are serving a more seriously ill population (Hawes, 1996; Johnson and Kramer, 1998). For example, many facilities have successfully reduced the inappropriate use of physical and chemical restraints. The focus of increased regulatory scrutiny on these two areas of care was a major contributing factor in reductions in both of these. Despite these improvements, serious quality-of-care problems persist in some nursing homes. Pain, pressure sores, malnutrition, and urinary incontinence have all been shown to be serious problems in recent studies of nursing home residents (GAO, 1998a; Mortimore et al., 1998). The committee recognizes that change in eliminating or reducing persistent and serious problems is a long process requiring diligent monitoring and enforced adherence to standards. In a paper prepared for the committee, Johnson and Kramer (1998)[1] noted that continuing problems include physical pain and insufficient attention to rehabilitation and restorative nursing. GAO (1999b) and the Office of the Inspector General of the Department of Health and Human Services (OIG, 1999c) reported that national data from the OSCAR system between July 1995 and October 1998 provide evidence of increasing problems with some aspects of care, including lack of supervision to prevent accidents, improper care for pressure sores, and inadequate assistance with activities of daily living.

Data based on state certification surveys of facilities indicate that problems occur in many nursing homes and that they are persistent in a smaller subset of facilities (GAO, 1999b). About one-quarter of nursing homes had deficiencies[2] in the highest-severity categories. Figure 3.1 shows the ten most frequent deficiencies for poor quality of care cited in the United States. In 1998, the most frequent deficiency was poor food sanitation (23.7 percent of the 15,401 facilities surveyed) (Harrington et al., 2000b). Failure to remove accident hazards was cited in 18 percent of facilities, poor general quality of care was cited in 17.2 percent, and failure to prevent or properly treat pressure sores was cited in 17.1 percent. Poor care planning, improper resident assessment, failure to prevent accidents, poor housekeeping, failure to protect the dignity of residents, and improper use of physical restraints were also problems in a significant proportion of homes.

GAO (1999b) also found that 40 percent of the facilities that had severe deficiencies in an earlier survey had deficiencies of equal or greater severity

---

[1]The committee commissioned this background paper from Johnson and Kramer for its use. Much of the analysis in this chapter on the quality of care in nursing homes draws from this paper.

[2]The Health Care Financing Administration (HCFA) defines a deficiency as a failure to meet a Medicare participation requirement. One or more deficiencies in critical areas result in a finding of substandard quality of care.

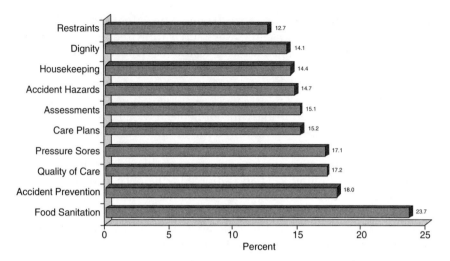

FIGURE 3.1 Top 10 deficiencies of nursing facilities and percent of facilities with the deficiency cited: United States, 1998.
SOURCE: Harrington and Carillo, 2000.

at the time of a later survey. In another study based on the federal and state survey process, GAO (1998a) found that serious and potentially life-threatening quality-of-care problems in the categories of neglect, abuse, malnutrition, and pressure sores occurred in approximately 30 percent of California nursing homes over a two-year period. This study found that another 33 percent of facilities had poor care that caused less serious harm, and 35 percent had more than minimal deficiencies. Overall, GAO found that only 2 percent of California facilities had minimal or no deficiencies, while one in nine was cited for causing actual harm or putting residents in immediate jeopardy (GAO, 1998a). GAO (1998a) also reviewed the medical records of a sample of 62 residents who had died. More than half (34 residents) had received unacceptable care that endangered health and safety. These problems included dramatic unplanned weight loss, failure to properly treat pressure sores, and failure to manage pain. Although problems in California nursing homes may not be representative of national problems, California's 1,370 nursing homes alone represent about 10 percent of the nursing homes in the United States.

Another study of 14 facilities documented significant problems with nutritional support, care for pressure sores, personal care, pain management, and personal environment and contracture care in 25 to 35 percent of the facilities studied (Kramer, 1998). Kramer also found significant problems with falls, functional losses, incontinence care, skin breakdown, use of physical restraints, avoidable deaths, antipsychotic drug use, and lack of functional rehabilitation in 10 to 15 percent of the facilities sampled.

Additional evidence comes from complaints to the Long-Term Care Ombudsman Program in some states (OIG, 1999a). The OIG and state ombudsmen link many of these complaints to inadequate nursing home staffing. Abuse, patient neglect, and the hiring of staff with criminal records have been widely reported in the media and by local ombudsmen, although the actual prevalence of such problems is unknown (Kauffman, 1996).

The current state of quality of care, based on some key indicators of quality, is summarized briefly below. This includes use of physical and chemical restraints, pressure sores, malnutrition, continence care, pain, and aspects of care related to quality of life.

Physical and Chemical Restraints

The greatest improvement in nursing home care is in the substantial reductions in use of physical restraints since the reforms in the Omnibus Budget Reconciliation Act of 1987 (hereafter OBRA 87). The Health Care Financing Administration (HCFA) defines restraints as mechanical devices, materials, or equipment that restricts freedom of movement or normal access to one's body. Restraints may cause decreased muscle tone and increase the likelihood of falls, incontinence, pressure ulcers, depression, and other problems. A number of studies have shown the value of reducing the use of restraints (Evans and Strumpf, 1989; Libow and Starer, 1989; Burton et al., 1992; Phillips et al., 1993a; Castle and Mor, 1998).

In the late 1980s, the prevalence of physical restraint use was an estimated 41 percent, with wide variability among facilities (Strumpf and Tomes, 1993). Using 1990 data, Phillips and colleagues (1996) reported a mean physical restraint use of 38 percent in 268 facilities in ten cities. Following the implementation of OBRA 87, Hawes and colleagues (1997b) reported a decrease in average restraint use to 28 percent for the same facilities. Other researchers also have reported declines in restraint use (Ejaz et al., 1994; Sundel et al., 1994; Graber and Sloane, 1995; Levine et al., 1995; Capezuti et al., 1996; Castle and Mor, 1998). OSCAR data show a 41 percent decline in restraint use since the early 1990s, from 21 percent of all residents in 1991 to 12.3 percent in 1998 (Harrington et al., 2000b).

Although the literature suggests an average decrease in physical restraint use since OBRA 87, Johnson and Kramer (1998) note that there is reason for ongoing concern. An average decrease in restraint use may mask persistently high use in some facilities. In 1995, for example, with the rate of restraint use at an average of 20 percent, 21 percent of the facilities had rates exceeding 25 percent of residents (Castle, 1998a; Castle and Mor, 1998). Moreover, evidence that facility factors such as staffing, occupancy rate, for-profit status, and Medicaid reimbursement policies affect restraint use more than patient needs raises questions about the appropriateness of restraint use (Phillips et al., 1996; Castle, 1998a).

The overuse of psychotropic medications, referred to as chemical restraints, was also targeted by OBRA 87. The average use of antipsychotic and sedative hypnotic medications appears to have declined, and there is no evidence that physical restraint reduction has been accompanied by increased use of chemical restraints (Siegler et al., 1997; Castle, 1998b). Garrard and colleagues (1995) reported a decrease in the use of anti-psychotic medications from a mean of 23 percent prior to OBRA 87 to 15 percent after OBRA 87 in all Minnesota nursing homes. Burton and col-leagues (1992) reported a 36 percent decrease in antipsychotic drug use in a sample of Maryland nursing homes between July and December 1990, when OBRA 87 regulations were being implemented. A longitudinal study of Tennessee Medicaid recipients in nursing homes showed a 26.7 percent decrease in antipsychotic drug use following implementation of OBRA 87 (Shorr et al., 1994).

Decreased use of psychotropic medications appears to have been accompanied by improved documentation of appropriate indications for psychotropic drug use. Llorente and colleagues (1998) reported that 70 percent of resident medical records were found to have appropriate docu-mentation, compared with less than 50 percent prior to OBRA 87. There is no evidence of improved behavioral management programs to replace the use of psychotropic drugs (Hawes et al., 1997b).

Quality concerns about psychotropic drug use persist, despite mean decreases in use. As Johnson and Kramer (1998) point out, psychotropic medication use is far more complicated. The arrival of multiple new anti-psychotic medications with improved side-effect profiles may result in increased use of antipsychotic drugs (Lasser and Sunderland, 1998). Few studies are available on the propriety of psychotropic drug use in indi-vidual patients.

Pressure Sores

Pressure sores (decubitus ulcers) are bruises or open sores on the skin, usually found on the hips, buttocks, heels, or other bony areas, from pressure or friction on the skin. They range from bruises in early stages to open wounds that may reach the bone at later stages. Severe pressure sores may result in pain or infection, and can be fatal. Because good nursing care can generally prevent pressure sores from occurring and ensure that the skin heals properly, the presence of pressure sores has been used for decades as an outcome indicator for quality of care in nursing homes (Zimmerman et al., 1995; Mukamel and Brower, 1998). Moreover, a study of three Department of Veterans Affairs nursing homes, with pressure sore prevalence ranging from 2 to 16 percent, found an association between prevalence and staffing patterns, after controlling for casemix, suggesting that pressure sores can basically be eliminated with appropriate nursing care (Rudman et al., 1993).

Data generally indicate, however, that pressure sores are a continuing problem in nursing facilities. They were reported for 7.1 percent of all nursing home residents in 1998, which was about the same as in 1991 (Harrington et al., 2000b). Other studies have reported prevalence rates from 7 to 23 percent, with wide variability among facilities (Zinn et al., 1993; Smith, 1995). In the most recent state surveys, 17.1 percent of facilities had deficiencies related to care for pressure sores (Harrington et al., 2000b), and in 10 states, the number of deficiencies had increased 21 percent from previous surveys (OIG, 1999b). Another study of 254 facilities in 10 states, however, showed some decrease in the prevalence of pressure sores following implementation of OBRA 87 (Fries et al., 1997). No increase in preventive skin care was evident in a pre- and post-OBRA cohort of 268 facilities (Hawes et al., 1997b).

As stated above, the prevalence of pressure ulcers in the population of nursing home residents, as reported in the federal inspection survey and reflecting the residents in the home at the time of the survey, varies by state and by type of facility. Even within states and types of facility variability is noted in the prevalence of pressure ulcers. For example, one unpublished analysis of OSCAR data indicates that among freestanding, non-hospital-based facilities, an average of 6 percent of residents per facility have pressure ulcers on the day of the survey. This varies by state between 3 and 8 percent as the average for these kinds of facilities, but the averages may belie considerable variability. Across the 50 states, 17 percent of facilities had greater than 10 percent of their residents with a pressure ulcer, varying from 1 percent of the facilities in one state to 27 percent in another. Even more variation is observed when these same figures are examined for hospital-based facilities which admit almost all of their patients from hospitals and where most residents do not remain for an extended stay. The risk of acquiring a pressure ulcer is strongly affected by the clinical characteristics of the resident as well as the nursing care provided, and residents entering a hospital-based facility are likely to be more impaired and have more serious medical problems (Vincent Mor, personal communication, May 9, 2000). However, a vast majority of nursing home residents are not such "short-stayers."

Since 1995, HCFA's OSCAR data have captured two measures of the rate of pressure ulcers: (1) the number of residents with a pressure ulcer on the day of the survey; and (2) the number of residents in the facility on the day of the survey who had a pressure ulcer at the time of their admission to the facility. In general, these two figures are highly correlated (0.72), but they are more correlated among hospital-based facilities (0.87) than among freestanding facilities (0.53) (Vincent Mor, Personal Communication, May 9, 2000). This is not surprising because one predictor of pressure sores is previous pressure sores.

Malnutrition and Dehydration

Nutritional problems and dehydration are considered to be serious—and commonly underreported—problems in nursing homes. Inadequate food intake has been found to be a major determinant of mortality in frail elderly people in nursing homes (Blaum et al., 1995; Frisoni et al., 1995). Blaum and colleagues (1995) found that needing assistance with eating was significantly associated with undernourishment among nursing home residents. Malnutrition, starvation, and dehydration have all been documented in recent studies (Kayser-Jones, 1996, 1997; Kayser-Jones et al., 1997; Kayser-Jones and Schell, 1997). Moreover, commercial dietary supplements are being used inappropriately as substitutes for food, perhaps because of insufficient staff for oral feeding and perhaps because of undiagnosed dysphagia or poor oral health (Kayser-Jones et al., 1998). Kayser-Jones et al. (1999) reported that in two nursing homes, fluid intake was inadequate for 39 of 40 residents, contributing to dehydration. (See Chapter 6 for further discussion of this subject.)

Continence Care

Incontinence is a common problem for nursing home residents and requires that they receive assistance in toileting and care to prevent accidents. Incontinence can be reversed in almost half of the individuals who develop it and can be improved in other individuals (Ouslander and Kane, 1984; Ribeiro and Smith, 1985; Palmer et al., 1991, 1994). Bladder incontinence was reported for 50.7 percent of residents in 1998, a 7.8 percent increase since 1991 (Harrington et al., 2000b).

Bowel incontinence, which declined only slightly (3 percent) during the 1991–1998 period, was reported as a problem for 41.6 percent of residents in 1998. In recent nursing home inspections, 10 percent of facilities were cited for deficiencies in incontinence care (OIG, 1999b). Because this problem is reversible in many cases, high prevalence of incontinence suggests poor care.

Research studies help illustrate the problems. In interviews, residents have indicated a preference for assistance in toilet use or changes of wet linen two times per eight-hour day (Simmons and Schnelle, 1999), but observational studies found that residents were changed less often than this and received toileting assistance even less frequently, an average of only 0.4 to 0.5 times in 8- or 12-hour periods during the daytime (Schnelle et al., 1988a,b; Bowers and Becker, 1992; Simmons and Schnelle, 1999). Residents who were demented and physically or verbally agitated were likely to receive lower levels of assistance (Schnelle et al., 1992b). The low frequency of toileting assistance has been attributed to its being more time-consuming for staff than simply changing residents' wet clothing or bedding. In fact, one study found that "usual" daytime toileting and mobility care required about 11 minutes of staff time per resident over a 12-hour period compared to 46 minutes per resident for a toileting assistance protocol (Schnelle et al., 1995a).

Urinary catheters are sometimes used to control bladder incontinence, but they should be used only when medically necessary because they are associated with infection and discomfort (Ribeiro and Smith, 1985). OSCAR data indicate that urinary catheter use declined by 10.6 percent between 1991 and 1998 for all nursing home residents in the United States (to 7.6 percent of nursing home residents in 1998) (Harrington et al., 2000b). Others examining catheter use following OBRA 87 reforms also found a decline. One study of pre- and post-OBRA period nursing home residents in Virginia found that less than 1 percent of the residents were inappropriately catheterized (Moseley, 1996). Hawes and colleagues (1997b) reported a statistically significant mean decrease in indwelling urinary catheter use from 9.8 percent to 7 percent following implementation of OBRA 87. The decline observed in catheter use may be viewed as a positive development in quality of nursing home care.

Pain Management

Despite widespread agreement that much pain can be ameliorated by appropriate use of medications, undiagnosed and untreated pain has been a widespread problem in many health care settings (AHCPR, 1994; IOM, 1997). Prevalence of chronic pain is estimated in 45 to 80 percent of nursing home residents (Ferrell, 1995; IOM, 1997). A study of Oregon nursing homes found that of the residents suffering from pain, 39 percent were inadequately treated for pain (Wagner et al., 1997), and another study found that more than one-quarter of nursing home residents suffering from cancer received no pain medication even though they had daily pain (Bernabei et al., 1998).

Levels of pain can be particularly difficult to determine, especially among people who cannot easily communicate in words, and methods to identify and assess other signs of distress need further development. In addition, people in general—and nursing home residents and staff in particular—may have low expectations, believing that pain but not pain relief is to be expected. More effective pain management techniques should be a priority for nursing homes, using, as appropriate, palliative techniques developed by hospices and others.

Hospitalization

As Johnson and Kramer (1998) point out, nosocomial infections, pressure ulcers, and deterioration of functional abilities because of bed rest are common iatrogenic complications of hospitalization of nursing home residents. A potential indicator of improved resident assessment and quality of care would be decreased overall hospitalizations and improved selection of patients for hospitalization. However, appropriate rates of hospitalization are difficult to determine (Castle and Mor, 1996). Mor and colleagues (1997) in a study of 250 nursing homes reported decreased odds of hospitalization of residents between 1990 and 1993, following implementation of the resident assessment system called for in OBRA 87. (See Chapter 4 for more details.) The effect was more pronounced among residents with cognitive impairments. Demonstration projects are now in place and will explore whether enhanced payments and provision of geriatric care through nurse practitioners and other personnel can reduce hospitalizations and lead to improved outcomes.

Quality of Life

Quality of life is difficult to conceptualize, let alone measure. Some commentators view quality of life as the sum of all other domains including physical health, cognitive status, and functional status as well as psychological, social, spiritual, and economic well-being, whereas others make a sharper distinction between quality of life as a psychosocial phenomenon apart from health status (Birren et al., 1991; Frytak, 2000). Quality of life has an inevitable subjective component, necessitating direct input from the persons most concerned—the long-term care consumers—to provide feedback on quality of life domains and to suggest how they should be weighted. But for long-term care consumers, especially residents in nursing homes, several problems require that information on quality of life be sought from multiple sources. Low expectations or fear of being critical of those on whom they are dependent may affect response. Also, some residents are too cognitively impaired to provide reliable information or, in some cases, any information at all. Their quality of life must be inferred from observation and other sources (e.g., family).

The literature contains many statements about what residents find important for the quality of their lives. Such statements are variously derived from empirical studies using focus groups (NCCNHR, 1985; Abt Associates, 1996), questionnaires to residents or family members (Kane et al., 1986; Kane et al., 1997), "Q-sort studies" with staff (Sano et al., 1999), systematic observations of residents (Lidz et al., 1992; Lawton et al., 1996), anthropological and ethnographic studies (Shield, 1988; Tellis-Nayak and Tellis-Nayak, 1989; Schmidt, 1990; Savashitsky, 1991; Gubrium, 1993), and psychologically oriented research dealing with the search for identity and meaning among nursing home residents (Tobin, 1991). Others have written autobiographical or fictional accounts of life in nursing homes from the perspectives of residents (Tulloch, 1975; Laird, 1985) or nursing aides (Bennett; 1980; Tisdale, 1987; Diamond, 1992: Foner, 1994; Henderson, 1995).

In addition to their emphasis on various aspects of staff behavior and choice, cognitively intact residents have also cited other features that make their lives better or worse in nursing homes, including the quality of food and the ambience at meal time; having a private room or having a compatible or at least not incompatible roommate (Lawton and Bader, 1970; Kane et al., 1997; 1998a); getting outside during pleasant weather; being able to maintain contacts and communicate readily with relatives and friends outside the facility (Kane et al., 1997); getting a good night's sleep; and for some cognitively intact residents, being spared frequent close contact with residents with dementia, particularly those whose behavior and demeanor are frightening or disturbing (Teresi et al., 1993). Residents with advanced cognitive disabilities are unable to report reliably and completely what affects the quality of their lives. On their behalf, observers comment on some things that seem to afford pleasure (e.g., music, other sensory stimulation) and those that bring misery (e.g., forced baths, being physically tied down).

Measuring Quality of Life. One approach to measuring quality of life for nursing home residents, called real experiences and assessment of life (REAL), was developed by researchers at Vital Research in California and tested in facilities under the auspices of a small business grant from the National Institutes of Health (Vital Research, 2000). The REAL is composed of yes-no questions and, in the resident version, generates six factors: help and assistance; communication with staff; autonomy and choice; companionship; safety and security; and food and environment. The survey is administered by staff of the research agency. The Confidence Satisfaction Survey was developed by Life Services Network of Illinois (1997) and uses many of the same items as REAL. This survey is administered by facility staff and sent for interpretation by the network. No standards have been published yet on either of these tools.

In recent years, considerable emphasis has been given to measuring well-being, including quality of life, for people with dementia in nursing homes (Albert and Logsdon, 1999). Some of these measures concentrate on behavioral symptoms exhibited by the person with dementia that tend to render caregiving difficult but may not always equate with a poor quality of life as experienced by the person with dementia (Cohen-Mansfield, 1989). Most of the approaches for examining functioning of the person with dementia rely on the summary reports of paid or family caregivers. Rabins and colleagues (1999) have developed a multidimensional instrument for measuring the quality of life (QOL) of people with dementia through reports from caregivers; it contains five domains: social interaction; awareness of self; feeling and mood; enjoyment of activities; and response to surroundings.

More recently, QOL measures gathered by direct interviews with people with dementia have been developed and tested. Examples include the quality of life–AD scale, a brief 13-item measure, each with a 4-point response set (Logsdon, et al., 1999); and the D-QOL, a longer self-report tool developed by Brod and colleagues (Brod et al., 1999); the latter tool also has five domains: aesthetics, positive affect, negative affect, self-esteem, and feelings of belonging. The work with these three direct-interview tools, as well as work with the REAL mentioned above, gives encouragement to the idea that data can be gathered by direct report from many nursing home residents with dementia.

Finally, the apparent affect rating scale (Lawton et al., 1996, 1999) has been developed as a way of making systematic observations of four mood states in people with dementia: pleasure, sadness, anxiety, anger, and interest. The instrument has been shown to be reliable even, under proper training conditions, when administered by nursing aides. It also has been shown to be sensitive to interventions of the nursing home and changes in staff behavior.

In 1998, HCFA awarded a contract to the University of Minnesota to develop and test measures and indicators of quality of life. The researchers are attempting to measure 11 quality of life domains: dignity, autonomy, individuality, privacy, enjoyment, meaningful activity, relationships, comfort, sense of security and order, spiritual well-being, and functional competence. The first wave field test, underway in 40 nursing homes in five states, is expected to be completed by June 2000 and include data measuring quality of life for about 2,000 residents, half with substantial cognitive impairment. The investigators are collecting data on individual residents from four sources whenever possible: the residents themselves, line staff members caring for each resident, resident observations, and family questionnaires. Analyses will examine the congruence of each data source as well as the psychometric properties and the reliability and inter-temporal stability of the measures (Kane et al., 1999).

Status of Quality of Life. In the past, several studies had found the circumstances of life in nursing homes limited (Diamond 1992; Gubrium, 1993; Henderson and Vespari, 1995). As shown in the previous pages, since the implementation of OBRA 87, quality of care in nursing homes has improved in some categories of care, but in other categories persistent problems remain. For quality of life in nursing homes, the situation is not as encouraging. On the positive side, improvements in care, such as reduced use of physical and chemical restraints, also improve aspects of quality of life, including autonomy and dignity. On the negative side, evidence of deficiencies in care, such as the high prevalence of incontinence, is not consistent with high quality of life. Even though OBRA 87 had beneficial effects on several measures of quality, Kane and colleagues (1997) for example, found that it was difficult for nursing home residents to exercise desired choices or for nursing assistants to enhance residents' choices. Poor quality of life in many nursing facilities continues to be a concern. Until sufficient trained staff is available to allow time and skills to provide the care and personal attention, and until the standards of quality of life included in OBRA 87 are rigorously enforced, problems with quality of care and life will persist in some facilities.

In recent years, efforts have been made to improve the quality of life in nursing homes as well as the ability to measure it. For example, Rader and colleagues have been developing approaches whereby bathing can be a more individualized and pleasant experience for residents (Rader et al., 1996; Hoeffer et al., 1997). Efforts to measure quality of life for nursing home residents with dementia have accelerated in the last few years; the available tools include scales administered to residents, staff, and or family (Lawton et al., 1996; Logsdon, et al., 1999; Rabins et al., 1999).

Innovations. In recent years, new approaches are beginning to be developed to restructure social and physical environments intended to support quality of life in nursing homes. These models represent a departure from the traditional institutional physical environment of nursing homes. A number of architects specialize in nursing home design. For example, they are removing the nursing stations from view, providing lounge space instead of being shared by residents and staff, and using alcoves in the hallways for medicine carts and work space for the nursing staff. To break the monotony of the environment, aquariums and pianos are being introduced (Ouslander et al., 1997). A loose consortium—whose members refer to themselves as "the nursing home pioneers"—is working to improve life in nursing homes, which they consider to require a culture change

(Fagin et al., 1997). Among their strategies are approaches that engage all residents as a community when feasible (Barkan, 1995), give nursing assistants more responsibility and flexibility, and emphasize processes of care that minimize dependence and promote more independent functioning as far as possible (Lustbader, 2000). For example, residents may serve on committees that interview and select staff or attend staff meetings whatever the subject (Burger, 1999).

One well-known innovative experiment, called the Eden Alternative, has brought plants, birds, and a variety of animals, and visits by children into nursing homes. This approach also moved towards empowering staff and developing caregiving teams that would make nursing homes more amenable to individualized care (Thomas, 1994). However, its effectiveness and transferability to other nursing homes with varying leadership, ownership, and casemix have not been rigorously evaluated. Some also fear that it has been grasped too quickly and that facilities introducing it may not be committed to the steady, persistent change needed to alter the quality of life in a nursing home.

Quality of life is also affected by the physical surroundings, which can be pleasing or depressing and can promote independence or dependence. In particular, most residents, prospective residents, and families consider a private room and bath important to independence, dignity, and social interaction (Kane et al., 1998a). A few new facilities are being designed entirely or almost entirely with private rooms.

Another model involves redesigning a facility, emphasizing small neighborhood concepts, or changing staffing patterns to promote continuity and the idea of the universal worker who can perform a variety of tasks (Fagin et al., 1997).[3] Variants of this neighborhood approach are found in other facilities.[4]

---

[3]For example, Fairport Baptist in Fairport, New York, now consists of *several* nine-resident "neighborhoods" with five single rooms and two L-shaped double rooms that maximize privacy. With no central hallways, each neighborhood has laundry facilities, a residential kitchen (where residents have access to the refrigerator), a dining area, and a sitting room but no nursing station. Meals are prepared in the centralized kitchen but are served in each neighborhood. All bedrooms and bathrooms have been decorated with features selected by the residents moving in. Most staff are assigned to neighborhoods to perform a range of tasks (e.g., personal care, housekeeping, serving meals), rather than operating centrally with responsibility for performing a smaller range of tasks for a larger number of residents. The nursing assistants, known as resident assistants, perform a wide range of tasks, including personal care, housekeeping, laundry, serving meals, and washing dishes in the kitchen's dishwasher. Centralized staff have been drastically reduced or eliminated (including housekeeping and wait staff), and staff ratios on the neighborhoods have increased (e.g., each neighborhood has one full-time staff at night). Residents are actively involved in planning their activities and their lives, including the design of the stained glass

An example of a successfully restructured nursing facility was reported to the IOM Committee on the Adequacy of Nursing Staff in Hospitals and Nursing Homes (IOM, 1996a, p. 255–256). The model of nursing care delivery implemented at the facility changed nursing care from a task-oriented system to a resident-oriented system by assigning primary nurses and their associates ongoing responsibility to care for a designated group of residents. The number of hours of care did not increase, but the skill mix did; the amount of licensed staff coverage over a 24-hour period increased from 24 to 45 percent. The increase of licensed staff is perceived as having improved the quality of care and the quality of life for residents and quality of work for staff, while remaining cost-effective. Ongoing data collection at that time supported this assertion, documenting notable reductions in the use of restraints and antipsychotic drugs, decreases in hospitalization rates, high resident satisfaction rates, reduced staff turn-over rates, and high levels of success with various forms of rehabilitation despite a continuously rising acuity level and an average age of 91 years.

At present, many of these innovative programs are relatively recent and rare. These and other similar examples, however, suggest that cultural change may be possible in nursing homes. Also, current federal and state regulations, despite their many strengths in defining standards of care, are not conducive to these types of changes. For example, the presence of birds or animals could violate state regulations, and some of the staffing arrangements could skirt the boundaries of regulatory acceptability. A facility may also be at risk of violating rules related to food service when residents cook or when residents and staff together determine ways to enhance their meals and snacks. More than 50 waivers of regulations were required in one model to implement its demonstration unit (Wolfe, 1999).

These approaches are intuitively very appealing and appear to avoid some of the quality-of-life problems common in traditional nursing homes. Given this, defensible data describing how life or care is better for residents living in these homes should be collected so that the quality implications of these models can be understood. Although the concepts behind the new care models are very appealing, details about how they work and, more specifically, for whom they work best are still unknown.

---

windows for a large central chapel under construction. A day care center is prominent in the facility, and the children interact with the residents.

[4]Some examples are: Evergreen in Wisconsin (Fagin et al., 1997) and Lyngblosten Home in Minneapolis (Wolfe, 1999). The latter is experimenting in a small portion of its facility with a Swedish model called the "service home" to assess if it can be applied to a certified nursing facility. Each resident has a private room and private bath, and all cooking is done in the experimental neighborhood of nine people.

Research, demonstration, and evaluation studies are needed to carefully describe the new interventions, and to evaluate their cost-effectiveness and their impact on quality of life and quality of care, when casemix is taken into consideration.

Limitations of the Evidence

Several limitations exist in the empirical evidence reviewed on quality of care in nursing homes. Averaging facilities is problematic—failure to improve in some facilities may be masked by large improvements in others, and vice versa. Average rates do not measure quality of care for individual residents.

As is common with studies using self-selected samples, some believe that the literature on nursing home quality may have problems with bias if results are based on sampled facilities willing to participate in the studies. The assumption is that willing participants are likely to be more receptive to regulatory and nonregulatory efforts aimed at improving quality. Others contend that there is no empirical evidence to support this concern. They advance the argument that many facilities regarded as poor performers are willing to participate in studies; they may be unaware of their relative performance. Also not all studies use convenience samples. Many use random samples of facilities with high participation rates. Other published studies have used data from OSCAR, the survey process, or the MDS. The validity and reliability of these data have been questioned by some. Since much of OSCAR and MDS data rely on reporting from facility staff, underreporting of problem areas is possible. Some items from the first version of the MDS showed adequate reliability; others did not perform as well (Phillips et al., 1993b; Crooks et al., 1995; Hawes et al., 1995b). Validation studies of the MDS version 2.0 found that new and revised items have both reliability and clinical utility (Blaum et al., 1997; Hawes et al., 1997b,c; Morris et al., 1997; Phillips et al., 1997). Problems with state survey reliability have been reported (Abt Associates and CHSRA, 1996; CHSRA, 1997; GAO, 1998a). In the state survey process, measures are derived from assessments by surveyors, pointing to the need for better training for surveyors.

In summary, there is sufficient cause for concern about poor quality of care in a number of nursing homes in the United States. Although care has improved in many facilities since OBRA 87 and there are some interesting models evolving to improve the physical environment, the configuration of staff, and the overall quality of life of residents that should be evaluated, the attention of policy makers must continue to be focused on those facilities that provide inadequate quality of care.

Community-Based Residential Care

As discussed in the previous chapter, a wide range of residential care facilities house people with long-term care needs of multiple levels. As many as one million people live in all types of board and care homes (Newcomer and Grant, 1990; Clark et al., 1994). The area of quality in these settings has received little research attention in the past.

No uniform definitions or criteria exist for judging the quality of care provided in these settings. Given the variations within and across states, comparisons among even similarly labeled facilities can be difficult. Moreover, assessments of the quality of residential care can be further complicated by the inclusion of measures of the physical environment, the ability of residents to remain in place following declines in functional status, and the delivery of services by facility staff versus external agency staff. If these factors are not uniformly incorporated into quality assessments, comparisons of and judgments about the quality of care delivered in these settings can be difficult.

Various studies have indicated that residents in nonmedical residential facilities were not receiving adequate care or protection (GAO, 1989, 1992a,b; Avorn et al., 1989). These studies showed unsafe and unsanitary conditions, improper use of psychotropic medications, and many other problems. These problems are heightened by rising resident acuity and high use of medications, questions about capacity of existing supply of professional staff to meet the needs of more impaired resident populations, and wide variations in regulatory approaches and concern about adequacy of most states' regulatory systems.

Board and Care Homes

Board and care homes have been around for many years and have filled an important need in long-term care for many elderly people and people with disabilities.

The main purpose of the 10-survey of board and care homes described in the previous chapter was to determine whether regulatory systems had an effect on the quality of care provided (Hawes, 1995a). The researchers found that the widespread perception that board and care homes are small, and therefore more "homelike," is somewhat misleading. Although most homes were small with 2–10 beds, more than three-quarters of the residents lived in homes with 11 or more beds. The majority of homes provided access to a range of services, but most were unable or unwilling to accommodate changing resident needs.

About 99 percent of the licensed homes and 76 percent of the unlicensed homes reported providing medication storage and supervision; 71 percent of the residents reported receiving assistance with mediations and 41 percent were taking psychotropic medications. Yet only 21 percent of the homes had a licensed nurse (RN or LPN) on their staff. Nearly 20 percent of the operators in licensed homes and 33 percent in unlicensed homes reported that they did not require any training for staff. Of staff who reported passing medications, 28 percent of staff giving injections were not licensed nurses. The staffing patterns, training of staff, and a lack of appropriate staff knowledge, and some care practices raise concerns about the quality of care provided in board and care homes. There is particular concern regarding the quality of care in some board and care homes that serve people with developmental disabilities and mental illnesses.

The study (Hawes et al., 1995a) found positive effects of regulation on safety, quality of life, and quality of care. States with extensive regulations had fewer unlicensed homes, and operators of the homes were better trained and with prior experience in providing health care and quality of life. Extensive regulation was associated with lower use of psychotropic drugs and use of fewer contraindicated medications, and positively associated with several quality-of-life measures such as preventing a very institutional environment, and the availability of social and recreational aids and supportive aids and devices. The study found no effect of extensive regulation on staff training, availability of licensed nurses on the homes' staff, knowledge of basic procedures and appropriate monitoring of health conditions and medication administration, availability of services, cleanliness, prevalence of safety features, and availability of physical amenities.

Assisted Living Facilities

Assisted living has become a popular subset of residential care facilities. They have been marketed as an option that could combine a capacity for high-quality individual service with physical environments that promote consumer choice, autonomy, dignity, privacy, and continuity with preferred lifestyles. Evaluating success or failure in meeting this objective is difficult because of limited data and the enormous variation among facilities and services. Hawes and colleagues (1999), reporting on the results of a large national probability sample survey of assisted living facilities having 10 or more beds and serving primarily older adults, found that 65 percent of facilities offered low levels of service (e.g., no full-time registered nurse on staff), with another 5 percent offering minimal services (see Chapter 2 for a description of the survey). Thirty-one to 34 percent of the facilities offered high levels of privacy, 40 percent offered low levels of privacy, and 26 to 28 percent offered only minimal levels of privacy.[5] Only 11 percent of the facilities provided high levels of both privacy and service.

Assisted living facilities on a multilevel campus with nursing homes and other programs (45 percent) were more likely to express a willingness to retain residents with greater health care needs and to offer more nursing care; however, they did not report having a more demanding casemix than freestanding programs. Almost half of the administrators interviewed indicated that their assisted living facility would not admit or retain a person with moderate to severe cognitive impairment.

The researchers concluded that there is a gap between the assisted living services currently offered and the philosophy of assisted living, which aims to combine private, residentially oriented buildings with high levels of service and "aging in place," regardless of changes in health or physical and cognitive functioning. Many facilities that call themselves assisted living fall short on one or more of these criteria. They also concluded that most assisted living in this country was not affordable for the moderate- and low-income elderly population and that affordable facilities were more likely to offer low or minimal levels of service and privacy (Hawes et al., 1999).

In Oregon, the regulatory model for assisted living requires high privacy and autonomy-enhancing features (e.g., locking doors, private-occupancy apartments with bathrooms equipped with roll-in showers, capacity for cooking and refrigerating food, and individualized care plans), and high service capability (e.g., three meals a day and personal care to enhance aging in place).

Quality-of-care problems, however, are reported for some assisted living facilities. A GAO (1999c) review of assisted living services in California, Florida, Ohio, and Oregon found that 27 percent of the facilities reviewed had been cited for five or more quality-of-care or consumer-protection deficiencies or violations during 1996 and 1997. The types of problems identified included providing inadequate or insufficient care; having insufficient, unqualified, and untrained staff; administering or storing medications improperly; and not following state admission and discharge policies. Another issue is holding assisted living settings responsible for developing plans of care. For example, Yee and colleagues (1999) found a need for more social activity and community involvement for residents in a congregate housing-type setting. Other factors that may

---

[5]High privacy facility is defined as one in which 80–100 percent of the units were private; low privacy facility is one that had no bedrooms shared by three or more unrelated persons, but in which fewer than 80 percent of bedrooms were private; minimal privacy facility is one that housed three or more unrelated individuals in the same bedroom (whether in a room or apartment).

make the situation more challenging are overbuilding leading to lower occupancy, problems with fiscal solvency, and incentives to accept and retain residents with greater care needs but pressure to preserve high rates of return by containing staff costs.

Among the various potential quality-of-care problems in assisted living settings discussed above, two conflicting concerns are raised. Some observers are concerned that assisted living offers a false promise to consumers of aging in place and that providers will be unwilling and unable to retain residents when their care needs become substantial. Others fear that assisted living settings will retain residents but fail to offer them needed services or, in the worst case, fail even to discern their deteriorating condition and need for services. One potential aid against either problem is ensuring that consumers have accurate and complete information about services available and allowed, policies regarding access to care and changing care needs, and charges. GAO (1999c) concluded that the variation among facilities and services designated as assisted living means that consumers must rely primarily on providers for information about services and policies. Currently, however, consumers often have inadequate information to use in selecting a facility and admission agreements often are misleading about what consumers can expect regarding continuing stays, discharges, services, and costs; and sometimes inconsistent with state law.

Adult Foster Care Homes

Another type of residential care is the adult foster home that typically provides care for a small number of residents (usually three to six) in private homes with a live-in care provider. They are licensed by states under a variety of names, with regulatory differences among states in terms of requirements and options (Folkemer, 1996). In most states, adult foster homes generally serve a low-income clientele, often with mental health problems.

In Oregon, the adult foster care model, introduced in 1982, has proved to be a popular mainstream program. By 1989, two-thirds of the foster home clients were privately paying individuals with higher levels of disability than those covered by Medicaid who, by definition, were eligible for nursing home care (Kane et al., 1991a). Controlling for casemix, a cross-sectional study found more socialization and satisfaction among foster home clients than nursing home residents (Kane et al., 1991a). A longitudinal study comparing Medicaid beneficiaries in adult foster care and nursing homes found no change in functional status for more than 85 percent of the clients, but among those with changes, the nursing home group showed more improvement and the foster care group more decline

(Stark et al., 1995). Although critics question how to interpret these data (e.g., whether functional status was the right outcome to assess), the study seems to suggest that foster care is a viable choice but could be improved by better access to medical and nursing care.

In terms of quality of life, adult foster care homes offer advantages related to homelike settings, but they also have disadvantages related to their small scale and reliance on the live-in caregiver for personal care, cooking, housekeeping, and recreational services, with little margin to cover additional help. In the Oregon program, for example, if one resident is bedridden or needs intensive nursing care, the foster care provider is less likely to be able to devote attention to activities for other residents. It seems probable that consumer satisfaction with adult foster care will depend not only on the intrinsic quality of the home but also on individual lifestyle preferences. Some people welcome the friendliness of a good adult foster home, whereas others prefer the privacy of a residential care setting over joining a stranger's household.

Residential Care for People with Developmental Disabilities.

During the mid-1980s, approximately 70 percent of people with developmental disabilities were cared for in institutional settings. OBRA 87 included a requirement that people with developmental disabilities living in nursing facilities be transferred to alternative settings if they did not need skilled nursing care. Since then, approximately one-quarter of the more than 50,000 people with developmental disabilities who had been living in nursing homes have moved to other facilities (Braddock et al., 1998). In addition, a growing number of states are providing services to people with developmental disabilities under Medicaid home and community-based services (HCBS) waivers. The majority of long-term care users with developmental disabilities now receive their formal care in the community.

Community-based living and smaller facility size have been associated with benefits such as increased community integration, adaptive behavior, choice making, mobility, family satisfaction, improved health, and decreased challenging behavior (Rotegard et al., 1983; Wilson et al., 1991; Heller et al., 1995; Conroy, 1996; Tossebro, 1996; Stancliffe, 1997; Stancliffe and Abery, 1997; Heller et al., 1998). Even for older persons with developmental disabilities, evidence indicates a positive long-term adjustment following movement from nursing homes to community-based settings (Heller, 1985; Heller et al., 1995, 1998). Smaller, community-based facilities are more likely to have policies and practices that support individual choice, to provide more individualized services with increased opportunity for variety and stimulation, to support community participa-

ɔ involve residents in policy making (Conroy, 1996; Tossebro, ...ncliffe, 1997; Heller et al., 1998).

However, some investigations have found problems with both poor quality and inadequate access to services in Medicaid waiver programs. A study of 1,878 persons with developmental disabilities in California found an elevated risk-adjusted death rate following deinstitutionalization, particularly for the highest-functioning individuals (Strauss et al., 1998; Shavelle and Strauss, 1999). The higher death rates for individuals with developmental disabilities were in part due to problems such as aspiration of food into the lungs or bowel impaction. HCFA investigations determined that similar problems existed in other states, many of which seem to be due partly to states providing inadequate case management services for monitoring quality of care.

Because the few studies that have been undertaken have found quality-of-care problems in all types of residential care, it is suspected that problems are widespread but generally unobserved. In any case, it raises the issue of the need for research on quality of care and particularly outcomes of care.

Home Health Care

Data on the quality of home health care are much less voluminous and systematic than those available for nursing homes. Most of the available data derive from HCFA's National Home Health Agency Prospective Payment Demonstration and from its support of research and demonstration projects using the Outcomes Assessment and Information Set (OASIS), which is now mandated for use by Medicare-certified home health agencies.

Few research studies have actually examined the quality of home health care. Most of the information about quality is available from the state survey agencies under contract by HCFA to regulate home health care. Research funded principally by HCFA has produced some data on processes of care and some on patient outcomes. Because a substantial percentage of home health care is financed by Medicare and because Medicare home health care services have grown rapidly over the past decade, research has focused on Medicare certified home health agencies, and many of the studies have centered around predictors of use and expenditures.

In recent years, GAO has conducted investigative studies of home health care agencies. In a study of home health agencies that had been certified, GAO (1997b) found that very poor care was provided by a number of agencies. Several examples were cited showing problems such as agency administrators with no health care experience, and agencies serving ineligible patients and falsifying records and staff credentials. On the other hand, GAO investigators found that only 3 percent of all certified agencies are cited by HCFA for being out of compliance with one or more conditions (GAO, 1997b).

In recent surveys by HCFA's Operation Restore Trust which reassessed certified home health agencies in California, HCFA found significant quality-of-care problems that led to the termination of many agencies from the Medicare program. In resurveys of 44 agencies providing high numbers of services and receiving high levels of Medicare payments, HCFA found that 80 percent were out of compliance with at least one of the federal conditions, and 21 of the 44 either voluntarily withdrew from the program or were terminated by HCFA. In these surveys, HCFA found agencies that could not provide lists of active patients, and did not know which patients were receiving care on a particular day, staff that were providing patients with medications not ordered by a physician, therapists who were not qualified, and laboratory services that were not monitored. They also found failures to provide nursing care as ordered and failures to initiate changes in patients' care plans (GAO, 1996a, 1997b, 1998b,c).

On the other hand, a retrospective review of Medicare patient records undertaken for agencies participating in HCFA's prospective payment demonstration revealed problems with potential adverse patient impact in only about 4 percent of the cases (Phillips et al., 1994). In the process of developing OASIS, a prospective study was conducted to assess the care provided for new patients by 44 Medicare-certified agencies in 27 states with approximately 2,600 patients, particularly related to six activities of daily living. The study compared rates of stabilization and improvements in functional status for two groups—those admitted for home health care from the hospital and those admitted from the community. Overall functional status was stabilized for 79 and 92 percent of patients in each group, respectively (Shaughnessy et al., 1994a). Rates of improvement in function ranged from 26 percent for ambulation among patients admitted from the community to more than 54 percent for bathing among those admitted from the hospital. Consistently lower rates of improvement among the group admitted to home health care from the community were attributed to the greater prevalence of chronic functional impairments in this group. Patients admitted from the hospital were more likely to have acute problems for which functional stabilization or improvement would be expected (Shaughnessy et al., 1994a).

Appropriateness of Services

In another major HCFA-funded study, Kane and Finch et al. (1994) examined the costs and outcomes of 2,100 elderly Medicare patients from three cities who were discharged from hospital to post-acute care settings with one of five diagnoses: stroke, chronic obstructive pulmonary disease, congestive heart failure, hip procedure and hip fracture. They found that in general patients who received home health care had better functional outcomes than those who went home without home health services. Subsequent analyses stemming from this study concluded that at six weeks, six months and one year post-hospital discharge, patients who received home health care experienced significantly higher functional improvement than patients discharged to other post-acute care modalities (rehabilitation facilities, skilled nursing facilities or home without home health care) (R.L. Kane et al., 1998). This study, however, did not examine the nature of home health care provided. Thus, no information is available on the type of personnel who provided care, their level of training, or the degree of physician involvement.

Findings on Process of Care

Under contract to HCFA, Abt Associates conducted the largest empirical assessment to date of process of care deficiencies in Medicare certified home health agencies (Phillips et al., 1994; Jette et al., 1996). The study reviewed retrospectively the records for 4,000 patient episodes drawn from 47 agencies participating in HCFA's prospective payment demonstration. To each episode of care nurse reviewers applied 10 quality-of-care screens, including adequacy of baseline assessment and care planning, addressing all documented problems, addressing all acute problems immediately, delivering all prescribed nursing or therapy services, deterioration of ulcers/wounds, deterioration of ADL status, and adequacy of discharge plan. In cases where reviewers determined failure on a particular screen, they made an additional determination involving three levels of problem: (1) a problem without potential for significant adverse effects on the patient, (2) a problem with potential for significant adverse effects on the patient, or (3) a problem with confirmed significant adverse patient effects.

Overall, reviewers identified no quality problems in 57 percent of cases and at least one quality problem in 43 percent of cases screened (Jette et al., 1996). Two-thirds of cases failed only one quality screen, 28 percent failed two screens, and the remainder failed three or more. Four percent of total cases were judged to have a quality problem with the potential for (3.9 percent) or actual (0.4 percent) adverse effects on patients. However, the researchers estimated that the proportion of cases with potential adverse effects might have reached 14 percent if all records that failed an initial screen had been reviewed by two different nurses. The most frequently failed screens in this study were delivery of all prescribed nursing or therapy services (33 percent of cases) and addressing all documented problems (20 percent of cases). Within the first area, inadequate evidence of patient teaching was the most commonly cited problem and within the second, inadequate evidence of follow-up on cardiovascular problems. As with all record review studies, the researchers could not separate inadequacy of documentation from actual lack of appropriate action on the part of the nurse or agency.

The Abt study revealed "considerable variation in level of quality care observed among the participating agencies" (Jette, 1996: 499). However, agency ownership was not significantly related to the frequency or severity of quality problems identified. Controlling for agency and reviewer characteristics, the likelihood of observed quality problems increased as patients' condition became less stable and as the number of different services provided to the patient increased. When agencies' status as fee-for-service versus prospective payment providers was considered, the study found no significant difference in the existence of confirmed quality problems with a potential to adversely affect patients (Phillips et al., 1994). Although the study agencies contained a mix of ownership status and geographic representation, the researchers cautioned that as volunteers for a national demonstration, the agencies might not be representative of the home health industry as a whole.

Many of the concerns regarding Medicare-funded home health care are related to the amount and appropriateness of service use and to agency business practices. A GAO (1996a) report highlighted variations in home health service provision by region and agency ownership. Nationally, the number of home health visits per beneficiary per year in 1993 was 57; regionally, the average varied from 79 visits in southern states to a low of 36 visits in states in the Northwest. GAO suggested that some of the regional variation might be explained by the availability of substitute services or by the beneficiary casemix. Variations by agency ownership were equally striking. Proprietary agencies provided an average of 78 visits per beneficiary in 1993, compared to 46 each for government and voluntary nonprofit agencies (GAO, 1996a). A similar pattern was found at the regional level and when patterns of service use were compared for four common diagnoses (diabetes, heart failure, hypertension, and hip fracture). The variations in service use by agency type were greatest for patients with diabetes, a chronic problem, and least for those with hip fracture, an acute problem.

GAO (1996a) did not directly examine the effectiveness of various care plans but suggested that weak oversight might be leading proprietary agencies to provide more services than were needed by beneficiaries. Possible overuse of services was attributed in part to Medicare fee-for-service payment methods (since modified), in part to limited physician review of the primarily nonmedical home health services, and in part to reduced funding for review of claims and on-site audits. Other GAO (1995, 1998b) investigations have documented financial irregularities and improprieties by specific agencies, including excessive skilled nursing visits, exaggeration of the severity of patient conditions, and services to patients of questionable eligibility.

Although little has been documented about the quality of home health care, many concede that the reports of these problems may not be isolated cases. Because of the rapid growth of home health agencies, with nearly 10,000 certified agencies in the beginning of 1997, the oversight problems are enormous (GAO, 1997b). The committee speculated that individuals living at home are reluctant to complain about poor quality of care for fear of losing their home care workers and receiving no services. Thus, oversight cannot rely simply on individual complaints about quality.

Home and Community-Based Services

Adults

Studies of HCBS usually concentrate on unmet need and its consequences (Allen and Mor, 1997) or satisfaction (Benjamin, 1998; Applebaum et al., 1999). Geron (1996, 1997) looked at satisfaction in terms of a number of issues that members of ethnic-specific focus groups said were important—for example, compatibility with providers, reliability of providers, task competence of providers, and adequacy of total service provision. Adequacy refers to getting enough services; competence refers to how services and care are performed; compatibility refers to the fit between the consumer and caregiver and the consumer's sense that the caregiver cares about him or her personally; and competence refers to the way personal care and homemaking tasks are literally conducted. Typically those who use home and community-based care of all types report high satisfaction (Geron, 1996; Benjamin, 1998; Kane and Huck, 2000). Such satisfaction is also reported for home care and day care delivered as respite services for dementia, though in these instances the respondents are typically family members. Reviewing empirical studies on respite care, Montgomery and Kosloski (1995) stated that "the most pervasive finding in the literature regarding the impact of respite services is that caregivers like the service and generally find programs to be valuable" (p. 50). Satisfaction is also high among general users of adult day care (Weissert et al., 1990).

The extent to which the availability of HCBS actually accounts for keeping people out of nursing homes has been hotly debated and is the subject of decades worth of research (Applebaum et al., 1986; Kane and

Kane, 1987; Weissert, 1997). In some of his writing, Weissert (1997) terms home care a failure because its users enter nursing homes at the same rate as the control groups. This also presupposes that the worth of home care is to be measured by its substitution for some other form of care (e.g., nursing home care or hospital care). These kinds of findings beg the question about the quality of home care itself. For the most part, critiques of home care for older people (Estes and Swan, 1993), as well as for persons with serious mental illness (Horowitz and Reinard, 1997) and for children with chronic illness (Perrin et al., 1997), chronicle lack of third-party payers and poor coverage of care rather than problems in care itself. There are no systematic studies in the literature to suggest that home care is of good or poor quality. The subject has been examined largely in relation to satisfaction, unmet need for care, or burden on family caregivers (which in some ways is another index of unmet need for care). Research on outcomes and other information on which to judge quality of these services is lacking.

Personal Care Services

Researchers have begun to describe the breadth and depth of Medicaid HCBS programs more fully, typically offering statistics on state and national trends (Litvak and Kennedy 1991; Burwell 1999; Miller et al., 1999a,b; Harrington et al., 2000d). Although the Medicaid personal care services (PCS) and HCBS programs have grown significantly over the past two decades (Miller et al., 1999a; Harrington et al., 2000b), the combined Medicaid PCS and HCBS waiver participants are less than the number of Medicaid institutional participants (Harrington et al., 2000a, LeBlanc et al., 2000a).

Wide variation exists among states in the total number of Medicaid PCS optional state plan benefit and 1915(c) HCBS waiver participants, ranging from 10.5 participants per 1,000 population in Missouri to less than 0.7 participant in Louisiana and Indiana (see Table 2.5). When Medicaid officials surveyed were asked if they had an adequate number of HCBS waiver slots or funding allocated for slots to meet the demand, only eight state officials replied that they had enough slots while 42 state officials said they either did not have enough slots or funds to fill the slots (Harrington et al., 2000a). The eight states that reported having adequate slots were: Missouri, Michigan, Rhode Island, North Dakota, Maine, Massachusetts, Alabama, and Arizona. Washington DC was just starting its waiver program so officials stated they did not know if they had adequate slots. Inadequate slots were most often reported for the mental retardation–developmental disabilities (MR/DD) programs. Of the 42 states reporting waivers with inadequate numbers of slots and funds, 37 states had inadequate numbers of slots and funds for individuals with MR/DD. In other states, there were inadequate numbers of slots and funds for the aged, those with disabilities, those with traumatic brain injuries, children with special health care needs, and those with HIV/AIDS.

Twenty-eight states report waiting lists in the waiver program, but 14 states could not report and the numbers ranged from 20 physically disabled in South Dakota to 11,000 on the aged and disabled waiver waiting list in Wisconsin. Louisiana reported 7,063 on the MR/DD waiting list and the wait for services was estimated to be 5 years in length. Although states reported that some legislators were sympathetic to the need to expand HCBS, most states with waiting lists had been unable to obtain adequate state funds for the program from the state legislature. Seven other states reported being involved in state litigation cases pertaining to waiting lists for HCBS services (California, Florida, Montana, New Mexico, Oklahoma, Texas, and West Virginia). Two states were under court rulings to either downsize the state facilities for individuals with MR/DD (Tennessee) or provide HCBS services for the mentally ill aged 22–64 (Colorado).

One of the most important reported barriers to the expansion of PCS and HCBS waiver services was the shortage of direct care workers, particularly those working in the home. States with large rural populations faced particularly imposing challenges. State officials identified these shortages as being related to the growing competition in the labor market and the low state Medicaid reimbursement rates for HCBS providers. Wage, benefit, and working condition studies may be needed to assist states in establishing market-based rates for home care providers. Perhaps special federal financial support could be designed to assist state Medicaid programs in increasing their state reimbursement rates for HCBS providers.

In summary, both PCS and HCBS programs appear to be expanding to meet the growing needs of Medicaid participants who are aged or disabled. The problem is that there is a large unmet need in many states based on the reports of state officials and waiting lists. Two major questions remain to be addressed. One is how to ensure that Medicaid participants are offered a choice between institutional and HCBS services and have access to appropriate services in the least restrictive environment. The second is how to ensure equity in access to PCS and HCBS services across states. Should the federal government require states to offer alternatives to institutional care for all Medicaid participants? Alternatively, should special programs be established to give incentives to states to expand access to PCS and HCBS services, while at the same time controlling the growth and expenditures for institutional care? A Blue

Ribbon Panel on Personal Assistance Services (1999)[6] reviewed federal and state statutes and regulations for personal care services and home and community-based services. The panel produced several recommendations and strategies for the federal and state governments to implement and promote consumer choice in community-based placement for people with disabilities who require routine, ongoing personal assistance services. The panel also urged HCFA to abandon the link between Medicare and Medicaid certification requirements for providers of home and community-based services.

The committee concludes that *research is needed to identify the need for PCS and HCBS services and to examine policy options that would remove the barriers and constraints that states are facing to meet the need for services. The committee believes that HCFA and state governments should work with providers and consumers to undertake research towards developing an appropriate array of community-based long-term care services to meet the needs of consumers and assess the quality of the service and outcomes.* At the same time, access to and choice of appropriate services can be argued to be essential to quality of care and quality of life for individuals with disabilities.

Department of Justice regulations implementing the Americans with Disabilities Act (ADA) now require that "a public entity shall administer services, programs, and activities in the most integrated setting appropriate to the needs of qualified individuals with disabilities" (28 C.F.R. 35.130(d)). In the recent *Olmstead v. L.C.* case, the Supreme Court held that institutional placement of individuals who could live in less restrictive settings may violate the ADA. The Court indicated that states are required to provide community-based services for persons with disabilities when state professionals determine that such placement is appropriate for the particular individual, the affected person does not oppose such treatment, and the placement can be reasonably accommodated without altering the program through which services are provided. The Department of Health and Human Services issued a letter to state Medicaid Directors regarding the Olmstead decision and informing states about ways to comply by preventing inappropriate institutionalization and providing home and community-based alternatives. Most states have much work that needs to be done to change their programs to ensure choice and access. The challenge is to reduce the reliance on institutional care and to shift services to the home and community when such care is appropriate.

---

[6]The panel was funded in 1997 by the Robert Wood Johnson Foundation through a grant to the Independent Living Research Utilization Program at The Institute for Rehabilitation and Research.

Home Care for Children and Adolescents

Children with major medical and technological needs often leave the hospital with careful plans for care and supervision from nurses and other caregivers with expertise in pediatric care. Difficulties often arise for families in providing or arranging long-term care at home and in the community with the loss of connections to hospital programs, limited communications among key providers, changes in home nursing care providers, and changes in the child's health situation. Moreover, many home care providers (mainly nurses) have little training or experience in the care of children. Instead, they may come from a background of providing care for older patients with very different conditions and know little about children's medication doses or equipment needs, or appropriate ways to monitor a child's condition or progress (Feinberg, 1985). At the point of discharge, hospital staff typically choose the nursing team to help the family at home or in the community based on their capabilities in caring for younger patients, but over time as staff change, later nursing personnel may have much less relevant experience. Nursing staff providing home care also have less supervision than hospital staff, and again agencies or programs may lack personnel equipped to supervise home and community care for children. Parents also report that equipment suppliers provide too little information regarding the use of their devices in the home, making it difficult for families to determine when the machine is malfunctioning or what to do about it.

Parents also complain about the interference of some home service personnel in their daily life routines. Although having complex equipment and additional care providers will change any household's activities, at times agency staff interfere inappropriately in how parents discipline their children or indicate disapproval of aspects of the family's living situations (Perrin et al., 1993).

Children and adolescents receiving long-term care services typically interact with a large number of service providers, including primary and subspecialty medical providers, nursing staff, equipment suppliers, and specialized therapists. A lack of coordination of these services can lead to conflicts among service providers, duplication of some services, and lack of access to others. Although families often learn over time how to coordinate services themselves, problems persist for many. Several programs (see Stein, 1998) exist to help families coordinate services, improving the quality and extent of services received (Stein and Jessop, 1984, 1991). Care coordinators may offer direct care, financial counseling, coordination among medical providers, teaching about the child's care needs, emotional support, coordination among the medical, education, and home nursing systems, help in finding services for the child, and guidance in teaching families to provide care coordination on their own. Few standards for training and qualifications of care coordinators exist, making assessment of these activities particularly difficult (Perrin et al., 1993).

Parents further report that care plans and services may not change frequently enough, leaving outmoded arrangements in place when the child's and the household's needs have changed. Most conditions leading to long-term care needs for children and adolescents are dynamic, requiring changes in treatments, technological assistance, and monitoring over time. The ability of family members to contribute to a child's care also may change. For example, family members may be able to provide an increased amount of care because they have developed the skills to provide certain services or a decreased amount of care because of changes in employment or family status. Other problems facing families caring for children at home include increased risk of depression and financial hardship (Quint et al., 1990; Thyen et al., 1999).

These shortcomings in home care services, especially for children, point to several likely opportunities to improve the quality of this care. In particular, efforts should be made to ensure that professionals involved in care have appropriate training and skills. Coordination of care should be viewed as an important component of the services available to families, either through trained care coordinators or through opportunities for family members to become care coordinators. Care plans can be used to establish goals for care, select measurable indicators of progress toward those goals, and allocate responsibilities among caregivers. With a person-centered approach to care, families should have the opportunity to participate as full partners in the formulation, implementation, and monitoring of such plans. In addition, family support services should be viewed as part of the array of services contributing to the quality of care.

Emerging Consumer-Directed Service Models

Consumer-directed service models have a brief history compared to traditional institutional and home care. They provide varying levels of consumer involvement and varying mechanisms of support for consumer direction (Flanagan and Green, 1997). Choice is typically between programs that provide cash payments and leave all service management to consumers or programs that allow consumers to delegate all of their service management to an agency. Formal evaluations of consumer-directed service models are still limited. The studies reviewed by the committee vary considerably in their size, methodological rigor, and vulnerability to biases. Nonetheless, the committee believes that taken together, the findings of the evaluation studies to date suggest that a consumer-directed approach may benefit a significant proportion of individuals with disabilities. Some studies have examined the impact of consumer-directed models on factors such as quality of life, control, productivity, use of preventive health care, and cost. Others have examined the impact of cash payment models. The findings from these evaluations are summarized below.

Impact on Users of Services. As noted in other parts of the report, the oldest consumer-directed service benefits are the Housebound and Aid and Attendance Allowance Program, operated by the Veterans Administration (Cameron, 1993). More than 200,000 veterans and surviving spouses received—by choice—cash benefits in place of formally provided homemaker, personal care, and other services. Funds may be spent on whatever consumers believe best meets their health and personal needs. An evaluation of this program suggested that participants received similar hours of care and were no worse off with regard to acute health care utilization than a comparison group receiving traditional services (Grana and Yamashiro, 1987). This evaluation unfortunately did not include measures of quality of care or life.

Most consumer-directed services and their evaluation have focused on personal care services. For example, a 1993 poll of 800 Medicaid beneficiaries who hired independent providers, rather than using agency providers, reported higher levels of satisfaction with care, provider stability, and quality of life (Harris and Associates, 1993). Two studies of personal assistance models in Virginia and California show increased productivity and satisfaction for individuals with physical disabilities. In Virginia, evaluations of consumer-directed personal assistance services compared outcomes for very small samples of individuals who received consumer-directed services through state Centers for Independent Living and those on the waiting list for such services (Beatty et al., 1998a). Consumer-directed services, including funding for personal assistance, as well as assistive technology, home modification, and adaptive equipment, were associated with greater reported control over one's life, greater satisfaction with services, and greater availability of services (Beatty et al., 1998b); increased productivity and employment (Richmond et al., 1997); and greater use of preventive health care (Adams and Beatty, 1998). The individuals on the waiting list tended to have less service needs, as assessed by the Center, than did individuals receiving the services. Although receipt of these services was based on need, it is possible that the frustration of waiting could have been reflected to some extent in the satisfaction scores for those on the waiting list.

In California, Benjamin (1998) interviewed by telephone 1,095 low income people who were aged or disabled or blind and who participated in either a consumer-directed or professionally directed program. Approximately half of the users of consumer-directed services were 65 years of age and older, and 52 percent had severe disabilities compared to 13 percent of the other group. Generally, users of consumer-directed services scored higher on variables related to service choice and satisfaction and preferred role of provider than did the users of professionally directed services. Also individuals who participated in consumer-directed service to pay for services from family members reported a significantly greater sense of security and interpersonal satisfaction. On dimensions of consumer safety and unmet need, neither model showed a significant advantage over the other.

Tilly and Bectel (1999) reviewed Benjamin's study and four European studies of consumer-directed cash payment service models in Australia (Badelt et al., 1997), Germany (Runde et al., 1996), the Netherlands (Miltenburg et al., 1996), and France (Gilles et al., 1995; Simon and Martin, 1995). They found that in these studies the receipt of cash subsidies was associated with enhanced perceptions of control over services and supports compared to agency services, allowed consumers to compensate relatives for care and to purchase more services, and enhanced overall quality of life. Simon-Rusinowitz and colleagues (1997) interviewed about 490 Medicaid personal assistance clients to assess predictors of consumer interest in the cash option model. Almost one-third of the respondents reported an interest in the cash option. They found that the greatest predictor of interest in a cash option was the individual's willingness to perform employer tasks, followed by a desire for involvement with one's own caregiving. Of those who expressed interest in the option, over half would use the cash to purchase more hours of service, followed by equipment and transportation.

Some studies report a positive association between perceptions of control and quality of life for individuals with disabling conditions (Rodin, 1986; Hofland, 1988). Other research has linked perceived control to health, disability, and quality of life among older adults (Salomon et al., 1998). Nosek et al. (1995) found a similar association between ratings of life satisfaction and control over long-term care, regardless of whether the care was provided in an institution, by an independent provider, or by a paid or unpaid care provider.

Although these consumer-directed options are relatively untested, preliminary evidence suggests their viability for people with disability receiving personal care services. Long-term care service users may be more satisfied with consumer-directed services and may benefit from other aspects of the arrangement, but from a quality perspective, there is little evidence-based research for concluding that consumer-directed services result in better quality of care. There is also a lack of an evidence base regarding the relationship between consumer-direction and consumer risk, both increased and lack of risk. In the absence of such research, those who want to promote or curtail self-direction fall back on beliefs, anecdotes, and assumptions. More research is needed that focuses on the benefits and risks of these models, and on the association between choice and participation in decision making and the quality of care.

> **Recommendation 3-1: The committee recommends that the Department of Health and Human Services, with input from states and private organizations, develop and fund a research agenda to investigate the potential quality impact associated with access to, and limitations of, different models of consumer-centered long-term care services, including consumer-directed services.**

CONCLUSION

Characterizing the quality of long-term care requires coming to grips with different criteria for quality and determining how to make trade-offs among various features of quality. Much more work is needed on these issues, including how to consider safety in comparison to other concerns; whether and how much to consider the quality of the physical environments in residentially based long-term care; and how to incorporate consumer choice and direction into quality assurance and quality improvement efforts. Moreover data and research are very scant for residential care and home care compared to information for nursing homes. Much of the long-term care literature other than nursing homes has focused more on adequacy of access and consumer satisfaction than on quality of care.

Allowing for these current limitations in characterizing quality, the committee's review of the available literature points to several general conclusions about the quality of care in various long-term care settings. Since the enactment of OBRA 87, nursing home care has improved in some areas with less use of physical restraints, better use of psychoactive drugs, and less use of urinary catheters. In other areas, such as prevention and treatment of pressure sores and incontinence care, quality problems remain and appear particularly persistent in some facilities. The quality of life in some nursing homes has been improved by the adoption of more consumer-centered approaches to care, but features such as lack of privacy continue to be problematic.

Residential care presents a mixed picture in terms of both quality of care and quality of life. Some small group homes and assisted living facilities offer high-quality care in settings that afford maximum privacy and dignity. However, others appear to lack adequately trained staff and to offer neither sufficient amounts of care nor "homelike" settings and the privacy that goes along with it. There are also indications that consumers may receive too little information to make informed choices regarding assisted living services.

Evidence regarding the quality of home health care is more limited than that for nursing home care, but also points to a mixed experience. Moreover, most of the research in this area measures satisfaction and unmet need, and not quality of care. Medicare-funded home health care generally appears to be of adequate quality in terms of the transactions between caregivers and care users. However, the program has suffered from problems of overuse and inappropriate use, leading to new constraints on payments that may adversely affect the availability of services for those with the most complex care needs. Access to HCBS and especially personal care services for people with disabilities needs to be improved and an array of options need to be developed and tested.

This review of the current quality of long-term care has highlighted for the committee several areas of concern, including lack of standard measurement tools and data to use in more systematic assessments of the quality of care in various long-term care settings, evidence of persistent problems in certain aspects of care (e.g., treatment of pressure sores) and in certain facilities, and indications that some problems can be traced to insufficient staff training or inadequate staffing levels. Subsequent chapters address various strategies for responding to these concerns with specific recommendations for improvements. Since no single strategy will be appropriate or sufficient to achieve the broad range of quality improvement goals in long-term care, the aim must be to find the mix of strategies that will most successfully balance differing views and goals.

4

Information Systems for
Monitoring Quality

Information based on valid, reliable, and timely data about the care
provided, the recipients of care, the facilities, and the caregivers providing care is fundamental to all strategies for monitoring and improving the quality of long-term care. Such information is of interest to many
constituencies, including consumers, caregivers, provider organizations,
managers, regulators, purchasers, and researchers. *Consumers* and their
advocates want information to guide the selection of care providers, monitor current care, inform efforts to encourage and promote system-wide
improvements in long-term care, and work with their providers to improve
quality of care. *Providers* want such information to target their efforts
toward improving care processes and outcomes. *Regulators* need this information to identify quality problems, target monitoring and enforcement
processes, and confirm corrective actions. *Purchasers* of care, such as Medicare, Medicaid, or even managed care plans, might use this information to
decide who should care for their beneficiaries or subscribers.

Over the last decade, the long-term care field has moved to develop
and implement uniform, universally required individual level data collection systems that can form the basis for measures of quality performance. The 1986 Institute of Medicine report recommended a uniform
minimum data set for nursing home resident assessment. However, such
a recommendation would never have been made without a general consensus that nursing home quality was poor and that the provider community was neither willing nor able to make the changes needed to improve
the quality of care without specific direction. As is described below, the

nursing home Resident Assessment Instrument was introduced early in 1990 and has become the basis for various payment and quality monitoring initiatives. The perceived policy "success" of the nursing home system prompted the Health Care Financing Administration (HCFA) to mandate the introduction of a measurement system for Medicare in order to reimburse for home health care. A number of states have had long-standing patient assessment systems of their own for users of assisted living facilities, senior centers, and non-Medicare home care providers. Numerous states are now struggling with the adoption of common, clinically relevant data elements pertinent to all long-term care clients that are applicable across all provider settings in order to facilitate and track Medicaid-managed care reforms tentatively being applied to the long-term care population.

The notion that information about care recipients and care providers, all linked into a single database, can be used to monitor and improve care is consistent with the extensive literature emanating from the continuous quality improvement field. The same data that make it possible for providers to identify current care practices that contribute to undesirable patient outcomes, can also be used by regulators to identify providers that may manifest care practices associated with problematic outcomes. Presumably these data could be used also to classify providers as "poor performers," which information then could be made available to the public.

This chapter discusses the current state of the major information systems in long-term care, their implementation status, their reliability and validity, and their application for clinical assessment, quality monitoring, and reimbursement. The discussion primarily focuses on the federal systems that provide basic information on monitoring compliance with regulations and on the quality of long-term care offered by nursing homes and home health agencies. These are the On-line Survey and Certification Assessment Reporting (OSCAR) System for nursing homes and home health, the minimum data set (MDS) for the Resident Assessment Instrument (RAI) for nursing homes used in developing quality indicators, and the Outcome and Assessment Information Set (OASIS) for home health care. The chapter then briefly describes the need to improve these existing information systems in light of their extensive use for policy and quality monitoring; state assessment systems for home and community-based service; and the measurement and implementation issues involved in efforts to extend their use to other long-term care settings and to include consumer perspectives in assessments of the quality of life and satisfaction with care. Because most existing data systems in long-term care have been developed primarily for adults, and the elderly in particular, some of the special challenges in assessing children's care also are discussed.

ON-LINE SURVEY AND CERTIFICATION ASSESSMENT REPORTING SYSTEM

The OSCAR system is a computerized national database for long-term care facilities used for maintaining and retrieving survey and certification data for providers and suppliers that are approved to participate in the Medicare or Medicaid programs. OSCAR also is used as a quality assessment tool. The database contains information entered by state survey agencies or HCFA regional offices during periodic inspections for certification of health care facilities.

OSCAR provides information on how well a nursing home has met the regulations in the past and provides on-site surveyors with background information on past performance. As such, it serves as a quality assessment tool. It has five major components of interest: facility characteristics, resident characteristics, staffing, survey deficiencies including scope and severity, and complaints (see Chapter 5 for more details). The data are collected and updated on a regular basis by state licensing and certification agencies under contract with HCFA to conduct Medicare and Medicaid certification surveys. At the time of state surveys, nursing facilities complete information on their facility characteristics, resident characteristics, and staffing on HCFA forms. Staffing data include the number of full-time equivalent positions in the facility—employees or contract workers—over the previous 14 days. The deficiency data are based on the findings from the state survey when a state surveyor, using protocols specified by HCFA, judges that a facility has not met a regulatory standard. Deficiencies are classified by scope and severity. These data are entered by state offices into the OSCAR database. It should be noted that there is often a lag (on average, 5–6 months) between the facility's survey and when the data can be accessed and aggregated for analysis. The system retains up to a four-inspections history of deficiency information and resident census data for the same period.

Each facility must have an initial survey to verify compliance with all federal regulatory requirements in order to be certified for Medicare or Medicaid. Once certified, nursing homes are resurveyed annually in order to continue certification. States are required to survey each facility no less often than every 15 months, and the state average is about every 12 months. Follow-up surveys may be conducted to ensure that facilities correct identified deficiencies. In addition, surveys are required when there are substantial changes in a facility's organization and management. Finally, surveys may be conducted to follow up a complaint that alleges substandard care.

OSCAR facility data, as recorded, include information on: type of certification, bed size, occupancy, the name and address of the corporation, ownership type (profit, nonprofit, or government), whether the facility is part of a chain, percent of residents on Medicare and Medicaid, information on special units for those with Alzheimer's disease, and other information. Information on the number of residents in the facility with particular problems (e.g., pressure sores, incontinence) or receiving special services (e.g., rehabilitation, tube feedings) on the day of the survey is also included. Staffing data reported includes the number of full-time equivalent positions in the facility—employees or contract workers—over the previous 14 days.

Resident characteristics also are reported by nursing facilities. These include activities of daily living (ADLs), restraints, incontinence, psychological problems, and other special care needs of residents. Nurse staffing (registered nurses, licensed practical nurses, and nursing assistants) hours per resident are reported by facilities for a two-week period prior to when the survey is conducted. These data are the only major source of information for all facilities on staffing levels. Finally, data on facility deficiencies are based on state surveyor evaluations of the process and outcomes of care in the facilities. Deficiencies are given on resident rights, admission, transfer and discharge rights, resident behavior and facility practices, quality of life, resident assessment, quality of care, nursing services, dietary services, physician services, rehabilitation services, dental services, pharmacy services, infection control, physical environment, and administration. OSCAR does not include claims, use, or expenditure data.

The instructions for completing the various components of the OSCAR data are included in HCFA's *State Operations Manual*, which guides the survey protocol to be followed by state officials for inspecting nursing homes during the annual certification and re-certification visits. Much of the information on facility and resident characteristics is initially compiled by facilities and then checked by surveyors against medical records, staffing records, and resident observation (Harrington and Carrillo, 2000).

OSCAR information can be used by federal and state survey agencies to examine a facility's survey results and patterns of deficiencies over time. The data can also be used to provide information to consumers. As part of President Clinton's nursing home initiative in 1998, HCFA has made much of the OSCAR data available to the public through its Medicare nursing-home-compare website, which presents OSCAR data[1] on every nursing home in the United States (HCFA, 1998a). In addition, several commercial firms have Internet-based systems that use OSCAR data in ranking nursing homes on the basis of their designated deficien-

---

[1]The site includes selected facility characteristics, resident characteristics, and deficiencies. HCFA is in the process of adding more OSCAR information to the website.

cies, as well as on the basis of the compatibility of the facility with the needs and preferences of residents. As part of a project for the Agency for Health Care Policy and Research, researchers have developed a prototype consumer information system based on OSCAR data.

HCFA periodically modifies the OSCAR system to include new data elements or provide new instructions to make the assembly of the OSCAR information consistent with other sources, such as the MDS. HCFA is planning on another major revision of OSCAR in the near future in order to accommodate new types of structural and process information that will better characterize the clinical resources available in and to the nursing home.

Limitations of OSCAR

There are several sources of concern about the limitations of OSCAR data, some of which emanate from a lack of explicit audit procedures. For example, the data on facility characteristics and staffing are not routinely audited by state surveyors to ensure the accuracy of the data. Data on facility ownership are not detailed enough to identify the owners of facilities for tracking and enforcement purposes, and information on changes in administrative leadership of facilities, although required by HCFA and reported to states, are not built into OSCAR.

OSCAR data about residents are based on aggregated resident characteristics summarizing the resident census taken by the provider before submission to the surveyors. Such data make it impossible to disaggregate the information to look at subsets of residents within a facility. With increased segmentation and specialization in the nursing home industry, a simple count of the number of residents with particular characteristics is increasingly misleading. For example, the severity of a facility's casemix is reflected in indicators such as the proportion of residents who are incontinent or are being tube-fed on the day of the survey. Interpretation of these data could be difficult without individual-level data that can be used to differentiate, at a particular point in time, between residents who acquired these characteristics while in the facility and residents who entered the facility with these characteristics. Moreover, the data collected on resident characteristics are not audited by state surveyors.

OSCAR data on staffing also are not audited by state surveyors, and analyses of staff-to-resident ratios show some facilities reporting data that are likely to be inaccurate (Harrington et al., 1998a). One reason for this may be that the instructions for completing the information are not easy to understand. Also, because nursing homes can often predict when surveys will be conducted and because the surveys report only the previous 14 days of staffing, facilities can "staff-up" before the inspection. Thus the usual staffing levels for a facility may differ from those reported during inspection, making it difficult to use OSCAR data to identify quality problems that may be related to staffing levels. Staffing data would be more useful if they covered longer time periods (e.g., a quarter) and were audited by conducting a check of personnel records. OSCAR data do not include information on staff turnover or continuity (length of employment) or on the education and training of staff. This information would be valuable in monitoring facilities with high turnover and poor staff continuity.

The OSCAR data on deficiencies are considered to be valid in part because deficiencies are generally scrutinized carefully and often contested by nursing facilities. However, variability within and between states in the consistency of adherence to survey "interpretive guidelines" in deficiency citations is problematic, at least on the basis of interstate variability in the number and types of deficiencies cited in the survey process (see Chapter 5 for further discussion) (Harrington and Carrillo, 1999).

Finally, the OSCAR system does not include cost data. Cost data are currently available only from the annual Medicare cost reports filed by nursing homes with the fiscal intermediaries (contractors that pay Medicare claims) and from the annual cost reports filed with state Medicaid agencies. The lack of national financial data and of standards for reporting these data impedes research on the relationship between the cost and the quality of nursing home services.

An additional source of information about long-term care in nursing homes is complaint data. OSCAR also includes data from surveys conducted as a part of complaint investigations. The General Accounting Office (GAO) (1999c) and HCFA have reported that some states have not been conducting systematic investigations of nursing home complaints and have not been entering complaint data into the OSCAR system. HCFA is working to improve the complaint investigation and reporting system.

THE RESIDENT ASSESSMENT INSTRUMENT AND THE MINIMUM DATA SET FOR NURSING HOMES

An important requirement of the nursing home reforms in the Omnibus Budget Reconciliation Act of 1987 (OBRA 87) was the development of uniform resident assessment for all nursing home residents. The resident assessment instrument (RAI) includes a set of core assessment items, known as the Minimum Data Set (MDS) for assessment and care screening and more detailed Resident Assessment Protocols (RAP) in 18 areas that represent common problem areas or risk factors for nursing home residents. Its primary use is clinical, to assess the functional, cognitive, and affective levels of residents on admission to the nursing home, at least annually thereafter and on any significant change in status and to develop individualized, restorative care plans. The RAI was designed as a structured approach to assessing a nursing home resident's needs for care and treatment in preparation for the development of a plan of care. The assessor is directed to examine certain issues or ask about certain aspects of the resident's condition; the instrument was designed to be completed by a trained nurse and not as an interview or survey to be completed by the resident.

Based on the advice and consultation from relevant professional and provider groups, researchers, and state and federal regulators, the MDS was created, tested, modified, retested, and then implemented by the end of 1990 in all Medicare- and Medicaid-certified nursing homes in the United States. The final version has 15 domains: cognitive patterns, communication and hearing patterns, vision patterns, physical functioning and structural problems, continence, psychosocial well-being, mood and behavior patterns, activity pursuit patterns, disease diagnoses, health conditions, nutritional status, oral and dental status, skin condition, medication use, and special treatments and procedures (Morris et al., 1990).

Extensive testing and analysis of the MDS has been undertaken to examine the reliability, validity, and sensitivity of individual MDS data elements, as well as composite scales constructed from these data elements. By and large, items characterizing patient's physical functioning were found to be reliable, valid, and sensitive to change. However, measures of depression and other psychosocial indicators have been shown to be less reliable and valid. For example, interrater reliability levels were significantly lower for residents with serious cognitive impairment, indicating the importance of being able to speak with residents (Phillips et al., 1993b).

Design of a revised instrument was initiated almost immediately after implementation of the initial version to account for the rapidly changing mix of people entering nursing homes and to make improvements based upon feedback from the evaluation on both clinical and empirical sources. Version 2.0 of the RAI's MDS was introduced in January of 1996 in most nursing homes across the country. Since June 1998, all nursing homes are required to transmit the MDS information electronically to HCFA on a quarterly basis.

The reliability of both the modified items and new items in MDS version 2.0 were tested and found to out-perform the previous version (Morris et al., 1997). A 4-year evaluation was conducted to assess RAI's impact on the residents' functional, cognitive status, and psychosocial well-being. A quasi-experimental design was used involving the collection of longitudinal data on two cohorts of nursing home residents. Two-thousand nursing home residents in a random sample of 267 facilities located in 10 geographic areas were assessed during the pre-RAI period. In the post-RAI period, 2,000 new residents in 254 of the same facilities were assessed. The researchers found that implementation of the RAI was associated with significant improvements in the quality of care in nursing homes by reducing overall rates of decline in important areas of resident function, in a variety of measures of processes of care, and in reduced hospitalization (Hawes et al., 1997a,b; Morris et al., 1997; Phillips et al., 1997).

HCFA initiated a multi-state Nursing Home Casemix and Quality Demonstration project using the MDS and other measures. The data from this project were used to develop the Resource Utilization Groups-III (RUGS-III) to determine the amount of resources needed for 44 different homogenous types of residents. They are now being used to classify residents in terms of the intensity of nursing and other services needed for the purpose of paying facilities differentially based upon the mix of residents in their home. A strong positive relationship was found between resident characteristics (casemix) and nurse staffing time needed to provide care (Fries et al., 1994). The RUGS-III system now forms the basis for the newly implemented prospective payment system for Medicare Skilled Nursing Facility admissions mandated under the Balanced Budget Act of 1997.

Concerns About Use of the MDS

The rationale for using the MDS to obtain data related to the quality of care is that the information collected is integral to the care process, forming the basis for the individualized care plan. Furthermore, state regulators are supposed to check the internal consistency of the MDS data in a resident's chart and their conformance to the picture of the resident as described in the medical chart and in nursing notes. A major assumption made by those who propose using these types of clinical data for quality monitoring is that, since the data have utility for the care process, facilities and nursing staff have a vested interest in their accuracy. In 1998, HCFA awarded a contract specifically to examine the accuracy of MDS data. An earlier study had found that the accuracy of 23 data items in patients' records increased significantly with the advent of the MDS (Hawes et al., 1997b).

The committee notes that such studies are not necessarily conducted under "real world" circumstances, and the test environment does not always match that for routine use of the instrument. Thus, these trials demonstrate the reliability of the MDS items themselves when used by trained staff, but may not necessarily reflect how the data are assembled in the average facility, raising the issue whether nursing homes have adequate staff with sufficient training and knowledge to perform accurate assessments.

Some concern has been expressed by providers about the institutional burden that use of the MDS imposes in terms of staff time, skills, and energy required. Although the committee heard from some providers that the burden was disproportionate to the value, most providers agreed that the MDS was useful in both resident care planning and internal quality improvement efforts, especially as computerized access to the assessment and related data became more available (AAHSA, 1998; ACHCA, 1998).

As stated above, the MDS is used to classify residents into 44 different RUGS for purposes of Medicare prospective payment. The new prospective payment system was developed using the amount of time needed to provide care to the different RUGS. Thus Medicare's higher rates are paid for residents in higher RUGS groups. One can speculate that as with the effect of the hospital prospective payment system on coding practices for hospital discharge diagnoses, higher payment rates for care of more seriously ill nursing home residents potentially could create incentives for nursing homes to "upcode" that might distort the MDS data. HCFA is conscious of this possibility and is currently pursuing the development of automated programs to monitor the accuracy and consistency of MDS data.

Development and Use of MDS Quality Indicators

Using data from the MDS, Zimmerman and colleagues (1995) developed quality indicators (QIs) as a part of the national Nursing Home Casemix and Quality Demonstration Resident Status Measurement study funded by HCFA. The QIs are designed to monitor the changes in residents and the outcomes of care (Zimmerman et al., 1995) for use by state surveyors to identify problem areas in individual resident characteristics and in services within facilities. Twenty-four QIs have been developed using the revised MDS (version 2.0), including accidents, behavioral and emotional problems, cognitive problems, incontinence, psychotropic drugs, decubitus ulcers, physical restraints, weight problems, and infections (Zimmerman et al., 1995). The QIs were designed to identify residents with the potential for receiving poor quality or high quality of care based on their prevalence rates in comparison nursing facilities. Some of the QIs were adjusted for those facilities with more high-risk residents; other QIs were based on a general standard and not risk adjusted by design. These measures were found to have high validity (Karon et al., 1999).

HCFA is using the QIs to bolster and systematize the quality monitoring process. QIs for individual facilities are now used by state surveyors in the survey process. This allows the observed rates of QIs in a facility to be contrasted to a statewide rate. These reports are provided to both the state surveyors and the facility being inspected. In addition, the software generates a listing of the individual facility residents who met the criteria for possible quality-of-care problems. This roster of residents is being used as the starting point for the selection of records for review during the inspection to determine whether a quality-of-care problem can be confirmed. The QIs have also been aggregated to create a set of facility-level quality indicators that characterize the quality of care in the nursing homes in which those individuals live (Zimmerman et al., 1995).

HCFA is currently funding a contract to identify those QIs that need additional validation testing and modification and to develop new sets of quality indicators for special nursing home populations, such as those receiving post-acute care over a short-term period and residents receiving palliative care. In addition, HCFA has commissioned the development of a new set of facility performance measures that will supplement MDS data with data from residents and their families that capture their values, preferences, and satisfaction with the care received.

These facility-level quality indicators can be valuable for targeting internal quality improvement activities by nursing facilities. These data could also be used as indicators of quality to guide decisions by purchasers or consumers. In spite of these concerns about the use of resident assessment information (originally designed to improve care planning) for policy and regulatory purposes, the committee believes that the general notion of using information about the performance of a facility should be encouraged. HCFA should continue to test and validate the systems of quality indicators now being planned and implemented for nursing facilities.

In the short term, HCFA plans to introduce quality indicator software into states' existing systems for uploading computerized MDS data from all facilities in the state. The plan calls for the software to generate quality indicator reports describing the proportion of the residents of the facility that, based on the most recent MDS assessment, meet criteria for potential quality problems ranging from having pressure ulcers, to taking antipsychotic medications in the absence of specific diagnoses, to declining in an area of activities of daily living. The observed rate of each facility will be contrasted to some "benchmark" that has yet to be determined. These reports will be generated both for the surveyors scheduled to inspect a facility as well as the facility itself.

HCFA is moving toward a more information-intensive approach as an outgrowth of the short-term plans mentioned above. It has awarded four major contracts to advance past work on quality indicators in the nursing home field. All are designed to further HCFA's goal of using the MDS, in both aggregated and individual-level format to bolster and systematize the quality monitoring process. HCFA's vision of this process is that the MDS data constitute the basis for directing survey and certification activities, setting payment levels, and developing information about the quality of long-term care providers to consumers and purchasers.

OUTCOME AND ASSESSMENT INFORMATION SET FOR HOME HEALTH CARE

The perceived utility of the nursing home resident assessment system, particularly its use in developing a Medicare casemix reimbursement method based on resident data, has prompted HCFA to mandate the introduction of a similar data system for Medicare-certified home health care agencies. The **O**utcome and **AS**sessment **I**nformation **S**et (OASIS) is a group of data elements that represent core items of a comprehensive assessment of an adult home care patient and form the basis for measuring patient outcomes for purposes of outcome-based quality improvement. OASIS is a key component of Medicare's partnership with the home health care industry to foster and monitor improved home health care outcomes and is proposed to be an integral part of the revised conditions of participation for Medicare certified home health agencies. HCFA regulations require that as of mid-1999, all certified home health agencies start systematically using OASIS to measure the functional status and medical conditions of all eligible Medicare beneficiaries receiving home health care. The state agencies have the overall responsibility for collecting OASIS data in accordance with HCFA specifications.

OASIS was developed by researchers at the University of Colorado (Shaughnessy et al., 1997a,1998b) over a 15-year period on the basis of work funded by HCFA and the Robert Wood Johnson Foundation. It was designed primarily to produce data that could be used in assessing the outcomes of care provided in the home setting, not as a comprehensive assessment instrument for use in planning patient care, although it does represent core items for an assessment of an adult home health care patient. The objective was to produce a data collection and quality improvement system that would be of primary utility to the home health care industry and the patients it serves. A secondary purpose has been to meet the needs of payers, regulators, and government.

The outcomes-based quality assessment approach represented by OASIS assumes that the quality of care provided by a home health agency can be evaluated on the basis of the outcomes its clients experience relative to similar persons served by other agencies or by the same agency over time (Shaughnessy et al., 1994a,b, 1998a). OASIS includes 89 items covering demographics and patient history, living arrangements, supportive assistance, sensory status, integumentary (skin) status, respiratory status, elimination status, neuro/emotional/behavioral status, activities of daily living, medications, equipment management, and other information collected at inpatient facility admission or agency discharge. Most OASIS data items are collected at the start of care and every 60 days thereafter until and including time of discharge (Shaughnessy et al., 1997a).

During the development of OASIS, several different reports were designed, tested, and refined by having home health agencies collect, computerize, and transmit OASIS data, and then use the resulting reports for clinical and administrative decision making, and, most importantly, quality improvement (Shaughnessy et al., 1998a). The three principal reports are (1) outcomes reports, (2) adverse event reports, and (3) casemix reports. The outcomes reports aggregate patient-level data to produce agency-level performance data on more than 40 outcomes, such as changes in ambulation or locomotion, speech or language, status of surgical wounds, and acute-care hospitalizations. Agency performance is compared to a national reference or benchmark sample and to the agency's own past performance. Risk-adjusted measures are included. The outcomes reports are typically produced annually to have an adequate number of cases for statistically meaningful results. Adverse event reports focus on low-frequency outcomes that may point to problem areas requiring attention. Casemix reports describe the demographic and clinical characteristics of patients admitted to an agency during the previous year.

OASIS was tested extensively for its soundness as a measurement tool and its usefulness in practice. Reliability and validity testing was undertaken with a view toward enhancing the precision and utility of the OASIS data set and the outcomes measures. For inter-rater reliability, for example, studies using either simultaneous or sequential ratings have demonstrated the reliability of the components of the OASIS instrument (Shaughnessy et al., 1994b, 1997a). In a recent study, with nurses independently visiting a patient's home on successive days, the reliability for core data items was 0.62 or above, with most items having reliability coefficients above 0.75 (Shaughnessy et al., 1997b).

Because it is likely that client outcomes are associated with clients' clinical condition on admission or their history of medical problems, the OASIS designers created reasonably homogeneous "casemix" groups of clients thought to be "at-risk" of experiencing a given outcome (whether positively or negatively defined). The developers of OASIS created 25 Quality Indicator Groups that encompass acute medical problems such as acute pulmonary conditions, as well as chronic conditions and impairments (not just medical diagnoses). Some end result outcome measures apply to all QI groups while others are specific to a particular group and the likely therapeutic goals that home health staff would set for these patients. Agencies can be compared on the percentage of the clients in a given QI group that improved, stabilized, or deteriorated between enrollment and the designated follow-up period.

OASIS has been adapted to meet the needs of various audiences, including home health care patients, Medicare beneficiaries, Medicaid clients, home health care clinicians, referring physicians, home health care administrators and managers, agencies that provide home health care, Medicare and other payers, Medicare Survey and Certification agencies, voluntary accreditation agencies, and the research community, policy makers, and consumers. Some of the applications of OASIS data that serve these various groups include the following: evaluating outcomes of home health care at the agency level; assessing quality of care across multiple provider settings; adjusting prospective payment rates for casemix differences; determining the impacts of payment and regulatory policies on home health care casemix and outcomes; detecting discrimination and access barriers to home health care; increasing efficiencies and effectiveness of Medicare and Medicaid survey and certification; facilitating voluntary accreditation; informing consumers; and marketing successful home health care programs. OASIS is being studied for use in Medicare prospective payment systems. For the National Prospective Payment Demonstration (Goldberg et al., 1998), 91 home health agencies in California, Texas, Florida, Illinois, and Massachusetts collected a subset of OASIS data for purposes of evaluating the impact of prospective payment on outcomes, and to selectively monitor and assure the quality of care in the context of the demonstration.

Despite its broad applicability to both Medicare and Medicaid populations, OASIS has developed no application for younger populations including children and young adults in home health care, or working age adults in various long-term care and personal assistance arrangements. Thus, the ability of OASIS to provide meaningful information regarding these populations is untested and unknown. Indeed, no current measurement systems provide useful data about quality of care for these populations.

CHALLENGES IN USING ASSESSMENT DATA

Several technical and methodological challenges exist in using individual-level assessment data successfully for policy purposes such as reimbursement and quality monitoring. Many relevant events of interest are relatively rare, particularly for individual nursing homes or home health agencies. For example, the number of individuals with incidence of pressure ulcers served by a facility or agency might easily vary quarterly from none to three, even in an excellent facility. This small number makes it difficult to calculate reliable estimates of the incidence rates of such events for a standard observation interval. However, as discussed in the previous chapter, prevalence data can be used in such cases to eliminate small numbers problems.

QI values are expected to change over time, but to be a good indicator of quality, they should be reasonably stable over "short" periods. In a study of 512 nursing facilities from two states, Kansas and South Dakota, Karon and colleagues (1999) examined the stability of QIs over each of two 3-month periods and one 6-month period. Results of the study indicated high levels of stability for most QIs. The authors concluded that QIs are reasonably stable over "short" periods of time. All QIs are not of the same type and depending on the characteristics and definition of each QI, the stability has to be examined with caution. Another study using resident-level data from 500 nursing facilities in Massachusetts examined the stability *over time*. As would be expected, they found only moderate to poor correlations *over time* within several quality indicators (Porell and Caro, 1998). This was particularly true for outcomes like change in ADL functioning simply because change rates varied over time, unlike the prevalence of restraint use, which was more stable.

Another concern is the accuracy and completeness with which data are collected and the uniformity of data reporting over time and across providers. This is a concern in most large data collection programs. One way to address this problem is to provide detailed guidance on the data collection and reporting processes. Evidence from the use of individual clinical assessment instruments indicates that explicit instructions and training in how to assess patients or clients improve the reliability of clinical data (Bernabei et al., 1997). Federal government agencies, such as the National Center for Health Statistics in the Centers for Disease Control and Prevention, in collaboration with states have spent decades refining uniformity of data elements reported in state vital records. The importance of similar collaborative efforts for long-term care quality measurement is clear.

An issue that must be considered in using assessment data on long-term care across settings is the effect of casemix differences among various groups of long-term care users. Residents of nursing homes are generally more disabled than people using home health care services, and nursing home residents may, therefore, be at greater risk for certain adverse health outcomes regardless of the quality of care they receive. Even within a single care setting, the populations served by some providers may have more serious health problems than those served by other providers.

Statistical "risk adjustment" techniques are used to help compensate for casemix differences, and the need for such adjustments has been shown in various studies of long-term care outcomes (e.g., Arling et al., 1997; Ooi et al., 1999).[2]

There are limits to what risk adjustment can do. As in the case of acute care hospitals, in some markets there are relatively few long-term care providers of a given type and these tend to be associated with certain specialization areas (e.g., post-acute rehabilitation services or dementia care). Indeed, research evidence shows that in the most competitive markets, providers seek to differentiate themselves precisely by specializing (Banaszak-Holl et al., 1996). Such specialization results in different types of patients being referred to different providers. The more this differentiation occurs, the less risk adjustment can account for very substantial differences in outcomes.

As indicated earlier, however, despite these problems it is essential that continued refinement and evaluation of these data should continue, keeping in focus the concerns discussed above.

ASSESSMENT AND QUALITY MONITORING INSTRUMENTS FOR OTHER SETTINGS

Minimum Data Set for Residential Care

A variety of residential facilities offer room, board, and supervision to frail individuals without certification by the Medicaid or Medicare programs. Regulated entirely by states under an often confusing array of labels, these facilities vary widely in terms of their staffing levels and staff training, and the impairment levels and medical and nursing care needs of the population they serve (Mor et al., 1986; Spore et al., 1996). Several states have developed assessment systems for use in such residential care settings drawing on the RAI and MDS for nursing homes for assessing key functional status items. Other items, however, were developed specific to the population monitored.

The instruments developed by Maine and North Carolina are reviewed briefly here. Both states have tested their instruments in real-world settings and are at the point of introducing them statewide. In Maine, the RAI for residential care facilities was designed to provide a core set of

---

[2]Risk adjustment here refers to the process of statistically compensating for differences in factors that influence outcomes apart from care (e.g., age, functional abilities, cognitive impairments, emotional impairments, presence of a surgical wound, shortness of breath, and various other physiologic conditions) when comparing the outcomes of one provider or care setting with others.

elements for assessing high risk individuals, improving and assuring quality, developing plans of care, and adjusting payment rates for levels of need (Mollica, 1998). North Carolina developed an RAI for Domiciliary Care, to be used in conjunction with the physician's assessment or physician's orders, to create a plan of care and to provide information to facility staff about a resident's functioning levels and needs for assistance (Hawes et al., 1995b). This instrument was tested in 28 facilities where trained facility staff completed the instrument for 105 residents who were then independently assessed by registered nurses. Items on physical functioning achieved adequate reliability, but the items on instrumental activities of daily living (IADLs) and some of the behavior and mood items were found to have relatively low reliability in this type of setting.

State Assessment Systems for Home and Community-Based Service

Many states have developed assessment systems to guide their HCBS programs. Some states have been using, improving, and modifying such tools for 20–30 years. However, most states use these instruments only for Medicaid reimbursed clients. In some states, information systems differ by target populations or programs, but other states are consolidating the instruments across programs and target populations (Kane, 2000). For example, Florida (Kane et al., 1991b), Kansas (Mollica et al., 1994) and to a lesser extent, Vermont (Reinardy et al., 1994) have consolidated assessment forms and procedures from different programs. The Florida effort also tested the reliability, sensitivity, and specificity of their new procedures and instrument.

These assessments are for care managers to: determine initial and continuing eligibility for the HCBS program and, if applicable, the levels of services and benefits to which the consumer will be entitled; establish priorities for beneficiaries and services if availability is limited; develop and implement a care plan incorporating consumers' needs and preferences; evaluate the effectiveness, safety, and adequacy of the individual plans; determine and improve the quality of services; and provide information describing the clients, services, outcomes, and costs of the programs, including variations on these elements.

Assessment instruments vary from state to state but typically include functional status, a summary of health status, cognitive status, affective status (especially depression), and social well-being including social and economic resources. Assessments also may include the physical environment, behavior that puts the consumers at risk, and well-being of the family caregiver. Some states assess the extent of burden on the family caregivers and the dependability of informal care providers.

Some state assessments instruments include consumers' responses in addition to the impressions of the assessor. Not all states aggregate assessment data into a single score for selecting beneficiaries, specifying how much care to offer in the community, and deciding who should be considered for community-based services and who should receive nursing home care. Such scoring systems could be useful in assessing the reliability of care plans and appropriateness of placements. Eligibility for nursing home care also determines eligibility for Medicaid HCBS waivers which are limited for those consumers needing nursing home level of care. Reviews of these practices in all 50 states conducted in the last decade showed wide variations in how nursing-home eligibility is determined (Justice et al., 1991; O'Keefe, 1996).

Some care managers are provided decision protocols to assist them in moving from raw assessment data to care plans. For example, a project in Philadelphia identified and developed care protocols for situations that care managers commonly face, such as people with cognitive impairment who live alone, people with alcohol problems, people who fall, and people who may be victims of abuse. For each of 12 such situations suggested by the initial assessment, templates detail assessment protocols and possible action plans (Amerman et al., 1995).

Integrated Assessment Instruments for Long-Term Care

Several states have begun to restructure their long-term care assessment instruments to be more compatible with HCFA'S MDS because of the increasing proportion of the population that moves into and out of nursing homes, returning home in need of other long-term care services. Compatibility of the assessment instruments might ease the care planning process once patients are discharged into the community. Rhode Island's Department of Elder Affairs, for example, has created a case management assessment instrument largely modeled after the MDS to allow for compatibility of assessments for individuals returning from a post-acute nursing home episode, as well as for those who will ultimately require long-term institutional placement.

Most states also have Medicaid waiver programs for home and community-based services that pay for a variety of services depending on an individual's eligibility for Medicaid long-term care services. Assessment instruments are designed to determine an applicant's eligibility for services and then to guide the development of a plan of care and referrals to service agencies for those who are eligible. In 1996, the GAO conducted a study to better understand the role of assessment in planning home and community-based care for the elderly with disabilities. It found that all instruments record applicants' physical health but the nature of the information collected varies enormously both across and within domains

(GAO, 1996b). GAO concluded that, although all states use assessments to develop a care plan, the comprehensiveness of the assessment varies, and most states do not have standardized terms. Also, most states do not require training in the administration of the instrument despite its importance.

There is strong interest in the possibility of identifying an instrument or set of core assessment elements that is applicable to all users of long-term care regardless of setting. This interest stems in part from a growing recognition of the overlap among the characteristics of long-term care populations served in different settings, and from a desire to compare the quality and costs of care across settings. The availability of such assessment tools for long-term care settings might also help in monitoring individuals as they move from one care level or setting to another. The development of uniform definitions of various community-based services, common measures, and common sets of codes for categorizing care users' physical, cognitive, and emotional functioning would facilitate the adoption of a common language for assessing long-term care needs and the outcomes of care. Clearly, much work is needed first to examine the diversity across states of the services, service settings and service arrangements, and the infrastructure for monitoring quality; and then to develop agreements on common core data elements and uniform definitions of various community-based arrangements.

> Recommendation 4.1: The committee recommends that the Department of Health and Human Services and other appropriate organizations fund scientifically sound research toward further development of quality assessment instruments that can be used appropriately across the different long-term care settings and with different population groups.

The committee notes that the Agency for Healthcare Research and Quality has initiated some efforts in this area. For example, they have awarded a research grant to develop quality measures for residential facilities that can be used for multiple purposes.

INCORPORATING CONSUMER PERSPECTIVES IN MEASUREMENT OF QUALITY

Provision of long-term care should reflect the preferences of consumers. This suggests that data are needed about consumers' perspectives on the quality of their care, and that consumers should be included as a source of data on the quality of care. Although staff assessments are a necessary part of these individual evaluations, especially for the portion of the long-term care population with severe cognitive impairment, staff may not be able to accurately assess such subjective conditions as pain or mood, or individuals' preferences for or satisfaction with care. Even when families serve as proxies for individuals whose impairments prevent them from responding directly, families' perceptions of satisfaction with care are not necessarily consistent with those of long-term care users themselves (Lavizzo-Mourey et al., 1992; Norton et al., 1996). Consumer and professional responses may differ at levels as basic as whether assistance is needed. Professionals may, for example, know more about the range of possible services, allowing them to identify an "unfelt need." The training manual for the two federally mandated systems—RAI/MDS and OASIS—specifies the use of multiple sources of information for most items, including interviews with direct staff across all shifts, interviews with and observations of the resident, interviews with family members and, where relevant, review of other medical records. Although much of the work on measuring quality of life and consumer satisfaction with care has focused on primary and acute care, some efforts are being made to develop measures of consumer and family perspectives on quality of care appropriate for long-term care. For example, the major provider associations have developed data sets that they recommend to their members interested in assessing residents' and family members' satisfaction with care. Many of the larger nursing home chains have designed their own systems to measure satisfaction and might even try to use these data in the strategic planning process. Some studies have also demonstrated the feasibility of consumer assessments of in-home services (e.g., Freedman et al., 1995; Capitman et al., 1997), including reports on unmet needs for service and satisfaction with nonmedical services. The committee recognizes that quality of care is more than satisfaction. It is important, therefore, that these facilities and others do not stop with satisfaction measures but go the next step to develop and refine measures of quality of care in the assessment data sets.

Consumer Satisfaction Surveys

Consumer assessments of care generally address three separate dimensions: (1) consumers' experiences of care, based on reports about matters such as whether they used their call bell to seek assistance and how long the response took (Gerteis et al., 1993); (2) satisfaction with the care received; and (3) consumer preferences regarding care, elicited through questions about the aspects of care they value most highly or the kinds of assistance they would like. Responses to the last set of questions can then be compared to information on the care actually provided to

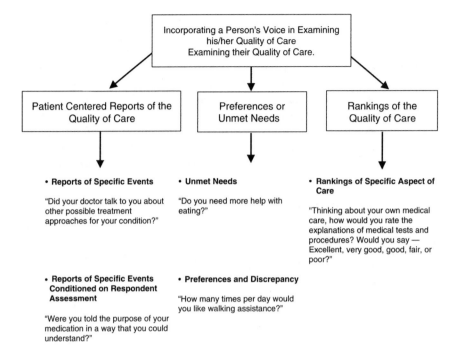

FIGURE 4.1 Proposed classification scheme for measuring a person's perspective about his/her quality of medical care.
SOURCE: Adapted from Teno, 1998.

identify possible unmet care needs. Figure 4.1 illustrates the kinds of questions that can be used to address these different dimensions of consumers' assessments of the quality of care they receive.

Some of the initial work on instruments for obtaining consumer-centered reports on medical care in acute care situations was done by Cleary and colleagues (1991). As shown in Figure 4.1, consumer-centered reports either ask a patient a factual question (e.g., Did someone speak to you about treatment for your concern?) or ask the person to judge one specific aspect of his or her medical treatment (e.g., Were you told of the purpose of your medications in a way that you could understand?). Cleary and colleagues noted that "questions were framed to be as specific as possible, to minimize the influence of confounding factors, such as the patients' expectations, personal relationship, gratitude, or response tendencies related to gender, class, and ethnicity" (Cleary et al., 1991, p. 255).

Traditionally, preference-based assessment (or indirect assessment of satisfaction) is based on a person's reports of unmet needs or desire for additional services (Hughes et al., 1988; Manton 1988; Wolinsky and Johnson, 1991). Satisfaction measures currently used in surveys rank a particular aspect of the care on an ordered qualitative scale (e.g., from "poor" to "excellent") or a numeric scale (e.g., from 1 to 5). The validity of measures of either satisfaction or preference may be affected by factors such as care user's reduced expectations, lack of choice, eagerness to please interviewer, unwillingness to complain, and fear of retaliation. Furthermore, preferences may be unstable. Some of these concerns about consumer assessment measures and methods are discussed below.

Issues in Collecting and Using Consumer Responses

Until recently, a consumer's perspective on the quality of health care was measured with satisfaction measures (or ranking of the quality of medical care). Such satisfaction measures can be problematic. The consumer must compare a recall or perceptions about the service provided with his or her expectation (or preference) about that service. These satisfaction measurement tools are questionable for several reasons. Many people use only the two best categories, even when medical care was less than optimal. For example, Williams and Calnan (1991) found that 95 percent of persons were satisfied with medical care, yet 38 percent reported that they had difficulty discussing personal problems with their physician and 35 percent felt that the physician did not spend enough time with them. Furthermore, the fundamental assumption is that the difference between "very good" and "excellent" is the same as the difference between "fair" and "poor." This assumption may not hold (Fowler et al., 1996). A midpoint response may reflect a serious concern.

Another important concern is the reluctance of consumers to discuss quality of medical care, even to an anonymous interviewer over the phone (Vouri, 1987). Persons receiving long-term care services may feel especially vulnerable because they are dependent on providers for basic needs.

Reduced expectations is another area of concern. In a study of seriously ill and dying patients, Desbiens and colleagues (1996) found that the majority of patients stated that they were "very satisfied" despite pain that was extremely or moderately severe for one-half or more of the time. In another study, family members who reported patients had severe pain before they died would state that "*the doctors did all that they could*" (Teno et al., 2000). Yet research indicates that between 70 and 90 percent of patients' pain can be palliated with sedation (Schug et al., 1990; Portenoy, 1994; Zech et al., 1995). Lowered expectations and the lack of knowledge about possible and appropriate care severely limits the validity of consumers' responses to questionnaires that ask them to rank aspects of their medical care. Furthermore, patient reports of quality of care may be overly based on the interpersonal skills of the provider and highly empathic skills may mask poor medical judgments. For example, caregivers with highly empathic skills may be described as "excellent" even when comparisons of their care with evidence-based practice guidelines or other criteria suggest significant concerns with the quality of that care (Callahan et al., 2000). However, the manner in which the caregiver relates to and interacts with the client is part of the quality of care. These and other important problems have been identified with satisfaction measurements (Cleary and McNeil, 1988; Rubin, 1990; Jackson and Kroenke, 1997; Rosenthal and Shannon, 1997; Kravitz, 1998; Teno, 1998).

Different strategies have been used in measuring the consumer perspective of the quality of care. Traditionally, patients' ranked or rated the quality of care. For the most part, these measures suffered skewed distribution, acquiescent response bias, and problems with reduced consumer expectations. Alternatively, preference-based assessment (or indirect assessment of satisfaction) is based on a person's reports of unmet needs or desire for additional services. But low or lowered patient expectations may limit both strategies. Furthermore, preferences may be unstable—both ethereal and ephemeral. Few studies have examined the stability or consistency of patient reports. Many researchers have questioned the appropriate use of consumer's responses in various areas of health care (Cleary and McNeil, 1988; Ware and Hays, 1988; Rubin, 1990; Aharony and Strasser, 1993; Zinn, 1994; Ross et al., 1995; Jackson and Kroenke, 1997; Rosenthal and Shannon, 1997; Kravitz, 1998).

Reliability and Validity of Responses. Several factors may influence the reliability and validity of consumers' reports regarding their care. Social desirability and acquiescent response biases are prevalent among dependent groups, such as the institutionalized elderly, in part due to fear of repercussions from caregivers (La Monica et al., 1986). Nursing home residents reported high levels of satisfaction with care at the same time that interviewer observations and resident's open-ended comments suggest dissatisfaction and a reluctance to criticize nursing home staff (Pearson et al., 1993) and describe other quality concerns (Callahan et al., 2000). Kinney and colleagues (1994) got similar responses from consumers of HCBS services in Indiana. Because older adults in general, and women in particular, as well as individuals in poor health, tend to report higher rates of satisfaction with health care services regardless of its quality (Locker and Dunt, 1978; Ross et al., 1995), long-term-care users may report high rates of satisfaction with substandard or inconsistent levels of care. The wording and sequence of the questions can also influence responses. Among the nursing home residents studied by Simmons and Schnelle

(1999), 80 percent reported satisfaction with care ("Are you satisfied with how often someone helps you to walk?"), but in response to a separate question on care preferences ("Would you like for someone to help you to walk more often?"), only 60 percent reported that they did not want more walking assistance.

Bias in Assessments. The cognitive impairments prevalent in long-term care populations, as well as some physical impairments, make the collection and interpretation of consumer information more problematic than in some other health care areas. Many cognitively impaired people are excluded from interviews assessing care or quality of life, based on the belief that these residents cannot accurately answer questions (Kruzich et al., 1992; Aller and Van Ess Coeling, 1995).

In summary, although consumer-centered measures of the quality of care are useful, poorly developed or improperly used measures of consumer satisfaction can be misleading. Careful attention to the types of respondents included as well as "proxies" for people who are cognitively impaired may mitigate many potential measurement biases.

Even assuming that consumer assessments provide reliable and valid information, they are not necessarily a guide to quality improvement interventions. With end-of-life care, for example, significant progress has been made in identifying the medical treatment preferences of residents and families, but using this information to change medical practice and achieve care that matches preferences has proved more difficult (SUPPORT Principal Investigators, 1995; Teno et al., 1995).

MEASUREMENT CONSIDERATIONS FOR CHILDREN AND YOUNG ADULTS

Measuring quality of care or outcomes of care for children and adolescents using long-term care presents particular challenges, mainly because of the complex problems of measurement in the context of children's growth and development. Many of the indicators used to assess disability among adults are related to limitations in the ability to live independently (e.g., the need for assistance with paying bills or bathing and dressing), but such indicators are generally not suitable for children and adolescents for whom independent living is not an appropriate goal, regardless of the presence of any disabling condition. Moreover, the normal developmental process means that expectations for younger children will be quite different from those for adolescents. At the age of 2, children cannot dress themselves, usually have limited control over toileting, and have limited verbal skills, whereas the typical 15-year-old can be expected to have more skills in all of these areas.

The dynamic nature of child development affects measurement in almost all domains and has made the development of measures of children's health status particularly difficult. For children, the domains of health status and quality of life that are particularly important include growth (mainly physical), development (mainly emotional, cognitive, and motor), and educational achievement. Indeed, for children, the important interaction with the educational sector—often affected by the demands of long-term care—has no equivalent in adult long-term care experience (Walker and Jacobs, 1985).

Another issue in measuring quality of care or outcomes for children concerns the unit of observation. Because of the dependence of children on the adults around them, especially their parents, to support their growth and development, assessments of long-term care programs should consider not only the effects on the child but also those on the child's environment. For example, parents of children with severe disabilities have a much higher rate of mental health problems, especially depression (Thyen et al., 1998; Thyen et al., 1999) and parents' poor physical or mental health negatively influences a child's development. Thus, programs aiming to improve outcomes for children with long-term care needs should address ways to strengthen families in general, rather than focusing only on the children, and assessment instruments should reflect these goals.

Current efforts to develop measurement instruments have resulted in a few general health status measures with some applicability across ages and stages of development, as well as numerous measures addressing more specific aspects of children's development (e.g., cognition or motor abilities); yet much more work will be needed to support careful assessment of the quality of long-term care for children. Current measures include: (1) the Functional Status II-R, a brief measure of general function applicable and tested across a relatively wide age range (Stein and Jessop, 1990); (2) the Child Health Questionnaire, similar to the Medical Outcomes Study SF-36 for adults, currently available in forms for children over age five (Landgraf et al., 1996); (3) the WeeFIM, a measure focused mainly on physical functioning of preschool-aged children with motor impairments (Msall et al., 1994); and (4) the Adolescent Health Status measure developed to gather adolescents' self-assessments of health status in several domains (Starfield et al., 1993). A version of this last measure applicable to younger school-age children has had extensive testing and will be released for general use shortly.

One of the health care industry standards for quality assessment, the Health Plan Employer Data and Information Set (also known as HEDIS), has only limited numbers of measures addressing quality of care for children and almost none addressing children with chronic conditions (Kuhlthau et al., 1998). The work of a child and adolescent health measurement task force under the leadership of the National Council on Quality Assurance and the Foundation for Accountability, includes, as one component, the development of a set of quality measures to assess care for children with chronic conditions. This set has as its base a section of the Consumer Assessment of Health Plans survey designed specifically for households with children who have chronic health conditions.

CONCLUSION

This chapter has reviewed the basis for the measurement of long-term care quality relying on individual-level information to create aggregated measures characterizing provider performance. In differentiating between staff-provided data (based on codification of staff assessment information) and consumer-provided reports on the nature and quality of care provided, this chapter does not intend to imply that they are mutually exclusive. Both have strengths and weaknesses, and they should be regarded as complementary.

Despite the potential weaknesses inherent in using staff-reported data, such data are currently more readily available than consumer-reported data for both the institutional and the home health arena. A substantial amount of research is devoted to the application of these individual-level data to aggregated performance measures. To be sure, additional research is still needed to grapple with the numerous complex technical and substantive issues cited here, but these problems are being addressed and several should be substantially resolved in time.

5

Improving Quality Through External Oversight

Organizations providing long-term care are staffed with professional, paraprofessional, and support staff, and often volunteers. In the final analysis, the quality and safety of long-term care is dependent upon these individuals' actions, but their actions can be and are influenced by external forces. These forces can provide guidance, often in the form of standards that establish parameters for structures and processes, and can set expectations for outcomes. External forces can also provide incentives, financial or otherwise, for specific actions that will affect access to and safety of care, and the quality of care and life in long-term care settings.

These external forces include formal quality oversight mechanisms, purchasers of long-term care, and families. This chapter focuses on three formal oversight mechanisms:

1. regulatory oversight by federal, state, and local governments;
2. consumer advocacy programs; and
3. accreditation.

The committee recognizes that other forces—including mass media, care management and monitoring programs, and contractor standards set by purchasers—also influence provider behavior. The approaches of regulatory oversight, advocacy, and accreditation are somewhat different. Their relative strengths and weaknesses may make them differentially suited to different long-term care settings (e.g., nursing homes, residential care, and home health care) and the individuals receiving care in them. They may complement each other in various arrangements such as that of deemed status, complaint investigation and mediation, or independent confirmation of measures of satisfaction of individuals in long-term care and their families.

Beginning with the development of licensure for health workers in the nineteenth century to the current ongoing government initiatives to define and enforce quality standards, regulation and oversight have figured prominently in efforts to assess, protect, and improve the quality of health care. Basic quality standards define and specify the minimum acceptable qualifications for state licensure and for certification for participation in Medicare and Medicaid.[1] This chapter focuses on the government's central role in setting and enforcing standards of quality for formal long-term care. It highlights the current status of the basic standards, the survey process for monitoring and assessing compliance, and the enforcement of the quality standards for nursing homes, residential care, and home health care. Throughout the chapter the committee provides suggestions and recommendations for further improvements at both the federal and the state levels.

CENTRAL ROLE OF GOVERNMENT

Through legislation, regulation, and judicial decisions, federal and state governments play a central role in the definition and enforcement of basic standards of quality for long-term care, particularly for publicly funded services and institutional care. In addition, regulations involving such matters as contracts or disclosure of information to consumers and the public are components of quality strategies based on consumer choice and quality improvement.

Most federal regulations of long-term care are linked to federal funding of services through the Medicare and Medicaid programs, and are administered by the Health Care Financing Administration (HCFA) of the U.S. Department of Health and Human Services (DHHS). Both programs have requirements for participation that health care providers must meet to receive payment.[2]

Federal and state governments share regulatory responsibilities for long-term care. Overall, the federal government has a dominant presence in nursing home and home health regulation through certification for

---

[1]Those who meet specified standards may also have to meet other conditions, for example, payment of a fee to actually secure a license.

[2]Until recently, these requirements were known as "conditions of participation."

Medicare and Medicaid participation. States, however, play the major role in regulating other kinds of long-term care. For example, they set licensure and other standards for various kinds of residential care arrangements. States also perform many of the certification procedures under contract with HCFA.

Although basic standards for long-term care are often defined and enforced primarily through the legislative and administrative process, standards put forward from other nongovernmental sources are also important. Many professional societies, trade associations, accrediting bodies, and other organizations have set voluntary standards that operate in tandem with regulations through voluntary compliance. Voluntary standards are often intended to "raise the bar" by promoting and recognizing performance beyond a basic, legally established level. In some cases, an approved accrediting organization's standards can be "deemed" to meet certification requirements for participation in Medicare or Medicaid, as is the case with the certification of home health care agencies, discussed later in this chapter.

The central elements of long-term care regulation at the federal or state level are:

- establishing quality and related *standards* for service providers;
- designing *survey processes* and procedures to measure and monitor actual conditions of residents or clients and *to assess compliance*; and
- specifying and imposing *remedies or sanctions* for noncompliance.[3]

These three elements of a regulatory system have been likened to "the legs of a three-legged stool" (IOM, 1986, p. 69), with each leg equally important to the effectiveness of the system. In order to assess compliance with federal Medicare and Medicaid requirements, HCFA relies on a survey and certification process, which is administered by state licensing and certification agencies. HCFA's ten regional offices are charged with the oversight and monitoring of the state survey and certification efforts for nursing homes and home health agencies.

In recent years, reporting of assessments of compliance with standards and sanctions for noncompliance has become prominent as consumer groups and others have pressed for more complete public reporting. To the extent that such reports accurately reflect quality problems, they can be useful both for policy makers and for people facing personal decisions about long-term care. Moreover, the enforcement of govern-

---

[3]*Remedies* and *sanctions* are used interchangeably throughout this report to refer to enforcement actions against providers failing to comply with regulatory requirements.

ment standards does not depend solely on periodic inspections by regulators or on self-enforcement by the regulated. Complaints from residents, family members, facility or agency staff, formally appointed ombudsmen, and others may help identify violations and other problems that regular, formal inspections and reporting systems may miss. Many complaints and concerns related to basic standards of quality may be voiced directly to providers, ideally prompting a constructive internal response. Beyond this "oversight-by-complaint" role, family, friends, and other visitors to the long-term care setting also provide social and practical support to those using long-term care, help paid caregivers better understand the perceptions and preferences of those they serve, and build links between long-term care and the larger community.

Arguments for and Against Regulation

Major goals of long-term care regulation have been described as (1) consumer protection, specifically, ensuring safety, quality of the care received, and legal rights of consumers, and (2) accountability for public funds used for care (IOM, 1986). With government accounting for 61 percent of nursing home and home health care expenditures (Braden et al., 1998), it has a responsibility to hold providers accountable for fiscal integrity and for the quality of care provided to beneficiaries. Medicare and Medicaid requirements of participation for nursing homes and home health care services serve both goals. States also have an obligation under their police power functions to provide oversight over the public health and safety.

Most policy makers acknowledge a particular need for federal and state regulation of long-term care. The reasons are several:

- Regulatory protection is essential given the significant vulnerability of many of the people using long-term care, including the very old and frail, the very young, and those with dementia, mental illness, and developmental disabilities. Many people with severe chronic or disabling conditions are highly dependent on others and unable to protect themselves from abuses and neglect by caregivers. Moreover, many have no immediate family members, friends, or advocates who are able to oversee their care and protection.
- Individuals needing long-term care frequently have multiple diagnoses and chronic conditions that require a wide array of medical and nursing services, medications, and treatments. Although some individuals have the knowledge and skills to direct their own care, others do not.
- Those using long-term care rely heavily on nonprofessional and para-

professional workers, which typically means they rely on workers who have little training or expertise in providing care.

- Much long-term care is relatively invisible, either because it is provided in the home or because it is provided in facilities without much community observation.
- Users of long-term care often lack choice of providers or services, which limits the effectiveness of market forces in ensuring quality.

On the basis of the above, a strong argument can be made for an active government role in defining and enforcing basic standards of quality for long-term care providers. In addition, ensuring their enforcement protects those using long-term care from neglect, abuse, and mismanagement.

Critics of regulation as a dominant strategy for protecting and improving the quality of long-term care present several arguments. During public meetings, providers criticized overreliance on regulatory strategies contending that:

- It may encourage mediocrity. They believe that too many providers concentrate narrowly on minimum requirements instead of striving for providing quality care.
- Regulation may create barriers to innovation. What may be a necessary rule for those not motivated or able to provide quality care, could be an obstacle to others seeking creative ways to improve the quality of care and life and autonomy of those using long-term care.
- There is a possible danger for regulation to proliferate excessively. For example, regulators concerned about marginally performing institutions and egregious instances of poor quality of care may be tempted to multiply structure and process regulations without regard to their effectiveness or costs.
- They believe that regulations focus too single-mindedly on protection and safety as objectives. Other values such as the quality of life or autonomy of those receiving care may be underemphasized.

With regard to federal regulation of nursing homes, however, the nursing home reforms in the Omnibus Reconciliation Act of 1987 (OBRA 87) actually changed the focus from a nursing home's ability to provide care to the quality of care provided. OBRA 87 requires nursing homes participating in Medicare and Medicaid to comply with extensive standards and these standards include ensuring various residents' rights related to admission, transfer, and discharge, and the right to be free from restraints and abuse, and to promote residents' quality of life. The regulations also focus more than before on processes of care and resident outcomes. In common with most complex human endeavors a perfect regulatory system is likely to be beyond human reach. Nonetheless, it is important for policy makers, regulators, and advocates to consider and weigh both the expected benefits and the expected burdens of regulations. Moreover, by listening to the concerns of those subject to regulation as well as the beneficiaries of regulations, policy makers may be able to develop effective, yet less costly and less resisted ways of achieving their goals. The challenge is to design and implement a system that does what it is intended to do at an acceptable cost.

BASIC STANDARDS OF QUALITY

In principle, some basic standards for long-term care could be developed that apply regardless of the setting or provider of care. In practice, however, most standards are designed for specific categories of providers or services. In general, it may be useful for policy makers, providers, consumer advocates, and others to think about standards applicable across various care settings. Such thinking may become increasingly necessary if concepts of consumer-centered and -directed care are to be developed. Indeed, regulatory standards related to outcomes have become an increasingly important objective in long-term care. This approach, however important, is beyond the scope of what the committee is able to address in this report.

Reflecting the differences in current regulatory programs in various long-term care settings, this chapter focuses on selected settings separately. As is typical of most long-term care issues, nursing homes have been the focus of most attention in standard-setting and enforcement activities. This again reflects a long history of concern about abuse, neglect, and poor quality of care in nursing homes and public concern about this frail and vulnerable group of long-term care users, who are subject to the greatest degree of provider control over their lives. The discussion that follows focuses on nursing homes, residential care facilities, home health care, and home care and other home and community-based services.

Nursing Homes

Both federal and state governments employ regulation as a strategy to protect quality of care in nursing homes. The federal government has defined standards or requirements for provider participation in Medicare, and Medicaid relies primarily on the states for assessment. The federal government retains authority to enforce compliance with nursing home standards of care, but generally delegates enforcement authority to states for other health care providers. States also independently regulate nursing homes, for example, by licensing them to do business in the state. A few nursing homes operate only under state regulation because they choose not to seek Medicare or Medicaid reimbursement, but nearly all facilities depend on such reimbursement and, therefore, have all, most, or some of their beds certified.

This study was not intended to replicate or update the Institute of Medicine's (IOM) 1986 report by producing a detailed analysis of the implementation of that report's recommendations or generating another set of comprehensive recommendations about nursing home regulation. *This committee generally endorses the directions set forth in the 1986 report and in the legislative reforms enacted in 1987.* During 1998 and 1999, however, new reports and investigations of serious problems in nursing home quality and government regulation demanded the committee's serious attention. As context for the discussion of these problems, a brief review of the 1986 IOM report and subsequent nursing home legislation is useful.

The 1986 IOM Report on Nursing Home Regulation

In its 1986 report on nursing home quality, the IOM committee noted "serious, even shocking, inadequacies" in the enforcement of then-current nursing home regulations. It identified "large numbers of marginal or substandard nursing homes that are chronically out of compliance when surveyed . . . [and that] temporarily correct their deficiency . . . and then quickly lapse into noncompliance until the next survey" (p. 146). The report identified problems in four broad areas: (1) attitudes of federal and state personnel about enforcement objectives and processes; (2) federal rules and guidelines for states; (3) variation among states in policies and procedures; and (4) resources to support enforcement activities. It also addressed other problems with existing procedures for interpreting survey findings, weighting or scoring facility performance on individual standards, and aggregating performance on individual standards to determine whether a facility is in compliance with a condition of participation. It also addressed problems of the predictable timing of annual surveys and the reliance on record reviews and staff interviews, rather than interviews and observation of residents, to determine quality.

The report proposed that regulations "require, whenever possible, assessment of the quality and appropriateness of care and the quality of life . . . being provided residents, and the effects on residents' well-being" (IOM, 1986, p. 71). It called for new standards in three areas: residents' rights, quality of life, and resident assessment. The 1986 IOM report proposed regulatory reform to focus the survey and certification process more on persistent offenders; to clarify federal objectives and rules by improving training, reporting, and oversight activities for states; and to establish a wider array of sanctions related to the seriousness of problems discovered. The report and subsequent legislation made clear that government's role was one of enforcement and not consultation. The framework also called for less reliance "on unguided professional judgments by surveyors" in determining what constitutes good care for residents with differing service needs (IOM, 1986, p. 71).

Nursing Home Reform Act of 1987—Setting Standards for Care

The Nursing Home Reform Act, a part of OBRA 87, created the most far-reaching changes in nursing home regulation since the Medicare and Medicaid programs were created in 1965. It was supported by a broad coalition of consumer, professional, and nursing home industry representatives. The legislation was generally based on the detailed recommendations of the IOM committee (1986), and delineated five major components addressing (1) resident rights, quality of life, and quality of care; (2) staffing and services; (3) resident assessment; (4) federal survey procedures; and (5) enforcement procedures (Harrington, 1998). For example, it created a new outcome-oriented survey process with two options—a standard survey and an extended survey. The standard survey required a stratified sample of residents (based on the characteristics or casemix of residents) for examining medical, nursing, and rehabilitative care; dietary services; social activities; sanitation; infection control; resident rights; and physical environment. In facilities found to be providing substandard care during the standard survey, an extended survey was to be applied, with a larger sample of residents, intended to uncover the causes of substandard care.

Continuing past practice, OBRA 87 required HCFA to contract with state agencies to survey nursing homes to certify their compliance with Medicare and Medicaid requirements. Consistent with the changes in the standards, enforcement was to focus on both processes and outcomes of care. The new inspection procedures were, however, to go beyond "paper compliance" to investigate processes and outcomes of care; interview residents, families, and ombudsmen about their experience in the nursing home; and directly observe residents and care processes. Surveys were to be unannounced and conducted every 9 to 15 months following the initial survey (but no sooner than 12 months on average for all facilities taken together) to give survey agencies some flexibility to link survey timing to past performance and also make it easier to create more unpredictable scheduling of survey visits. States could also initiate a survey in response to a resident or other complaint at any time. Resurveys were authorized after any change of ownership.

The new standards and survey procedures were implemented

through a series of regulations and transmittals published by HCFA in its *State Operations Manuals*.[4] The first regulations implementing the act took effect in 1990; the last regulations (those related to enforcement of standards) were implemented only in 1995. The regulations established 15 major categories for compliance to cover the structure, process, and outcomes of nursing home care with specific requirements for each category.[5] Additionally, OBRA 87 requires nursing homes to provide certain services, including nursing, dietary, physician, rehabilitative, dental, and pharmacy services. It also included requirements for administrative standards including nursing aide training, a medical director, and clinical records.

The OBRA 87 standards for residents' rights included privacy, freedom from physical and mental abuse, restricted use of physical or chemical restraints, and opportunities to file grievances. The process of care and the environment should promote residents' quality of life, and services should help residents attain or maintain the highest practical level of physical, mental, and psychosocial well-being. The requirement that well-being be maximized "implied that *improvements* in health and functional status be achieved, when possible," which shifted the focus away from custodial care toward rehabilitation (IOM, 1996a, p. 134). OBRA 87 was notable for requiring individual resident assessments and care plans for each resident described in the previous chapter.

The committee concluded that these basic standards of quality set forth in OBRA 87 are generally reasonable and comprehensive. As discussed in Chapter 3, research studies suggest that these standards may have contributed to improved care and outcomes for nursing home residents. *Definitive, rigorous evaluation of their continuing impact on quality of care and outcomes is necessary.*

State Survey Process

To monitor and assess compliance by nursing homes with Medicare and Medicaid requirements for participation, HCFA relies on a survey and certification process administered under contract by state agencies. As specified by OBRA 87, nursing home surveys gather information

---

[4]The regulations were issued in 1988, 1989, 1991, 1992, and 1994, and the transmittals were included in the *State Operations Manuals* (HCFA, 1995a–c).

[5]The categories are (1) resident rights; (2) admission, transfer, and discharge rights; (3) resident behavior and facility practices; (4) quality of life; (5) resident assessment; (6) quality of care; (7) nursing services; (8) dietary services; (9) physician services; (10) rehabilitation services; (11) dental services; (12) pharmacy services; (13) infection control; (14) physical environment; and (15) administration (HCFA, 1995a–c).

through facility visits; observations of residents; reviews of records; and interviews with residents, family members, and facility staff and management. Thus, assessments are not dependent solely on facility records and reports. HCFA has developed standardized forms, sampling methods, and survey procedures to ensure the reliability, accuracy, and comparability of state surveys of nursing homes. In a further effort to achieve consistency, HCFA's *State Operations Manual* (HCFA, 1999c), including the Interpretative Guidelines, provides more detail and guidance for state surveyors.

After surveying each facility, state surveyors determine whether the facility has met or not met each standard. If a facility is judged to not meet a standard, it is given a "deficiency." Generally deficiency determinations are made by survey teams and reviewed by state supervisors. Facilities have the option to challenge the factual basis of deficiencies in an informal dispute resolution and to appeal decisions through an administrative review process.

State survey results showed a clear trend in declining numbers of deficiencies after the enforcement regulations were implemented in 1995, with a small increase in 1998. As seen in Figure 5.1, the average number of deficiencies reported per facility declined from 10.8 per facility in 1991 to 4.9 per facility in 1997, a 44 percent decrease (Harrington and Carrillo, 1999). In 1998, however, the average number of deficiencies per facility increased slightly to 5.2. At the same time, the percentage of facilities reported to have no deficiencies increased from 10.8 in 1991 to 21.6 in 1997, and then dropped to 18.9 percent in 1998 (Harrington and Carrillo, 1999; Harrington et al., 2000b).

Survey results also show substantial variation across states (see Table 5.1). In 1998, the average number of deficiencies ranged from 1.9 per facility in New Jersey to 14.2 in Nevada (more than a sevenfold difference) (Harrington et al., 2000b). Similarly, the percentage of facilities with no deficiencies varied from none in Washington, D.C., to 47.7 percent in New Jersey. For the most part, the higher the average number of deficiencies in a state, the lower is the percentage of facilities reported to have no deficiencies cited (Harrington et al., 2000b).

Weaknesses in the Current Survey Process

Although the declining number of deficiencies and increase in the number of deficiency-free facilities may indicate substantially improved care in nursing homes, the analysis presented in Chapter 3 suggests that taking too optimistic a stance may be unwarranted. Instead, it may suggest weaknesses in the nursing home survey process—specifically, its ability to reliably detect quality problems. The inability or unwillingness

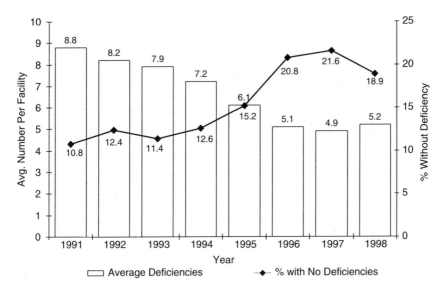

FIGURE 5.1 Average number of deficiencies and percent of facilities without deficiencies: United States, 1991–1998.
SOURCE: Harrington et al., 1999, 2000b.

of surveyors to detect quality problems may be one explanation, particularly following implementation of more vigorous enforcement regulations in 1995 (Johnson and Kramer, 1998; Mortimore et al., 1998; Schmitz et al., 1998).

Several studies support the conclusion that the current survey process fails to identify important quality-of-care problems. A study conducted by the University of Wisconsin in 1996, which involved 6 concurrent surveys and 23 survey observations performed by independent investigators, showed that state surveyors consistently cited fewer deficiencies in care and rated problems as less severe than did the researchers (Abt and CHSRA, 1996). Similarly, two concurrent surveys conducted for the General Accounting Office (GAO) in California also found that surveyors did not detect some serious quality-of-care problems related to hospitalizations, deaths, falls accompanied by fractures, restraint use, failure to dress and groom residents, malnutrition, infections, and pressure sores (GAO, 1998a; Johnson and Kramer, 1998). Forty concurrent surveys in ten states revealed that state surveyors were inconsistent in detecting problems related to outcomes of care, particularly those related to maintaining resident function, pressure sore prevention, and nutritional support (Johnson and Kramer, 1998). At the same time, state surveyors also cited some

TABLE 5.1 Average Number of Deficiencies per Certified Facility and Percent of Facilities with No Deficiencies, by State: United States, 1992–1998

State	Average Number of Deficiencies per Facility							Percent of Facilities with No Deficiencies						
	1992[a]	1993[a]	1994	1995	1996	1997	1998	1992[a]	1993[a]	1994	1995	1996	1997	1998
Alabama	6.8	5.4	7.4	6.7	6.4	6.1	5.9	5.3	6.7	7.9	7.1	12.0	7.1	7.4
Alaska	6.1	10.8	4.3	3.2	2.2	3.6	3.2	6.7	0.0	21.4	15.4	31.3	21.4	21.4
Arizona	5.5	3.6	7.1	7.1	5.7	5.1	6.0	22.8	23.7	11.9	2.7	4.9	5.9	6.2
Arkansas	10.5	7.6	7.5	8.1	8.2	7.5	7.3	2.6	4.6	4.1	5.8	6.6	3.9	4.7
California	16.2	17.8	16.2	11.7	10.7	10.7	10.4	2.8	2.4	1.2	3.3	4.0	3.0	1.8
Colorado	11.7	6.9	2.5	2.4	2.6	2.3	2.2	2.1	5.0	28.4	31.0	33.7	42.8	34.9
Connecticut	4.8	5.6	3.7	2.3	1.5	2.1	2.7	13.6	13.6	18.0	37.1	46.5	33.6	23.6
Delaware	5.8	6.3	7.2	6.6	9.5	7.3	10.1	12.1	21.6	7.0	12.1	2.7	11.9	7.4
Florida	6.3	5.7	6.8	7.0	6.1	6.4	7.2	16.2	16.4	10.9	10.5	15.2	11.0	10.5
Georgia	7.5	5.7	6.1	5.0	3.3	2.6	3.6	12.0	15.6	14.8	17.3	34.3	32.1	23.4
Hawaii	15.3	18.1	18.4	9.7	4.8	6.6	7.8	0.0	0.0	0.0	4.8	2.5	9.5	2.3
Idaho	12.1	10.9	8.5	6.1	6.3	7.1	7.1	4.8	3.1	7.7	7.5	10.8	7.8	6.3
Illinois	8.1	8.2	8.5	7.9	6.2	6.0	5.8	3.9	5.1	4.0	5.5	9.0	6.9	7.9
Indiana	5.8	7.3	7.7	7.4	6.5	6.8	7.8	12.3	11.3	8.2	7.5	11.9	9.5	7.4
Iowa	5.4	4.8	4.0	3.8	4.0	4.8	4.6	17.7	17.9	23.9	25.7	24.9	17.9	15.8
Kansas	13.0	8.9	6.8	6.5	6.2	5.5	5.1	1.0	4.6	8.6	5.4	11.3	11.4	19.5
Kentucky	5.3	4.2	3.1	4.1	2.3	3.2	6.0	33.9	39.0	37.8	44.9	56.4	49.2	13.8
Louisiana	11.8	11.7	7.8	6.3	4.7	4.2	3.7	6.3	8.8	14.1	15.6	20.3	23.2	30.4
Maine	2.9	3.6	4.5	4.0	2.4	2.7	3.3	37.6	35.2	13.0	10.4	32.0	32.8	13.6
Maryland	3.7	2.7	4.0	4.1	2.6	2.2	2.4	29.2	31.8	21.5	30.1	34.8	36.7	37.4
Massachusetts	3.2	5.7	4.7	4.6	3.2	2.6	2.8	22.8	13.5	16.7	22.9	36.0	47.8	41.3
Michigan	16.8	16.1	13.3	13.6	9.8	8.6	9.3	1.2	1.0	0.7	1.4	3.7	2.7	3.1
Minnesota	5.3	7.4	6.8	5.3	2.9	2.7	3.6	16.4	8.4	7.6	9.7	27.4	28.6	25.2
Mississippi	11.6	10.6	10.8	8.0	4.8	3.9	4.6	3.1	7.9	11.1	12.6	24.7	27.9	16.0
Missouri	9.0	7.9	4.8	4.1	4.2	3.6	4.1	12.0	14.2	27.4	25.8	28.2	29.6	23.0

State														
Montana	10.5	10.3	9.6	7.2	5.7	3.5	5.6	5.2	4.2	3.1	0.0	14.0	22.1	10.9
Nebraska	8.7	6.0	4.7	3.5	3.6	2.6	3.0	4.6	7.3	13.1	24.8	29.7	42.9	34.4
Nevada	18.8	19.2	17.2	15.0	12.7	14.3	14.2	0.0	0.0	7.5	0.0	0.0	0.0	7.3
New Hampshire	2.5	2.2	2.7	2.0	4.4	3.3	2.7	43.9	36.4	43.3	38.9	22.9	29.3	38.7
New Jersey	6.7	4.4	3.8	4.0	2.6	2.4	1.9	14.6	19.0	28.9	27.7	36.9	42.5	47.7
New Mexico	9.0	6.2	4.7	3.7	1.7	1.8	4.5	7.0	8.7	15.6	29.9	48.1	57.1	22.7
New York	v3.1	2.4	2.5	3.1	2.7	2.2	2.0	36.4	31.9	31.5	27.6	31.4	35.3	39.6
North Carolina	6.5	5.9	5.8	4.8	4.0	3.4	4.6	11.8	9.5	10.6	17.9	22.7	34.8	25.7
North Dakota	5.7	6.5	6.2	4.8	6.6	7.9	7.4	10.7	2.5	3.7	16.9	8.1	4.0	6.8
Ohio	3.8	7.4	7.3	6.6	4.8	4.0	4.6	22.6	8.4	7.1	10.6	17.2	22.2	22.9
Oklahoma	5.1	4.9	4.6	4.7	4.0	4.2	3.7	10.6	15.1	19.1	20.4	24.8	25.3	28.3
Oregon	13.1	7.6	5.9	5.6	5.2	4.7	4.6	3.2	8.3	15.3	16.0	24.0	26.3	21.9
Pennsylvania	6.3	6.1	5.4	3.8	3.1	3.2	3.8	14.0	12.9	11.6	21.4	27.8	25.0	19.5
Rhode Island	4.6	5.5	4.4	3.6	2.9	3.4	3.6	25.8	15.6	15.2	19.5	26.7	22.8	21.4
South Carolina	8.8	9.5	6.4	5.2	7.3	7.9	7.9	3.4	2.2	6.0	7.1	6.7	6.3	4.9
South Dakota	5.5	5.4	4.4	4.5	4.3	3.3	3.7	14.3	8.3	8.5	19.8	19.0	21.8	11.6
Tennessee	9.8	8.6	7.6	7.2	5.9	2.6	3.7	4.8	4.2	8.1	7.3	9.9	29.9	21.8
Texas	10.5	8.6	7.9	5.9	4.1	4.2	4.2	3.3	4.9	9.5	14.2	23.2	23.2	20.1
Utah	12.3	8.9	5.2	5.0	4.4	3.2	4.0	1.2	4.6	6.7	9.2	13.9	24.2	23.6
Vermont	5.5	7.9	7.1	7.2	2.1	1.8	2.0	4.6	2.4	5.6	5.0	21.6	37.8	32.4
Virginia	2.2	4.2	3.6	3.4	3.8	3.1	3.5	40.8	21.7	24.7	27.3	35.7	36.3	32.0
Washington	9.7	9.5	8.1	7.3	7.5	8.4	8.6	6.0	6.8	7.4	8.9	9.4	4.7	4.4
Washington, D.C.	6.4	10.8	9.4	6.1	6.1	4.6	4.7	13.3	0.0	5.6	0.0	11.1	9.1	0.0
West Virginia	17.1	15.4	8.3	6.5	4.5	5.7	5.7	0.0	0.0	3.1	9.0	14.6	10.3	7.3
Wisconsin	4.0	4.5	3.6	3.4	3.5	3.5	3.9	19.1	19.8	18.6	22.0	27.5	20.8	20.5
Wyoming	10.8	15.6	14.4	7.2	3.1	6.3	4.6	2.9	3.6	0.0	5.3	29.7	2.8	12.5
US	8.2	7.9	7.2	6.1	5.1	4.9	5.2	12.4	11.4	12.6	15.2	20.8	21.6	18.9

[a]Some facility data are not available from historical records.
SOURCE: Harrington et al., 2000b.

facilities for deficiencies that appeared to be a function of their high prevalence of seriously impaired residents rather than poor quality care (Abt Associates and CHSRA, 1996).

The failure of surveyors to reliably detect and cite quality problems has major implications. Quality problems will persist and residents will suffer in ways that could have been avoided if an effective survey program had detected problems and required their correction. Enforcement efforts may not be appropriately directed at the worst offenders, and some nonoffenders may erroneously be penalized (Johnson and Kramer, 1998). Survey information made available to the public may mislead consumers. Finally, facilities are not given adequate feedback about quality problems, which hampers facility-level efforts to improve care (Johnson and Kramer, 1998).

Strategies to Improve the Survey Process

Following the release of the GAO studies and the U.S. Senate Special Committee on Aging hearings on survey and enforcement activities in 1998 and 1999, DHHS responded by announcing a number of specific steps to improve the survey and monitoring process (HCFA, 1998a). HCFA regularly reports on these steps to the U.S. Senate Special Committee on Aging, and consumer groups are closely monitoring this process (e.g., the Center for Medicare Advocacy, the National Citizens' Coalition for Nursing Home Reform).[6] *The committee generally endorses HCFA's efforts to improve the current survey process.* The following section briefly reviews important areas in which efforts are being undertaken and identifies areas of potential further improvements.

Targeting Chronically Poor-Performing Facilities. In 1998, as a part of the President's initiative to ensure the health and safety of nursing home residents, federal and state regulators began to target a small list of about 100 nursing homes that had poor records of compliance with quality standards to ensure these facilities receive more frequent inspections. Targeting poor-performing facilities for more frequent surveys is consistent with OBRA 87. GAO (1998a) also recommended that HCFA target facilities with serious repeat deficiencies.

HCFA's approach to identifying poor-performing facilities is based solely on facilities with repeat violations that have caused serious harm. The approach could be improved by developing a more proactive, focused

---

[6]Additional information on this subject can be found at www.medicareadvocacy.org and www.nccnhr.org.

process. HCFA has statistical data that could be used to identify poor-performing facilities. These data include quarterly quality indicators (QIs) developed from the Minimum Data Set (MDS), described in Chapter 4, which identify individual residents with potential problems (such as weight loss and pressure sores) and those who have declined over time, indicating potentially poor quality of care. QIs can also be used to identify facilities with high percentages of residents that have negative QIs. HCFA also has data on staffing levels in facilities that show outliers with unusually low staffing per resident-day. Facilities with average staffing below a selected percentile—especially facilities with documented past problems—could be subjected to more frequent inspections because they are "at risk" of quality problems. The use of these types of statistical data could improve HCFA's ability to monitor facilities with potentially poor quality outcomes, without waiting for a facility to achieve two consecutive poor evaluations, each of which may cause actual harm or immediate jeopardy to residents. These proposals for more focused monitoring to target chronic poor performers do not require legislative action and generally have been accepted by government, consumer, and industry groups.

Another potentially high-risk situation that HCFA and state survey agencies should consider tracking and targeting for special surveys includes changes in key administrative and clinical staff. One recent report cited annual turnover rates of nursing home administrators at 30 percent (AHCA, 1998). Anecdotal reports reinforce the concern that leadership turnover is a problem. Logic also suggests that changes in leadership would increase instability and resident vulnerability in facilities, although there are no data to confirm this hypothesis.

Focusing on Poor-Performing Owners and Poor-Performing Chain Facilities. Although HCFA has identified some nursing home chains (multifacility organizations) that are delivering substandard care in multiple facilities, the current survey and enforcement procedures are primarily designed to survey and enforce standards in individual facilities. A multifacility chain is one that owns, leases, or operates more than one facility, according to the HCFA definition, and these account for more than half of the nation's nursing facilities (Harrington et al., 2000b). HCFA does not have an information system that accurately identifies ownership for use in monitoring performance of nursing home chains and targeting poor-performing chains.

Moreover states are required to conduct surveys whenever there is a change in ownership, but states are not always informed when there are new corporate owners. Regulations do not require the reporting of a change in ownership when a transfer of stock or the merger of another corporation into the provider corporation has occurred (42 C.F.R 489.18). However, HCFA (1998a) has announced steps in this direction by proposing to have the database of state survey results include major state enforcement actions (e.g., decertification) against individual and corporate owners of nursing homes. Although HCFA plans to target chains with bad records across states, it does not have a mechanism yet for taking enforcement actions against a chain even when a high percentage of the chain's facilities may be classified as substandard. *Improved data on ownership, changes in ownership and quality, and new survey and enforcement procedures would greatly enhance HCFA's ability to target and monitor poor-performing chains.*

Focusing on Resident Problems. After OBRA 87, state surveyors focused on physical and chemical restraints as important indicators of quality problems. However, they failed to identify serious problems of malnutrition, dehydration, undertreatment of pain, and pressure sores during the survey process (Johnson and Kramer, 1998). This situation occurred in part because surveyors were not trained to focus on these types of resident problems. HCFA now has revised its *State Operations Manual*, Appendix P (HCFA, 1999c), to add new investigative protocols on pressure sores, dehydration, malnutrition (unintended weight loss), and abuse prevention. These protocols should be valuable tools for surveyors to identify and evaluate problems and to standardize the survey process.

Improving Sampling Procedures and Sample Sizes. To focus adequately on serious resident problems, sampling techniques used for these surveys should be revised to target samples of higher-risk residents (including those who are newly admitted, bed-bound, or long-stay residents). GAO (1998a) specifically recommended that sampling procedures use electronic information becoming available from the MDS system on individual resident QIs to identify and sample records for "high-risk" residents. The QIs allow surveyors to detect serious potential resident problems such as malnutrition, dehydration, pressure sores, pain, and other conditions (Zimmerman, 1999). HCFA has asked surveyors to review the data for each facility and the QIs prior to conducting surveys, but the extent to which the QIs are being used by state surveyors is not known.

Another problem identified by GAO (1998a) was that the survey sample sizes were not large enough to detect problems of concern or to determine the scope of identified problems. Again, HCFA has instructed surveyors to take stratified samples to review enough residents to detect the prevalence of problems. Although HCFA has developed new instructions in Appendix P of its *State Operations Manual* (HCFA, 1999c) for sample size selection, the facility samples remain small (Kramer, 1999). (For a 100-bed facility, a total of 5 comprehensive resident reviews and 12 focused reviews are required.) *Sample sizes clearly have to be increased, and investigations of resident care problems have to be conducted to determine the full scope and severity of each serious problem.*

Reducing the Predictability of the Survey Process. When facilities are able to predict the timing of annual reviews and prepare accordingly, they can temporarily hide deficiencies in their usual performance and mask areas of poor-quality care. The problem of survey predictability was pointed out in the IOM 1986 report, and OBRA 87 attempted to address the problem by creating penalties for any individual that notified facilities about the time or date of a survey. In 1995, HCFA issued guidance to states to ensure that all surveys are unannounced but did not require that survey cycles be varied to reduce their predictability. The GAO (1999b) review of state survey activities identified the predictability of state surveys as a continuing problem and found that the timing of many surveys had not varied by more than a week for several cycles. HCFA (1998a) also reported that the surveys were highly predictable: almost all surveys were scheduled to begin on a Monday, and surveys were rarely conducted in the evening, at night, or on holidays. The main rationale for predictable schedules was to avoid overtime and have uninterrupted time on-site (HCFA, 1998a).

In 1998, HCFA took steps to make survey schedules less predictable and to increase the number of surveys conducted on weekends and nights (HCFA, 1998a). The new *State Operations Manual* (HCFA, 1999c, Section 7207) specifies that standard surveys must be unannounced and at least 10 percent of surveys must begin either on the weekend or evening or early morning hours. The month in which a survey begins should not coincide with the month of the previous survey. *The committee fully endorses actions by HCFA to make both the numbers of months between surveys and the days and hours on which surveys occur more variable, and supports further expanding the number of surveys that are conducted on evenings and weekends.*

Strengthening Consistency of Survey Determinations. As described earlier, states vary substantially in their survey and enforcement findings, and no evidence suggests that this variation is a function of corresponding variation in the quality of care provided in states. The implementation of OBRA 87 was only partly successful in improving protocols for assessing compliance, monitoring state survey agencies, and training and support for surveyors. HCFA has recognized that large differences in survey agency practices continue to exist. During the past two years, HCFA has increased its training activities of surveyors, training more than 600 federal and state surveyors to be trainers (HCFA, 1999a). Given the large number of surveyors nationally and the complexity of the survey system, more extensive, comprehensive federal training is needed to bring about consistency and competency in the survey process across states (Zimmerman, 1999). *The mandatory training of all federal and state surveyors should focus on survey techniques that will standardize the entire survey process, increase consistency across states, and enhance investigative and inferential decision capability.*

Some experts have argued that HCFA needs to substantially improve the survey process by making it more structured to reduce unwarranted variation (Kramer, 1999; Zimmerman, 1999). These researchers at the University of Wisconsin and the University of Colorado have a contract with HCFA to develop a more structured activity, with criteria and guidelines for determining compliance with the regulations.

Strengthening the Federal Oversight Role. GAO (1999e, p. 8) documented that HCFA's ten regional offices charged with the oversight of state survey agency performance have "limitations that prevent HCFA from developing accurate and reliable assessments." The use of comparative surveys (a federal survey completed within a few days of the state survey) is relatively minimal, even though this is inherently more accurate for oversight purposes than observational surveys of state agency staff, which are currently employed more frequently. GAO (1999e) also documented the uneven way in which regional offices monitor state agencies and the failure to hold states accountable for poor performance of their contracted survey duties.

HCFA (1999a,b) has responded with new guidelines to improve the regional office oversight of states. It has announced plans to review state performance, for example, by identifying states that report improbably high numbers of homes with no deficiencies. HCFA also proposed to take steps to correct lax enforcement processes, for example, through loss of funding and replacement of poor-performing state survey agencies. More intermediate sanctions may be necessary to ensure state compliance. HCFA, however, has not yet developed means of monitoring the performance of the regional offices in their oversight role.

Improving Complaint Investigations. In the past, HCFA survey procedures required states to investigate within two working days the most serious complaints that allege immediate jeopardy to the health and safety of residents. However, the time, scope, duration, and conduct of investigations of other types of complaints are determined by state survey agencies. GAO (1999c) found that states frequently understated the seriousness of the complaints (thus avoiding the requirement to investigate within two working days) and more generally failed to investigate serious complaints promptly. GAO (1999c, p. 3) also reviewed the nursing home complaint investigation process and found that "HCFA reporting systems for nursing homes' compliance history and complaint investigations do not collect timely, consistent, and complete information." In addition, some states used procedures or practices that may limit the filing of complaints (such as asking for written complaints). HCFA directions and oversight of complaint investigations were found to be minimal.

In response to the GAO (1999c) study, HCFA has agreed to undertake actions to improve the complaint investigation process and to establish a complaint category for allegations of "actual harm" and to investigate these complaints within ten working days. Complaints of immediate jeopardy are to be investigated within two working days. HCFA also agreed to strengthen the federal oversight of the state complaint investigation system and allow the regional offices to conduct verification surveys of complaint investigation. Also, the information system requiring states to enter all complaints into the On-Line Survey and Certification Assessment Reporting (OSCAR) System will be improved. HCFA has requested and the administration has proposed new funds for its nursing home initiative, including improvement of the survey system (White House, 2000). HCFA has also developed a contract to study the complaint investigation system and to improve the system. *The committee supports the importance placed by HCFA on improving the complaint investigation system. It is a key to protecting the health and safety of nursing home residents.*

Certifying the Accuracy of Nursing Home Data. Because surveys include reviews of residents' medical records, the accuracy of these records is essential to reliable and valid survey results. The GAO (1998a) report on quality problems in California nursing homes noted suspicious gaps in information and implausible entries in the sample of records it reviewed. A study of nursing home records on dietary intake found that nursing home staff often incorrectly record the amount of food consumed by residents (Kayser-Jones et al., 1997). Another study found that records on restraint use and removal were highly inaccurate (Schnelle et al., 1997). Nursing home staff have testified about requests or orders to falsify nursing home records (U.S. Senate Special Committee on Aging, 1998). Some errors undoubtedly arise from poor record keeping, which—although a problem in need of correction—is a lesser concern than deliberate falsification of records. In terms of the latter, at the present time no specific "severe" penalties exist for falsification of records or false reporting. *New penalties may be needed for deliberate falsification of medical records.*

Enforcement of Standards

The goal of the enforcement process under OBRA 87 was to achieve sustained facility compliance with federal requirements of quality care.

Prior to this legislation, the only sanction available was decertification, a penalty with such serious consequences for residents of a sanctioned facility that regulators were reluctant to apply it. The revised enforcement system was intended to give surveyors more flexibility in fitting remedies to the seriousness of deficiencies and to make the actual imposition of intermediate sanctions more likely.

The sanctioning authority under OBRA 87 allowed the imposition of civil money penalties, denial of payment for new admissions, temporary management, immediate termination, and other remedies or sanctions. The law required that all states enact the list of "intermediate sanctions" (sanctions other than decertification) and that they be imposed for violations of residents' welfare and rights as well as for health and safety violations. The statute required that mandatory remedies be imposed for repeated or uncorrected deficiencies and that the enforcement actions minimize the time between the identification of violations and the imposition of remedies. The law allowed all sanctions other than civil money penalties to be imposed before the administrative appeals were decided and barred HCFA from playing a consultative rather than an enforcement role.

The final enforcement rules were published in the Federal Register on November 10, 1994 (59 Fed. Reg. 56,116), and became effective on July 1, 1995 (HCFA, 1995b). In establishing the enforcement rules, HCFA was prescriptive in its rating system for the scope and severity[7] of violations and in terms of the intermediate remedies that should and could be applied. Beginning in July 1995, state surveyors were required to rate all violations based on their scope and severity, and then to link sanctions to the scope and severity of the violation identified (HCFA, 1995b). Deficiencies were to be given for problems that had resulted in or could result in a negative impact on the health, safety, welfare, or rights of residents. To guide states, HCFA established a graded system for classifying deficiencies and penalties by severity and scope. As shown in Table 5.2, each deficiency is rated in one of 12 categories labeled "A" through "L" depending on the severity and scope. Facilities that do not have deficiencies exceeding the first three category levels (A–C) are considered to be in "substantial compliance" with the regulations and they are not subject to sanctions, although they are expected to correct their deficiencies. Those with deficiencies in categories higher than C are "not in substantial compliance" and are subject to intermediate sanctions or termination from the program, depending on the scope and severity of the problem.

---

[7]HCFA uses severity to refer to the effect of a deficiency on resident outcomes; scope describes the number of residents potentially or actually affected (HCFA, 1999c).

TABLE 5.2. Level of Deficiencies, Based on Scope and Severity of Substandard Care, and the Remedy Categories Available to States for Each Level of Deficiency

Severity of Deficiency	Scope of Deficiency		
	Isolated	Pattern	Widespread
Immediate jeopardy to resident health or safety	**Level J** Required remedy category: 3 Optional remedy category: 1 or 2	**Level K** Required remedy category: 3 Optional remedy category: 1 or 2	**Level L** Required remedy category: 3 Optional remedy category: 1 or 2
Actual harm that is not immediate jeopardy	**Level G** Required remedy category: 2 Optional remedy category: 1	**Level H** Required remedy category: 2 Optional remedy category: 1	**Level I** Required remedy category: 2 Optional remedy category: 1 or temporary management
No actual harm, with potential for more than minimal harm, but not immediate jeopardy	**Level D** Required remedy category: 1 Optional remedy category: 2	**Level E** Required remedy category: 1 Optional remedy category: 2	**Level F** Required remedy category: 2 Optional remedy categories: 1
No actual harm with potential for minimal harm	**Level A**[a] Required remedy category: none	**Level B** Required remedy category: none	**Level C** Required remedy category: none

[a]All facilities receiving deficiencies are required to submit a plan of correction except for those with level A deficiencies only.

Remedy Categories:
Category 1:
- directed plan of correction,
- state monitor, and/or
- directed in-service training.

Category 2:
- denial of payment for new admissions,
- denial of payment for all individuals imposed by HCFA, and/or
- civil money penalties of $50–$3,000 per day or $1,000–$10,000 per instance.

Category 3:
- temporary management,
- termination of certification, and/or
- optional: civil money penalties of $3,050–$10,000 per day or $1,000–$10,000 per instance.

SOURCE: HCFA, 1999c.

Under HCFA guidelines, however, most facilities are given a grace period, usually 30 to 60 days, to correct deficiencies. The exceptions are for facilities with deficiencies in the highest severity categories (level J through L) that cause immediate jeopardy and for those that cause harm with severe repeat deficiencies. Facilities that cause immediate jeopardy are not given the opportunity to correct deficiencies before sanctions are imposed, whereas facilities with less serious deficiencies generally are given the opportunity to correct them. Regulations also require a notice period before the sanction can take effect. Remedies recommended by states must be sent to HCFA regional offices, and a 15–20 day notice for the facility to come into compliance must be issued (HCFA, 1999c). In cases of immediate jeopardy, the sanction can be put into effect after a two-day notice.[8] Civil money penalties can be assessed retroactively for noncompliance that occurred between surveys.

In addition, "substandard quality of care" is defined as one or more deficiencies that constitute either immediate jeopardy (of any scope), actual harm, or at a level of no actual harm but with a potential for more than minimum harm. For the latter two categories the scope of the harm must be a "pattern" or be "widespread." Substandard quality of care in these scope and severity levels is limited to deficiencies in the regulatory requirements under resident behavior and facility practices, quality of life, or quality of care (HCFA, 1999c). Facilities receiving a determination of substandard quality of care are subject to loss of their authority to conduct nursing aide training, which consequently may make the hiring of nursing aides difficult. In addition, the facility is subject to all of the above sanctions relevant to the scope and severity of the deficiency.

Enforcement Trends and Variability

Review of deficiency ratings over a three-year period show that few deficiencies (0.6 percent in 1998) were classified as causing immediate jeopardy (in the highest categories for scope and severity). Figure 5.2 shows that the percentage of deficiencies designated as having a minor or minimal impact declined over the period while the percentage of total deficiencies classified as having the potential for actual harm in isolated situations (level D) increased from 30.2 to 41.1 over the three year period, but levels E and L remained about the same. The percentage of deficiencies that were considered to have caused actual harm in isolated situations (level G) increased somewhat over the three years, but all other categories appeared to be about the same (Harrington and Carrillo, 1999;

---

[8]The new guidelines give states opportunity to impose some remedies directly.

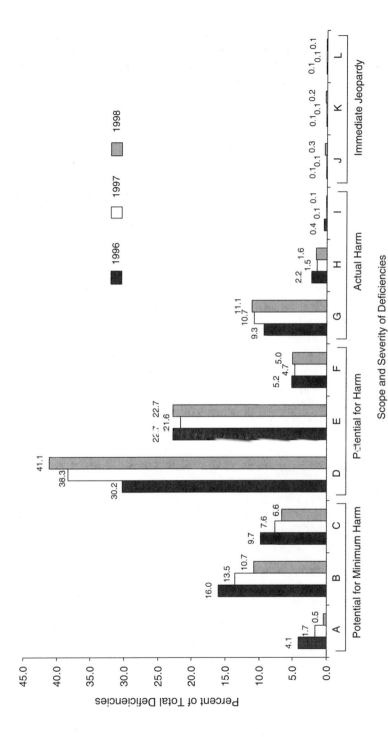

FIGURE 5.2 Surveyor evaluations of the scope and severity of deficiencies, as a percentage of total deficiencies, cited in all nursing facilities: United States, 1996 ($N = 79,925$), 1997 ($N = 76,291$), and 1998 ($N = 79,895$).
SOURCE: Harrington and Carillo, 2000.

Harrington et al., 2000b). Only a few facilities are being given deficiencies for immediate jeopardy at the level J or higher (about 0.6 percent of facilities) where sanctions would be imposed without the opportunity to make corrections.

Continuing Weaknesses in Enforcement of Standards

The U.S. Senate Special Committee on Aging (1998, 1999), GAO (1998a, 1999b,c,e), and HCFA (1998a) have identified a number of continuing problems with the enforcement of nursing home standards. The federal goals to achieve both compliance and continued compliance with federal standards have yet to be fully met. For instance, GAO (1999b) examined the enforcement of federal nursing home regulations and concluded that although HCFA has taken steps to improve the oversight of nursing homes, it is unable to ensure that nursing homes *maintain* compliance with federal health care standards. According to GAO, more than one-fourth of the facilities had deficiencies that caused actual harm to residents or placed them at risk of death or serious injury and many others had serious deficiencies.

GAO (1998a) reported that once the state survey agency identified deficiencies in the quality of care, it was ineffective in achieving the remedial state of consistent compliance with the law. Nearly 10 percent of California nursing homes serving thousands of residents were cited twice in a row for "actual harm" violations, strongly suggesting that these homes were not correcting problems identified by surveyors. California took relatively few disciplinary actions against facilities cited for repeated "actual harm" violations. Between 1995 and 1998, nearly three-quarters of the 122 facilities in California cited for serious deficiencies in at least two consecutive years never had federal intermediate sanctions take effect (GAO, 1998a). GAO (1998a) also found that over the course of two standard surveys conducted between 1995 and 1998, one-third of the nursing homes (407 out of 1,370) had serious violations that caused death, seriously jeopardized residents' health and safety, or were considered to be substandard.

Strategies to Improve the Enforcement Process

Reflecting recommendations from consumer groups, GAO, and others, HCFA has taken a number of steps to correct identified problems in the enforcement of federal nursing home standards.

Definitions of Facility Problems. Until recently HCFA's definition of poor-performing facilities applied to relatively few facilities. A facility had to be cited on its current survey and on one of its two previous standard surveys for substandard quality of care. HCFA now has expanded the definition to include facilities cited for isolated cases of actual harm in two or more surveys (HCFA, 1999c). Facilities are allowed to correct deficiencies, and sanctions are optional if only one such deficiency has occurred.

In addition, HCFA's definition of what constitutes a widespread deficiency has been limited and needs revision. "Widespread" was considered to take in situations where all or nearly all of a home's residents were affected by a problem, including those for whom the deficiency could not have occurred (e.g., those who were continent could not be characterized as lacking a plan for achieving continence) (Edelman, 1997). In a facility where most of the residents on a nursing care unit were negatively affected by poor care, the deficiencies would not be considered widespread, but rather would be classified as a pattern. This has the effect of limiting the ability to assess sanctions in situations where they may be indicated.

Elimination of the Grace Period Before Sanctions Are Imposed. HCFA (1998a) has recently issued a memorandum to the states phasing out the grace period that allowed time for facilities to achieve compliance with regulations before penalties were applied. Apparently at odds with OBRA 87 mandates, HCFA's 1995 enforcement regulations established a grace period, which allowed facilities with deficiencies to make corrections before being subject to intermediate sanctions (Edelman, 1998a–c). GAO (1998a) reported that grace periods were granted to 98 percent of facilities in California and to 99 percent of facilities nationwide. These grace periods often allowed 30–45 days before a penalty could be applied. Only facilities whose deficiencies posed immediate jeopardy to residents' health or welfare or those that were defined as poor performers were denied the opportunity to correct deficiencies before remedies were imposed. The revised HCFA *State Operations Manual* (HCFA 1999c, p. 7–27) states that facilities will not be given an opportunity to correct before remedies are imposed (1) when they have deficiencies of actual harm (at level G) or a more serious level on the current survey *and* on the previous survey; (2) when they received a per-instance civil money penalty; (3) when the deficiencies were for immediate jeopardy; or (4) when the facility had previously been terminated. Except in these instances, the opportunity to correct without sanctions remains unless a state chooses to establish additional criteria. *The committee urges HCFA to accelerate the schedule for phasing out the grace period.*

Revisiting All Facilities Before Sanctions Are Lifted. In principle, sanctions are supposed to remain in place until a facility corrects the deficiencies and a revisit has been completed. Until recently, HCFA did not require on-site revisits of facilities found to have deficiencies that did not cause serious harm or substandard care. Instead, these facilities were allowed to self-certify when they came into compliance (GAO, 1998a). As a result, only about 15 percent of facilities were subject to revisits, even though some of these facilities had repeatedly been designated as poor performers and as providers of substandard care.

Following the GAO (1998a) study, HCFA adopted a policy that all problem facilities with recurring serious violations should receive an on-site visit before a state was considered to be in compliance with the regulations. The HCFA *State Operations Manual* (1999c) has been revised to indicate that facilities with deficiencies causing actual harm or more must have an on-site revisit of the facility. This policy is a substantial improvement over the previous one.

Limiting the Use of Civil Money Penalties. In 1996, HCFA issued guidelines that urged states to limit the imposition of civil money penalties (CMPs) to situations of immediate jeopardy to the health and welfare of residents or uncorrected deficiencies at the time of a revisit of a poor-performing facility (Edelman, 1998a–c). This policy contradicted the intent of OBRA 87 for intermediate remedy provisions and the HCFA regulations. HCFA now has lifted the moratorium on the collection of certain civil money penalties but still limits CMPs to serious deficiencies which HCFA defines as levels G, H, and I, or as "substandard care." The penalty may be assigned retroactively for the number of days out of compliance since the last standard survey. The manual made clear that CMPs may be issued for up to $10,000 per day or per instance when a deficiency constitutes immediate jeopardy or involves actual harm.

Federal Procedures Create Lengthy Delays. Although the law says that all remedies other than civil money penalties can be imposed immediately pending an appeal, the notice of sanctions and the federal appeals process can result in lengthy delays in implementation of CMPs. The sanctions and civil monetary penalty system is seriously hampered by a backlog of administrative appeals that can last for several years and CMPs cannot be collected until the appeal is resolved (GAO, 1999b). The appeals may take two to five years and the weight of the administrative backlog has approached gridlock. The administration has requested additional funds from Congress to increase the number of hearing officers for appeals to speed the process, which appears to be needed. Even with more funds, the process set forth in the HCFA *State Operations Manual* (1999c) appears unnecessarily cumbersome and time-consuming. More work is needed to streamline the enforcement process.

Access to Information About Enforcement Actions Against Facilities. In response to requests by advocacy organizations, HCFA agreed to make deficiency reports, including the scope and severity of deficiencies and other information about individual facilities, available on the Internet in 1998. HCFA has established this information about nursing homes on its Web site at www.hcfa.gov/Medicare/NHCompare. This is an important first step toward making information more accessible to the public. The committee hopes that this information will be expanded and improved as experience is gained to include all sanctions, remedies, and appeal decisions.

Stricter Provisions for Decertification and Minimum Time Periods for Recertification of Terminated Facilities. One important additional step is to target facilities that move in and out of compliance ("yo-yo" facilities). As the IOM committee reported in 1986, many facilities have had repeated violations that have caused serious harm and injury to residents and these facilities generally have escaped the imposition of any sanctions because they were repeatedly allowed to correct the violations. This problem has not gone away, as documented by GAO (1998a). In addition, terminated facilities can fairly easily gain recertification without a specific waiting period. For example, of the 16 facilities terminated in California between 1995 and 1998, 14 were reinstated and 11 were reinstated under the same ownership as before the termination. Of the 14 reinstated homes, 6 were cited for new, serious violations (GAO, 1998a).

HCFA has explained that termination from the Medicare and Medicaid programs is an option when there is a condition of immediate jeopardy or when there is a history of noncompliance and other remedies have failed to bring about compliance (HCFA, 1999c). Facilities that are decertified can immediately reapply for certification and must be admitted back into the program if they meet the compliance requirements. Facilities are required to pass two surveys within a one- to six-month period verifying that the reason for termination no longer exists and that the provider has maintained continued compliance. HCFA termination procedures have not been effective in eliminating those facilities that are chronic poor performers from the program. In December 1999, HCFA changed the rules about readmitting facilities that are terminated. It now requires a "reasonable assurance" process for facilities terminated from Medicare (Transmittal 13, § 7321, pp 7–43).

Temporary Management. Despite provisions in OBRA 87, for a wide range of sanctions, states still find it difficult to apply temporary management to persistent serious offenders. Use of temporary management would avoid decertification, which results in relocations causing distress to residents and families. Temporary management or receivership is a serious alternative sanction against a poor-performing provider, but it is less disruptive than decertification. Yet few temporary managers have been imposed (HCFA, 1998a), and it is not clear why. HCFA should consider studying the barriers to using these procedures and streamlining its procedures so that they could be more quickly and easily applied in appropriate circumstances.

Informal Dispute Resolution Process. In 1995, HCFA adopted an informal dispute resolution process that allowed nursing facilities to challenge the imposition of deficiencies in a process separate from the formal appeals process (HCFA, 1999c). This process was not mandated by OBRA 87 and was opposed by consumer advocates as a method of delaying the imposition of intermediate sanctions. The process may be a significant factor in the decline in deficiency citations and associated sanctions, and it may also be adding to state agency costs. On the other hand, the process may be resolving misunderstandings and reducing the number of formal appeals. *HCFA has not evaluated the informal dispute resolution process, but such an evaluation should be conducted.*

Recommendations for Nursing Home Assessment and Enforcement

The above discussion of federal and state enforcement of nursing home regulations in this chapter has identified problems with both the identification of quality care and the enforcement of compliance with quality standards. The committee also reviewed and made suggestions throughout the discussion for needed improvements in the various federal and state survey and enforcement activities. HCFA's recent initiatives are welcome and should be sustained and expanded. The following recommendation provides major directions for continued improvement of the assessment and enforcement of regulatory quality standards:

Recommendation 5.1: The committee recommends that:

- **Federal and state survey efforts focus more on providers that are chronically poor performers by surveying them more frequently than required for other facilities, increasing penalties for repeated violations of standards, and decertifying persistently substandard providers;**
- **HCFA's monitoring in all areas of state survey and sanction activities be improved by ensuring greater uniformity in state surveyor interpretation and application of survey regulations, and be reinforced by assistance and sanctions as necessary to improve performance; and**

- An analysis be commissioned to examine if increased funding is needed to HCFA to improve the state survey and certification processes for nursing homes.

RESIDENTIAL CARE FACILITIES

Standards for Residential Care

The regulation of residential care occurs primarily at the state level. The federal regulation directly affecting residential care is the 1976 Keys amendment to the Social Security Act. This law was passed to protect Supplemental Security Income (SSI) recipients from substandard board and care homes. States are required to certify that all facilities in which significant numbers of SSI residents reside meet appropriate quality standards. In general, the states have broad discretion in carrying out this oversight. The state role includes licensing and monitoring compliance with health and safety regulations, such as building codes, food handling, medication storage and distribution, and staffing requirements. A GAO (1999a) study found that oversight by HCFA was limited and that states rarely sanctioned facilities for providing substandard care.

Medicaid is increasingly paying for residential care under its 1915(c) home and community-based service (HCBS) waiver program (Harrington et al., 2000f). It relies on each state to design and administer its own program. The Medicaid HCBS waiver program requires states to provide assurances that necessary safeguards have been taken to protect the health and safety of beneficiaries receiving long-term care—including residential services (other than room and board)—under the waiver. States vary in their regulation of the range of services covered by the Medicaid waiver program, and little is known about the specific nature or effectiveness of their efforts (Harrington et al., 2000d). The committee is seriously concerned about the lack of descriptive information and assessments of current state regulatory activities. A systematic approach to collecting and monitoring all aspects of state regulatory activities for residential care should be developed.

State Variability in Standards and Enforcement for Residential Care

Residential care arrangements have filled an important need in the continuum of care for long-term care. State standards for these care arrangements including assisted living facilities, a relatively recent subset of residential care, are highly variable (Mollica, 1998; Hawes et al., 1999). As described in Chapter 2, this variability begins with the very definition of the kinds of settings subject to particular regulations and extends to such matters as who can be served (admission and discharge criteria), what services can be provided, what staff are required, and how personal and social living spaces must be configured.

The complexity of the situation facing state regulators is illustrated by the fact that there are numerous levels and types of residential care including group homes, foster homes, assisted living facilities, residential care facilities, mental health facilities, mental retardation facilities, personal care homes, supportive living facilities, and habilitation facilities. Moreover, they are called by more than 25 different names with multiple categories and titles within states (Lewin/ICF and James Bell Associates, 1990; Hawes et al., 1993).

The lack of uniformity in names of programs is repeated in state regulatory standards for different types of facilities. A 1995 study of adult foster care, for example, found that just half of the 26 states with adult foster care required licensing by a state health licensing agency, and that public funds were used to pay for services for half or more of residents in 18 states (Blanchette, 1996).

State licensing survey activities are sometimes divided among agencies or divisions. For example, mental health programs may survey residential care for people with severe mental illness, developmental disability programs may survey facilities for people with mental retardation, and still other agencies may survey facilities serving primarily elderly people. Hawes and colleagues (1993) documented that there were 62 agencies in 50 states and the District of Columbia that license homes serving a predominantly elderly population. Many additional agencies license facilities serving residents with psychiatric illnesses or mental retardation and developmental disabilities, and some states require accreditation (Hawes et al., 1993). Other states license homes that provide treatment for those with serious mental illness and substance abuse problems.

In addition to conventional regulation by licensure, some state care management programs have public agencies operating more as contractors than as regulators. These programs may operate under Medicaid HCBS waiver provisions, which allow them to place individuals in residential care settings for certain services. In their oversight role, case managers review these settings for placement, and for removal of residents whose needs are not being met. Few studies, if any, have been conducted to evaluate state oversight of residential care settings through these types of case management mechanisms.

Concerns about the widespread belief that the current board and care homes have many inadequacies and are responsible for an increasingly frail population led the AARP, in 1990, to contract with the Research Triangle Institute to conduct a national study of state board and care regulations (Hawes, et al., 1993). Data were collected from state regulatory and funding agencies, and local ombudsman care management agencies involved in the provision of board and care. Some of the key findings place board and care homes in perspective. State agencies identified a total of 31,942 licensed homes that met the study criteria of serving a primarily elderly population and of being subject to licensing requirements. States varied from about 24 to more than 4,000 homes. The survey found that most states did little either to identify unlicensed homes or to require unlicensed homes to become licensed.

State inspection processes are fairly similar—most states inspect facilities once a year—however, enforcement actions are quite limited and generally only in the form of corrective action plans. Thirty-seven agencies had the authority to issue provisional licenses, usually as a sanction against homes with deficiencies, but only 17 reported using that authority three or more times in the year preceding the interviews. Fines and other more severe forms of sanctions, even when authorized, were seldom imposed (Hawes et al., 1993).

Such variations in state policies reflect different perceptions about whether congregate residential care is primarily a medical service or primarily a housing arrangement intended to allow people to age in place in a noninstitutional setting that is meant to emphasize autonomy and privacy. Unresolved questions remain about the acceptable role and extent of regulatory standards in residential care settings.

Weaknesses in State Regulation of Residential Care

Very little has been done to evaluate the effectiveness of current policy and regulatory practices in residential care. The few studies undertaken have raised serious questions about the effectiveness of state regulation and licensure promoting quality in residential care. As stated earlier, Hawes and colleagues (1993) found that state regulation and enforcement of standards were weak. Sanctions were used infrequently. Most states did not have the authority to ban admissions, and when they did have the authority, it was rarely used.

A GAO (1997a) study of assisted living reported problems with many facility contracts with residents, usually called admission contracts. Under these contracts, residents generally agree to limit the facility's potential liability for specific risks that the resident assumes, such as a fall when climbing stairs. However, the GAO (1997a) report stated that "a recent limited study of industry practices noted that contracts had no standard format, varied in detail and usefulness, and in some cases were vague and confusing" (p. 6). GAO's conclusion was based on findings reported by the American Bar Association and by Consumer Reports. "For example, none of the contracts examined mentioned how often services would be provided; a number of contracts stated only that services would be provided as the facility deemed appropriate. Furthermore, few specified what would happen when the resident's health declined, such as what needed additional services would be provided, whether there are additional charges for those services, or whether the resident would be asked to leave because needed services could not be furnished" (p. 6). GAO further stated "that little is known about the accuracy and adequacy of information furnished to individuals and their families. As a result, consumers may be at risk if they lack the necessary information to make informed decisions" (p. 6). A GAO study (1999a) of four states found that assisted living facilities were not routinely providing prospective residents with information on services, costs, and policies that were sufficient to make informed selections about facilities.

Some believe that residents have unequal bargaining power with facilities and that written contracts may place residents at risk of exploitation. Others argue that consumers may have cognitive problems that limit their ability to be fully informed in signing contracts for services. Contracts offered by facilities should be understandable to the layperson and generally specify the facility's responsibility to the resident, how the facility will respond to resident needs and changes in health status, how quality care will be maintained, and how the resident's rights will be protected.

The same GAO (1999a) study of four states found that assisted living facilities showed wide variation in state standards and the procedures for surveying facilities, which ranged from annual to biennial inspections. It also found that the results of state licensing and monitoring activities on quality of care and consumer protection varied. More than 25 percent of facilities were cited by state licensing or other agencies for five or more quality-of-care or consumer protection related deficiencies during 1996 and 1997, and 11 percent had ten or more deficiencies. State agencies also respond to complaints by conducting investigations of the facilities. Some of the problems cited were facilities (1) providing inadequate or insufficient care to residents; (2) having insufficient, unqualified, and untrained staff; (3) not providing appropriate medications; and (4) not following state admission and discharge procedures (GAO, 1997a).

Recommendation 5.2: The committee recommends that state agencies working with the private sector develop programs to disseminate information to consumers on (a) the various types of long-term care settings available to them, and (b) where applicable, information on the compliance of individual long-term care providers with relevant state standards.

Directions for Standard Setting for Residential Care

Based on the studies cited above, the need to focus attention on weak government oversight of these types of long-term care settings seems clear (Hawes et al., 1993, 1999; GAO, 1997a, 1999a). This attention provides an opportunity for federal and state governments to devise and evaluate appropriately balanced new approaches. Although residential care settings pose quality concerns, some committee members believe that consumers are choosing residential care over nursing homes because of quality-of-life issues and the greater flexibility these facilities provide to residents.

Little study of state enforcement actions has occurred and variation across states is enormous. If survey and monitoring are not combined with an effective enforcement process, then the impact of standards for residential care will continue to be limited. The committee believes that research examining the effectiveness of state survey and enforcement activities for residential care especially in terms of quality of care, quality of life, staffing and other related measures should be given high priority. Although not all committee members are in agreement on the specifics, there is general agreement that at this time regulatory mechanisms for residential care do not need to mirror the extensive federal regulatory system that is in place for nursing homes.

Recommendation 5.3: The committee recommends that all states have appropriate standard-setting and oversight mechanisms for all types of settings where people receive personal care and nursing services. The committee recognizes that before this recommendation can be implemented, research examining the effectiveness of state survey and enforcement activities for residential care must be undertaken.

Any oversight mechanism should recognize that one of the strongest preferences of most people with functional limitations is to avoid disruption in their living arrangements. For example, some argue that standards for assisted living should allow for admission or continuation of residents as if they were receiving similar services in their own homes. That is, regulations should not bar the admission, nor require the discharge, of people needing skilled nursing care as long as the care is of the sort that home health care agencies provide in personal homes. Others argue that regulations should guarantee that residents' health and safety is protected in these settings, and that when such health and safety protection cannot be ensured, residents and their families should be informed and alternative living arrangements should be made (Kane and Wilson, 1993). Still others recommend that there should be at least some minimum regulation of medication storage and administration in board and care homes because many of the residents are elderly, frail, and vulnerable (Garrad et al., 1997). They also recommend a specific minimum level of training for staff who set up and/or administer medications. Some states have allowed nurses to delegate nursing services to unlicensed personnel in residential care and consider that this approach can be safe and effective (Kane et al., 1995).

In general, the committee believes that state regulatory standards should include a requirement for a care or service plan based on an assessment of each resident's needs and preferences, and a means of monitoring the plan's application; a process for identifying medical problems and health changes and securing appropriate medical attention; and an expectation that there will be appropriately trained staff on duty and awake 24 hours a day, seven days a week. Minimum protections for fire and life safety, for example, are also necessary. These requirements should be standardized across facilities and states.

One important concern is comprehensible definitions of the boundaries of the various kinds of residential settings and services within a state. Such definitions will help people needing long-term care and their families understand their options and choose among them. For example, state regulations should distinguish between assisted living arrangements and smaller group home arrangements that typically serve fewer residents. Although policy makers need to establish clear boundaries and definitions distinguishing particular types of facilities or services, their decisions at times may come into conflict with preferences of patients, advocates, and families for smoother, less constrained transitions, from one level of dependency, and the associated service requirements, to another.

Because the public and policy makers are searching for an adequate understanding of the range of residential care options and appropriate boundaries for these options, they would benefit from more systematic information about state experiences with different care options and with different regulatory strategies and labels. Standard definitions and boundaries across states need to be developed in order to collect national systematic and comprehensive data on residential care settings, their characteristics, staffing, and care provided. A reasonable start toward the development of standards and definitions for some elements of residential long-term care has been made by the Assisted Living Quality Coalition (ALQC, 1998). The coalition has engaged in consensus building among representatives of consumers, providers, regulators, purchasers, and financiers of long-term care. Recently it set forth a framework for quality in assisted living that included a key role for basic regulatory standards as well as an emphasis on innovation, collaboration, and quality improvement structures (ALQC, 1998). The group agreed on the need for minimum standards related to care processes associated with desired resident outcomes and proposed that such standards should:

- define the service being offered and the practice processes and structural capacities necessary to operate;
- establish minimally acceptable practice guidelines; and
- provide the basis for corrective action when problems arise.

Although the coalition as a group did not endorse a set of basic standards, it reached a degree of consensus, except for disagreement in two significant areas: a requirement for private rooms and consumer options for pursuing judicial enforcement of perceived noncompliance with standards. Despite these two areas of disagreement, the coalition report included an appendix of guidelines for states developing standards (ALQC, 1998, p. 30).

HOME HEALTH AGENCIES

Standards for Home Health Care Agencies

Each area of long-term care presents different surveying and monitoring challenges. For home health agencies, a particular challenge arises from the lack of a facility setting in which staff and patients or residents are congregated and, thereby, more easily observed or interviewed. Services are dispersed across millions of "settings of care" (personal homes and congregate residences). Monitoring quality in home health care is complicated by the number of agencies involved, the growth of agency branch offices (nearly 5,000 in 1997 compared to just under 1,250 in 1993 [GAO, 1997b]), the reliance of agencies on contract and part-time personnel, the difficulty of making site visits to patient homes, and reductions in funding for state survey and certification activities.

As GAO (1997b, 1998b) pointed out, by 1996 the program was growing so fast that HCFA was attempting to certify about 100 new home health agencies per month. This growth in agencies actually reversed when HCFA placed a moratorium from September 1997 to January 1998 on the admission of new agencies into the Medicare program until new requirements could be implemented. More importantly, new Medicare payment rules have made the home health sector less financially attractive. According to HCFA, the number of agencies has dropped by about 1,000 since October 1997 (DeParle, 1999).

The federal government sets the requirements for home health agencies to participate in the Medicare and Medicaid programs, and most states use these requirements as the basis for regulating agencies for their state Medicaid programs. States administer certification and licensure programs that include inspections with sanctions such as fines, suspension of payments for care, and decertification from participation in Medicare and Medicaid. Officials also may respond to resident and other complaints about substandard care.

The federal government's concern about home health care has often been less focused on quality per se than on the escalating use and cost to Medicare of home health services. The expansion of the Medicare home health benefit as a result of judicial decisions (especially *Dugan v. Bowen*, 1989) contributed to an explosion in Medicare home health use and costs. The government has taken steps to rein in costs by tightening eligibility determinations, intensifying investigations of fraud and abuse, and revamping the system of paying for home health services. The payment changes are reviewed in Chapter 8.

As defined by OBRA 87, Medicare requirements of participation for home health agencies cover structure and process of care, administration, and required service capacities including home health aide services and physical therapy. Currently, standards are composed of 12 component areas including patient rights, acceptance of patients, plans of care, skilled nursing services, and clinical records. Most requirements are further subdivided into specific standards. For skilled nursing services provided by home health agencies, the 15 standards are divided into those that cover registered nurses and those that cover licensed practical nurses.

The survey guidelines for home health agencies require an initial or standard survey to assess whether the home health agency has the capacity to deliver services that meet minimum standards. Once an agency passes its initial survey, it should be recertified every 12 to 26 months following the same survey process, with the frequency varying depending on the results of prior surveys. Complaints can also trigger surveys.

Medicare standards of participation for home health agencies do not require that an agency provide all or even most of its services directly, and an agency can contract with noncertified agencies to provide services, including skilled nursing care. GAO has suggested that "excessive contracting may be an indication that [an agency] is exceeding its capacity to effectively care for its patients" (GAO, 1997b, p. 7).

Until recently, agencies could be certified before they had actually provided care to a sufficient number of patients to establish some kind of performance record. In 1998, HCFA required, as proposed by GAO, that agencies must have provided "quality" care to at least ten patients before being allowed to provide care to Medicare patients, and at least seven patients must be receiving active care at the time an agency seeks certification (HCFA, 1999b). Most states have additional requirements for licensure beyond Medicare–Medicaid certification, but at least ten states have no independent provisions for licensing home care agencies (Harrington et al., 2000e).

Improvements in Home Health Agency Standards

In 1997, HCFA proposed the first broad revisions in the home health agency requirements for participation since OBRA 87. One objective was to make requirements more "patient centered" and "outcomes oriented." Another objective was to encourage agencies to undertake internal quality improvement. Structure and process requirements were to be clearly related to achieving good, and avoiding bad, patient outcomes.

HCFA now requires the use of a uniform assessment instrument (the Outcome and Assessment Information Set [OASIS]) for Medicare home health beneficiaries for agencies to participate in Medicare. Rules for home health agency use of this instrument were issued in January 1999 and have since been revised, in part to respond to increasing industry consolidation and concerns about consumer privacy. The assessment instruments should be accompanied by specific guidelines for care planning and service provision. *The committee supports HCFA's efforts to make home health regulations focus on the processes and outcomes of care. It also supports research on care processes and outcomes and the development of practice guidelines to guide and improve home health care.*

Deemed Status

In addition to certification based on state surveys, federal law provides that home health agencies may meet Medicare participation requirements by receiving accreditation from either of two private organizations, the Joint Commission on Accreditation of Healthcare Organizations (JCAHO) or the Community Health Accreditation Program of the National League for Nursing. To qualify an accrediting organization for deemed status, HCFA has to compare the organization's standards and survey processes with those specified for Medicare; assess the organization's survey process, personnel, and resources; evaluate the process for monitoring agencies found out of compliance; and assess the adequacy for oversight and validation purposes of the organization's data reporting capacities. Recent analysis is not available on whether the deemed status approach is effective in ensuring quality care.

Weaknesses in Regulation of Home Health Agencies

Licensing and regulation of home health providers—other than Medicare- or Medicaid-certified providers—is uneven across states. For example, some states rely on federal home health care standards, whereas others have adopted additional state regulations for agencies not seeking federal certification. One result is that gaps exist in information about the number and kinds of entities that are providing home-based health care. Even less information is available about the adequacy and appropriateness of the services provided.

GAO has been critical of HCFA's oversight of the Medicare home health benefit, particularly for lax fiscal oversight (e.g., see GAO, 1995, 1996a, 1997b, and 1998c). Some criticism has focused on problems in the survey and enforcement process that may affect the quality of patient care. One strong criticism was that the threat of termination from Medicare had little if any deterrent effect and that problem agencies continue to operate with impunity (GAO, 1997b). Similarly, when enforcement actions are not taken, it can encourage more disregard for public regulatory standards (Edelman, 1998a).

A GAO report (1997b) has criticized the initial certification process and the recertification process, both of which are meant to assess home health agency capacity to provide quality health services. The report stated that the certification process for home health agencies is easy— "probably too easy" (GAO, 1997b, p. 2). Initial surveys cover only 5 or 12 Medicare requirements for participation, which means surveyors cannot determine whether all standards are being met. Moreover, surveyors did not always conduct home visits to patients and therefore had no way of assessing whether care was being properly delivered. In addition, the number of patients that surveyors are required to survey is too small to adequately determine whether the agency is meeting standards.

GAO (1997b) also found that some agencies had never delivered services for which they sought certification under current HCFA procedures. Moreover, in numerous instances, home health agencies were certified without meeting minimum standards. In addition, GAO (1997b) found that agencies can continue as Medicare providers even if they have multiple deficiencies as long as they have an approved plan of correction. The same yo-yo pattern described earlier for nursing homes also characterizes home health agencies.

Under current HCFA procedures, once a home health agency is found to be jeopardizing patient health and safety and the violations are considered to be immediate and serious, the agency can be placed on an accelerated timetable for termination. However the agency is allowed to take corrective action or to establish a plan for correction, so that those with many substandard conditions can continue in the program. During the period 1994–1996, terminations initiated by HCFA affected only about 0.1 to 0.3 percent of the total number of agencies (GAO, 1997b).

As with most programs dependent on public funds, a problem with the survey process for home health regulations relates to budget constraints. Some states have reportedly not been conducting resurveys of home health agencies because of lack of funds and are only conducting surveys for new certification.

Directions for Regulation of Home Health Agencies

Several of the committee's suggestions for improvements in nursing home survey and enforcement activities also apply generally to home health regulation and are generally consistent with GAO recommendations for home health care. *In particular, as with nursing homes, federal and state survey efforts should focus more on chronically poor-performing providers by surveying them more frequently, increasing penalties for repeated violations of standards, and decertifying persistently substandard providers. Federal and state survey efforts should focus more on high-risk events such as rapid caseload growth and management changes.*

In addition, HCFA should make information about poor-performing providers more easily available to consumers, consumer advocates, state policy makers, and others. *The committee recognizes that adequate levels of funding are needed for HCFA to be able to improve state survey and certification processes for home health care providers in an effective and efficient manner.*

HOME CARE AND RELATED SERVICES

Home care services, including personal care services or personal care attendants are the responsibility of state agencies, even though many of these services are paid for by the Medicaid program. States have flexibility in designing these types of programs under Medicaid and may offer such services through home health care agencies or home care agencies, independent providers, or some combination of these. In a recent study, the majority of states allowed self-direction of personal care using independent providers, while the remainder used agency providers (LeBlanc et al., 2000a).

States vary in the monitoring of home care services. Where services are offered through home health agencies, federal and state licensing and certification rules apply. In a study by Harrington and colleagues (2000e), there were 14,045 licensed home health care agencies and 801 other licensed home (or personal) care agencies in the United States in 1998. Where services are offered through home care agencies, state licensing standards apply rather than federal certification rules. Only 59 percent of the total licensed agencies were certified for Medicare and Medicaid, meaning that 41 percent of the agencies followed state licensing laws only (Harrington et al., 2000e). Ten states, however, used only federal home health certification rules and did not have their own licensing requirements in 1998. A review of state licensing regulations found that they offered greater flexibility and were less stringent than federal rules. The one exception was that some states were more stringent than the certification rules in criminal background checks for staff. Thirteen states required criminal background checks for home health agencies and nine states required them for home care or personal care attendants (Harrington et al., 2000e).

LeBlanc and colleagues (2000a) found that care management was the primary means of monitoring personal care services in the states. Formal training of direct care providers was not a common requirement. Most states did mandate some type of supervision of personal care attendants. Some states also conducted client satisfaction surveys by telephone or mail, but most of these were not regularly administered.

The extent of actual state monitoring of quality in home care services for both agencies and independent providers is unknown. Nor is it known how effective the states are in ensuring quality in home care services. This is clearly an area that needs more research attention.

THE ROLE OF ADVOCACY

The roles of consumers, their families, and communities are essential in the design, implementation, and evaluation of long-term care. Historically, advocacy by consumers, family members, and committed community members has played a critical role in shaping long-term care policy and services (Shapiro, 1993). Consumer activists spearheaded the passage of key legislation, such as the Nursing Home Reform Act (OBRA 87), the Americans with Disabilities Act, and the Rehabilitation Act. They likewise spurred the development of federal requirements for state rehabilitation agencies to establish consumer advisory boards and the Medicaid program to grant waivers allowing states to fund community-based services and personal assistance services (Covert et al., 1994; Powers, 1996; Ragged Edge, 1997). Currently, hundreds of local, state, and national advocacy and self-advocacy organizations are active in monitoring and shaping the direction of long-term care for older and younger adults (Estes and Swan, 1993; Shapiro, 1993; Dybwad and Bersani, 1996). Groups advocating on behalf of children and their families frequently serve as advisers to state and local service providers. For example, most children's hospitals have family advisory boards that contribute to decisions ranging from facility design to assessing consumers' views of their care experience.

Depending on its purposes, resources, and circumstances, an advocacy program may work at the individual, organizational, or system (local, state, national) level, or some combination of these. The range of functions includes:

- assisting people with long-term care needs to work toward self-advocacy;
- assisting with individual complaints and mediating conflicts;
- working on behalf of a group of long-term care recipients;
- working with health care providers on resident or consumer protection and quality improvement;
- monitoring the application of regulations;
- educating individuals and communities about quality-of-care factors and consumer protections;
- mobilizing community efforts to reform ineffective or harmful programs and policies; and
- participating in local, state, and national advocacy efforts.

The advocacy models include the publicly funded Long-Term Care Ombudsman Program; resident representatives and councils in nursing homes, assisted living facilities, and other residential settings; family councils for both congregate residential and other settings; and independent state and national advocacy organizations.

Long-Term Care Ombudsman Program

Probably the best-known advocacy effort in long-term care is the Long-Term Care Ombudsman Program, which was mandated under the Older Americans Act in 1978. The program addresses concerns related to individual residents and broader system-level issues. Program staff investigate and resolve complaints made on behalf of residents living in long-term care facilities. They also help educate the public and facility staff on complaint filing, new laws governing facilities, and best practices used in improving quality of care and evaluating long-term care options. In addition to advocacy on behalf of residents, ombudsmen are typically involved in analyzing, monitoring, and recommending changes in the design and implementation of laws affecting residents. Ombudsman programs also support the activities of resident and family councils as well as citizen organizations. The program receives financial support from the federal government and many state and local jurisdictions. In 1998, it was responsible for consumers using 2,624,248 long-term care beds with total funding of almost $47,405,000 (AOA, 1998).

Many long-term care ombudsmen and other long-term care professionals argue that routine on-site presence of ombudsmen builds awareness of the program, establishes resident confidence, allows resident problems to be detected before they become serious, and promotes positive working relationships with facility administration and staff (IOM, 1995, p. 62). The regular presence of persons from outside the facilities has been identified as an important factor in improving quality of care and quality of life in facilities (IOM, 1986; Barney, 1987; Feder et al., 1988; Glass, 1988; Cherry, 1991, 1993; Nelson, 1993). The services provided by ombudsman programs are also relevant to the growing number of consumers of community-based long-term care services, including those directing their own services. These consumers now have no consistent access to external assistance in resolving their complaints and care problems. These programs are critically important, and will become even more so as the use of long-term care increases and relatively fewer resources are available for quality assurance.

Resident Councils

The Nursing Home Reform Act of 1987 provided for the right of residents and family members to organize resident councils in nursing facilities. Ideally these councils are organized, self-governing, decision-making groups of long-term care residents who meet regularly to voice their needs and concerns and to have input into the activities, policies, and issues affecting their lives in the facility. Through a resident council, residents can positively affect their facility, making it a reflection of their preferences and values (Clark and Brown, 1998). In recent years, family councils have taken a more active role in improving conditions in nursing homes because of the residents' impairments.

Independent Advocacy Organizations

Since the late 1960s, citizen groups have organized in many communities to improve conditions in nursing facilities. Similar groups have been organized at the state and national levels with a focus on public education and advocacy. These groups provide an important complement to consumer advisory teams, community councils, ombudsman programs, and quality improvement groups that function to promote the development of quality services within long-term care settings. They are typically directed and staffed by consumer activists and perform a variety of functions, including consumer education and support; monitoring and reporting facility and program adherence to regulations and quality standards; advocacy for care reform and policy development; and support of local advisory and governance groups within long-term care settings.

The range of advocacy groups reflects the diversity of long-term care users and their families. Some groups focus on specific populations, such as those with mental retardation, whereas others focus on particular service settings. For example, the National Citizen's Coalition for Nursing Home Reform (NCCNHR) and Consumers United for Assisted Living (CUAL) have been advocates for reform in these long-term care settings. American Disabled for Attendant Programs Today (ADAPT) has been active in the expansion of personal assistance services to people with disabilities. Various national groups, including Family Voices, Federation for Children with Special Needs, National Parent Network on Disabilities, and Pilot Parents have advocated in most states for improved services for children and assistance to families caring for children with chronic health problems at home. In addition, community-level groups teach advocacy skills, link families to necessary services, and help them navigate the health care system.

Despite their strengths, citizen groups are often limited by their reliance on volunteers and charitable contributions and their lack of guaranteed access to nursing homes and residential care settings. Fear of retaliation against residents often keeps families and other interested parties from protesting poor conditions and otherwise acting to improve quality of care (Monk et al., 1984; IOM, 1995).

Independent advocacy organizations have a unique and critical role as an independent voice for the consumers of long-term care. They are also essential partners of providers, state regulators, financiers, and third-party payers in monitoring and advancing the quality of services. Advocacy organizations are increasingly being integrated into comprehensive long-term care quality initiatives (ALQC, 1998).

Recommendation 5.4: The committee recommends that the federal and state governments encourage the development of effective consumer advocacy and protection programs by providing funding and support for the following types of activities:

- **consumer education and information dissemination initiatives; and**
- **complaint resolution programs and processes targeted at consumers of community-based long-term care.**

ACCREDITATION

Accrediting bodies are independent, not-for-profit, nongovernmental entities that are governed by boards composed of health care professionals, consumers, representatives of provider organizations, and purchasers. Through an evidence-based and consensus-building process, accrediting bodies set standards for quality and safety in health care provider organizations and make the standards publicly available. The accrediting bodies then evaluate provider organizations that volunteer to be assessed against these standards. Successful compliance with the standards leads to "accreditation" of the provider organization, and the accrediting organization's decision, as well as a summary of the findings that led to that accrediting, are made public. In the long-term care arena, accreditation programs currently exist for some nursing homes, home health care, adult day care, hospice, assisted living, and long-term care pharmacies.

Accreditation standards are usually intended to "raise the bar" by promoting and recognizing performance beyond basic, legally established levels, including through programs of continuous quality improvement. In some cases a government agency can grant an accrediting body "deemed status" for a specific accreditation program—that is, a provider organization accredited by that body is deemed to be in compliance with the quality-related regulations for the organization's participation in the Medicare or Medicaid program, or with state regulations for licensure. Under these circumstances, the provider organization does not have to undergo a separate government survey; instead, the government agency relies on the accrediting body's evaluation to make its Medicare or Medicaid certification or licensure decision, as described above for home health agencies.

The 1986 IOM report on nursing home quality discussed accreditation and deemed status at length and rejected it for nursing homes. At the request of Congress, HCFA (1998b) evaluated whether private accreditation of nursing homes would be preferable to the current system of public accreditation. HCFA secured an independent evaluation by ABT Associates. HCFA concluded that the private survey process done by JCAHO was not effective in protecting the health and safety of nursing home residents. According to HCFA, granting "deeming" authority to JCAHO may place nursing home residents at serious risk. As one example, in more than half of the 179 cases where both JCAHO and HCFA conducted inspections of the same nursing homes, JCAHO failed to detect serious problems identified by HCFA (HCFA, 1998b). Nevertheless, accreditation can play a role in encouraging providers to go beyond the basic governmental regulations and strive towards higher standards.

CONCLUSION

Governments have a central role in defining and enforcing basic standards of quality for long-term care. Professional, trade, consumer, and other organizations generally make a different contribution by going beyond minimum performance levels to set requirements that encourage excellent care.

Although OBRA 87 has achieved advances in the quality of care and life in some areas, the implementation of its survey and enforcement efforts has been less than satisfactory, as HCFA, the agency with primary responsibility for its implementation, has recognized. Although HCFA has moved to strengthen its oversight of state survey and enforcement activities and to improve their effectiveness and efficiency, these activities need to be sustained and revised in collaboration with state officials, providers, and consumers. This report was not intended as a full review of the implementation of OBRA 87; this chapter has focused selectively on problem areas in regulatory standards and made recommendations that would improve the reliability and validity of federal and state enforcement efforts primarily affecting quality of care.

Little information is available about federal or state performance in monitoring the quality of long-term care provided under Medicaid's home and community-based services waiver program. To guide decisions, policy makers need more information about how this program is working and, more generally, about how states are defining and regulating community-based long-term care services and supportive housing for different populations. The committee is concerned about reports of quality problems in community-based residential care. At the same time it believes that because of the complexity of the various settings, the inadequate information about quality, and the fragmentation of the various state regulations, the creation of a detailed federal regulatory system at this time is unlikely to bring about better quality of care and quality of life for users of these services. The committee believes that people using long-term care should, within certain broad limits, be able to make choices among alternatives that offer varying balances of autonomy, safety, and other values that sometimes conflict.

6

Strengthening the Caregiving Work Force

The previous chapter focused on regulatory standards and their enforcement. This chapter examines federal and state personnel standards for various long-term care settings. It reviews the literature on the relationship between staffing and quality of care, and presents recommendations for improvements. This chapter also examines the training and education of personnel; hiring and employment issues, including registries and background checks before hiring; and barriers to a stable workforce, with particular emphasis on wages and benefits. Finally, the chapter discusses the management and organizational capacity needed to improve quality of care.

Provision of formal long-term care to the population requires an adequate, skilled, and diverse work force. Registered nurses (RNs), licensed practical nurses (LPNs), and nursing assistants or aides (NAs) and home health aides represent the largest component of personnel in long-term care. Other professionals—including physicians, social workers, therapists (physical, occupational, and speech), mental health providers, dietitians, pharmacists, podiatrists, and dentists—provide many different kinds of essential services to at least a subset of those using long-term care. Non-professionals, who provide the majority of personal care services, such as assistance with eating or bathing, have a major impact on both the health status and the quality of life of long-term care users. In addition to direct care providers (or caregivers), administrative, food service workers, housekeeping staff, and other personnel play essential roles in long-term care.

As shown in Chapter 2, in 1998, nursing homes, personal care facilities, residential care, and home health and home care agencies accounted for nearly 3.2 million jobs. Of these jobs, 1.18 million, or 37 percent, were paraprofessionals (including nursing assistants, personal care aides, and home health care aides), 9 percent were RNs and 8 percent were LPNs (BLS, 2000). Approximately 57 percent of the paraprofessional workers were employed by nursing facilities, 28 percent by home care agencies, and 15 percent by residential care facilities or programs in 1998 (BLS, 2000).

Long-term care services are labor intensive so the quality of care depends largely on the performance of the caregiving personnel. Personnel standards vary considerably across long-term care settings. For purposes of this report, "staffing levels" include numbers of staff, ratios of staff to residents, and the mix of different types of staff in nursing homes and residential care facilties. In home care, staffing levels cannot be discussed in these terms since each client is served individually and agencies are staffed to meet client needs. Rather, the committee considered the amounts and types of services provided to clients with various needs. In a labor-intensive field such as long-term care, the numbers, training, and competence of staff are widely viewed as critical to the quality of services.

Most of the research on the relationship between quality of long-term care and the number and type of staff and their expertise and skills relates to nursing homes. Some studies have examined home health care workers, but few of these studies have examined the relationship between work force characteristics and quality of care. Little is known about the relationship of staff to quality of care in other long-term care settings.

In addition to staffing levels, a key issue is whether the work force in long-term care has adequate education and training to provide high quality of care to individuals. Federal standards have been set for some personnel in nursing homes and home health agencies, but not for personnel providing care in other types of long-term care settings. Some states also have their own requirements for personnel, particularly for the regulation of health professionals and long-term care administrators. These requirements vary across states.

This chapter discusses the caregiving work force separately for each setting. The committee examined existing standards and reviewed the available empirical evidence and research literature on the relationship of staffing patterns and quality. The committee deliberated on the need for changes in standards, education and training issues, and the work environment.

NURSING HOMES

Federal and State Nursing Home Staffing Standards

To participate in the Medicare or Medicaid programs, long-term care facilities must meet federal certification requirements established by the Health Care Financing Administration (HCFA, 1994). The Nursing Home Reform Act, embedded in the Omnibus Budget Reconciliation Act of 1987 (OBRA 87), included a number of provisions related to staffing, which were implemented by the HCFA in a series of regulations and transmittal letters (HCFA, 1994, 1995a–c). The legislation required increased nurse staffing and social work services and set minimum training requirements for nursing assistants. Specifically, OBRA 87 requires nursing facilities certified for Medicare and Medicaid to have licensed nurses on duty 24 hours a day; an RN on duty at least 8 hours a day, 7 days a week; and an RN director of nursing. The statute permits the director of nursing and the RN on staff for 8 hours a day to be the same individual. Furthermore, each nursing home is required to have a medical director responsible for the medical services of the facility residents. Facilities with 120 or more beds must have a full-time person with a bachelor's degree in social work or a related field. HCFA regulations also require social activities; medically related social services; dietary services; physician and emergency care; and pharmacy, dental, and rehabilitation services (including physical, speech, and occupational therapies, which are mentioned explicitly) (HCFA, 1995a–c).

More generally, the law requires "sufficient staff" to provide nursing and related services to attain or maintain the "highest practicable level" of physical, mental, and psychosocial well-being of each resident. The federal law and the implementing regulations, however, do not provide specific standards or guidance about what constitutes "sufficient staffing." Registered and licensed nurse requirements are not adjusted for facility size or casemix. The HCFA survey and certification program does not have procedures for auditing staffing levels or for monitoring the accuracy of staffing data reported by facilities.

In addition to federal requirements, some states have licensing requirements for staffing in nursing facilities that go beyond the federal staffing requirements, although they vary widely across states (NCCNHR and NCPSSM, 1998). In a recent survey, 21 states reported legislative action or interest in increasing staffing standards (NCCNHR and NCPSSM, 1998). California increased its minimum nursing home requirements for direct caregivers to 3.2 hours per resident-day (excluding administrative nurses) (California State Budget Act, 1999). *The committee generally endorses the*

OBRA 87 standards and the states' efforts to improve the staffing requirements in nursing facilities.

Current Staffing Levels in Nursing Homes

Staffing data are available from the On-Line Survey and Certification Assessment Reporting (OSCAR) System, the Medicare time studies conducted by HCFA, and periodic national sample surveys conducted by the federal government.

OSCAR System. OSCAR data, collected during the certification surveys by state agencies that verify compliance with all federal regulatory requirements, show staffing data reported by facilities for the two weeks prior to the survey. Figure 6.1 presents the available OSCAR data on all staff in nursing facilities in the United States during calendar year 1998. It shows that average total staffing hours were 5.9 hours per resident-day for all nursing facilities in the United States in 1998. Nursing staff represented 59 percent of the total personnel hours. Housekeeping and other staff was the second largest category, with 0.77 hour (46 minutes) per resident-day, and dietary staff had 0.71 hour per resident-day. The activity staff averaged 0.16 hour (10 minutes) per resident-day. All other staff were less than 7 minutes per resident-day.

Table 6.1 shows that the average number of hours for registered nurses (including nurse administrators) was 0.74 hour per resident-day. LPN hours were 0.69 hour per resident-day and NA hours were 2.09 hours in 1998. Total nurse staffing per resident-day was 3.52 hours. When the total hours are divided by three (8-hour) shifts per day, each resident was receiving about 15 minutes of RN time per shift, 14 minutes of LPN time, and 42 minutes of nursing assistant time per shift.

Averages for the country as a whole, however, mask substantial variation among states and among facilities within states. As seen in Table 6.1, there are wide variations in staffing levels for different types of facilities. Hospital-based nursing facilities had almost twice as many total hours of nursing care and 4 times as many registered nurse hours as freestanding nursing facilities. Skilled nursing facilities (SNFs) for Medicare-only residents had 2.3 times as many total nursing hours and 6 times as many registered nursing hours as facilities with Medicaid-only residents. Larger facilities had higher nurse staffing hours than smaller facilities. Some facilities report very low nurse staffing levels. Table 6.2 shows that of the total certified nursing homes, 2,701 facilities (19 percent) provide less than 2.7 nursing staff hours per resident-day.

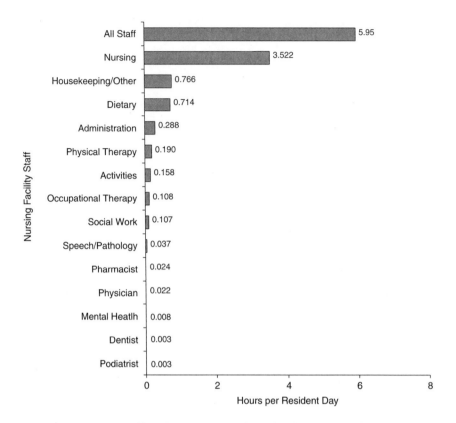

FIGURE 6.1 Mean staffing hours per resident day for nursing facilities in the United States surveyed in calendar year 1998. NOTE: Facilities with inaccurate resident data or incomplete staffing data (497 facilities) were removed. Facilities with staffing levels in the lower 1 percent and the upper 2 percent (1,211) (calculated separately for Medicaid only facilities and Medicare certified facilities) were removed.

Medicare Staffing Time Studies. In 1990, Congress passed legislation requiring HCFA to develop a Nursing Home Casemix and Quality Demonstration program (OBRA, 1990). This HCFA project developed a method for classifying nursing home residents into 44 different Resource Utilization Groups (RUGs) based on a study of resident characteristics in relation to the facility staff time expended to provide care, including nursing and therapy staff (Fries et al., 1994).[1] These studies were then used to develop

---

[1]For details of the methods, see Fries et al. (1994). For information about the quality indicators developed from Minimum Data Set data, see Zimmerman et al. (1995).

TABLE 6.1 Nursing Staff Levels per Resident Day, by Facility Type and Region for Nursing Homes: United States, 1998

Facility Characteristics	Number of Facilities	Percent of Facilities	Nursing Staff			
			Total	Registered Nurses	Licensed Practical Nurses	Nursing Assistants
			Mean Hours			
Total	13,396	100.0	3.52	0.74	0.69	2.09
Type of facility						
Hospital based	1,702	12.4	5.79	2.13	1.22	2.44
Non-hospital based	11,991	87.6	3.20	0.54	0.62	2.04
Certification						
Skilled nursing facilities for Medicare only	1,054	7.7	6.95	2.91	1.50	2.53
Skilled nursing facilities for Medicare or Medicaid	10,909	79.7	3.28	0.58	0.63	2.07
Nursing facilities for Medicaid only	1,730	12.6	2.98	0.43	0.58	1.97
Size						
1–99 beds	6,843	50.0	3.78	0.91	0.73	2.14
100+ beds	6,850	50.0	3.26	0.56	0.66	2.04
Region						
West	2,030	14.8	3.63	0.81	0.61	2.21
South	4,487	32.8	3.63	0.67	0.84	2.11
Northeast	2,481	18.1	3.62	0.84	0.62	2.16
North Central	4,695	34.3	3.32	0.72	0.62	1.98

SOURCE: Harrington and Carrillo, 2000.

a Medicare payment system for use by the five states participating in the demonstration starting in 1995. Ultimately, Congress adopted a Medicare prospective payment system (PPS), implemented by HCFA in 1998.

Prior to the implementation of the PPS, HCFA commissioned three major studies to measure staff time in nursing facilities. The purpose of these studies was to define the relationship between resident resource utilization and nursing and therapy staff time. The RUGs were derived in

TABLE 6.2 Distribution of Combined Nursing Hours per Resident Day in All Certified Nursing Facilities: United States, 1998

Percentile	Average Hours per Resident Day	Number of Hours	Cumulative Number of Hours
0–9	0.90–2.45	1,343	1,343
10–19	2.46–2.70	1,358	2,701
20–29	2.71–2.88	1,320	4,021
30–39	2.89–3.04	1,397	5,418
40–49	3.05–3.20	1,347	6,765
50–59	3.21–3.37	1,428	8,193
60–69	3.38–3.58	1,360	9,553
70–79	3.59–3.91	1,381	10,934
80–89	3.92–4.65	1,386	12,320
90–100	4.66–16.67	1,373	13,693

NOTE: Median (50th percentile) = 3.21 hours per resident day. Mean = 3.52 hours per resident day. N = 13,693 certified nursing facilities. Facilities with inaccurate resident data or incomplete staffing data (497 facilities) were removed. Facilities with staffing levels in the lower 1 percent and the upper 2 percent (calculated separately for Medicaid-only facilities and Medicare-certified facilities) (1,211 facilities) were removed.
SOURCE: Harrington and Carrillo, 2000.

part and updated based on these time studies. The 1995 and 1997 time studies were used primarily to set reimbursement rates for a Medicare prospective payment system (Burke and Cornelius, 1998; Reilly, 1998). From the perspective of staffing requirements, the major concern with these studies has been that nursing and therapy time was based on existing practices in facilities and not on the staffing time required to meet the needs of residents.

The average time per resident-day for different types of nursing staff from HCFA time studies in 1995 and 1997 (averaged together) includes direct and indirect (e.g., administrative) nursing time. Table 6.3 compares HCFA time study data with OSCAR staffing data. The average time, based on HCFA time studies, was 4.17 total nursing hours per resident-day (Burke and Cornelius, 1998). This figure was higher than the 3.52 hours reported on OSCAR, probably because the time studies focused on facilities with high numbers of Medicare residents rather than on those with only Medicaid residents.

The new Medicare PPS pays nursing facilities based on the resident casemix. The Medicare payment formula was based on the amount of time that nurses and therapy staff are expected to provide for Medicare residents with different types of impairments. Nursing facilities are not, however, required by HCFA to provide the hours of time for which they

TABLE 6.3 Comparison of Average Nursing Hours per Resident Day for OSCAR Data, HCFA Time Studies, and Time Proposed by Experts

Nursing Staff	OSCAR Data, 1998[a]	HCFA Time Studies 1995–1997[b]	Time Proposed by Expert Panel[c]
	Average Hours per Resident Day		
Total	3.52	4.17	4.55
Registered nurses	0.74	1.15	1.15
Licensed practical nurses	0.69	0.70	0.70
Nursing assistants	2.09	2.32	2.70

NOTE: times listed include all administrative nursing time and indirect care.
[a]Harrington et al., 1999.
[b]Burke and Cornelius, 1998.
[c]Harrington et al., 2000.

are paid under Medicare. Thus, payment is not tied directly to staffing levels in nursing facilities.

There are some indications that staffing ratios have increased somewhat in recent years. The total nursing hours per resident-day reported on OSCAR data for all facilities has gradually increased. Figure 6.2 shows that the total number of hours per resident-day in nursing facilities, as reported in OSCAR, was 3.0 hours in 1991. By 1998, this total was 3.5 hours per resident-day. Much of the increase in hours was due to increases in RN hours over that period. The slight increase (less than 10 percent) observed may be attributed in part to the requirements of OBRA 87 and in part to the increased acuity of residents and the consequent staffing required to care for residents who need specialized services.

Relationship of Staffing and Quality of Care

Many factors influence the quality of care provided to residents by staff and the quality of life of the residents. Staffing levels and staff characteristics are critical structural elements. In addition, education and training of staff, attitudes and values, job satisfaction and turnover of staff, salaries and benefits, and management and organizational capacity of the facility are all factors affecting quality.

As reviewed in the 1996 Institute of Medicine report on the adequacy of nurse staffing in hospitals and nursing homes (IOM, 1996a), a number of studies have shown a positive association between nurse staffing levels and the processes and outcomes of nursing home care (see for example

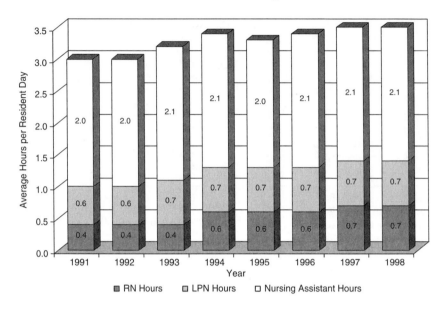

FIGURE 6.2 Average nursing hours per resident day in all certified nursing facilities: United States, 1991–1998.
SOURCE: Harrington and Carrillo, 2000.

Linn et al., 1977; Nyman, 1988b; Munroe, 1990; Cherry, 1991; Spector and Takada, 1991; Aaronson et al, 1994; Cohen and Spector, 1996).

Nyman (1988b) found that nursing hours per patient-day were positively related to three quality measures. Kayser-Jones and colleagues (1989) found that inadequate staffing resulted in poor feeding of residents and inadequate nutritional intake, which contributed to resident deterioration and hospitalization. Munroe (1990) found a positive and statistically significant relationship between the quality of care (measured by deficiencies) and higher ratios of RN and LPN hours per resident-day and lower turnover rates. Spector and Takada (1991) found that higher staffing levels and lower RN turnover rates were related to improvements in resident functioning. Lower staffing levels were associated with high urinary catheter use, low rates of skin care, and low resident participation in activities. Braun (1991) found that higher RN hours were related to lower mortality rates. Cherry (1991) also found that increased RN hours were positively associated with a composite of good outcome measures (fewer decubitus ulcers, catheterized residents, or urinary tract infections, and less antibiotic use). Cohen and Spector (1996) found that higher ratios of RNs to residents, adjusted for resident casemix, reduced the likelihood of death and that higher ratios of LPNs significantly improved resident functional outcomes. The relationship between inadequate staffing and malnutrition, starvation, dehydration, undiagnosed dysphagia, and poor oral health of residents has been documented (Kayser-Jones, 1996, 1997; Kayser-Jones et al., 1997; Kayser-Jones and Schell, 1997). Kayser-Jones and colleagues (1999) showed that nearly all nursing home residents studied in two facilities had inadequate fluid intake. They attributed this finding to inadequate staffing supervision to provide care to nursing home residents with dysphagia, severe cognitive and functional impairment, and aphasia or inability to speak English.

A study of Minnesota nursing homes found that in the first year after admission to a nursing home, the licensed nursing hours (but not nonlicensed) were significantly related to improved functional ability, increased probability of discharge home, and decreased probability of death. However, when limited to chronic care residents the role of professional nursing hours disappeared (Bliesmer et al., 1998). Harrington et al. (2000h) showed that higher nurse staffing hours, particularly RNs, were associated with fewer nursing home deficiencies. In contrast, one longitudinal study of nursing home residents in Massachusetts found that better health outcomes (e.g., survival time, functional status, incontinence, and mental status) were not related to higher RN staffing levels (Porell et al., 1998).

Bowers and Becker (1992) found that *nursing assistants* reported inadequate time to provide high quality of care and the widespread use of techniques for cutting corners required to manage the workload. Foner (1994) reported that workload demands for productivity in nursing homes were in conflict with the need to provide individualized care. Two studies identified reports of psychological and physical abuse of residents by nursing assistants, which were found to be related to the stressful working conditions in nursing homes (Pillemer and Moore, 1989; Foner, 1994). Some of the staff problems can be directly related to poor wages, limited or no health benefits, and high turnover rates (IOM, 1996a).

The most important factor in determining staffing levels should be the resident casemix within facilities. Previous studies have shown a strong positive relationship between casemix adjusted resident characteristics and nurse staffing time (Arling et al., 1987; Cohen and Dubay, 1990; Zinn, 1993a,b; Fries et al., 1994). Thus, facilities with higher casemix levels should require more nursing staff time to meet resident needs.

Several studies have shown the importance of nursing management by professional nursing staff and gerontology specialists in making improvements in quality of care (Schnelle, 1990; Schnelle et al., 1990; Hawkins et al., 1992). The knowledge, hands-on care, and leadership of RNs were essential to sustained quality improvement interventions (Schnelle, 1990).

Other studies have demonstrated the important role that *gerontological nurse specialists* and *geriatric nurse practitioners* play in improving quality (Kane et al., 1988; Mezey and Lynaugh, 1989, 1991). Improved outcomes of care and fewer hospitalizations with the use of gerontological nurses have been documented (Mezey and Lynaugh, 1989, 1991; Buchanan et al., 1990; Mor, 1999). Mor (1999) found lower rates of risk-adjusted hospitalization (but not mortality) for residents in facilities that have a nurse practitioner or physician assistant, but he did not find an effect of RN staff ratios on hospitalization rates. The 1986 IOM Committee on Nursing Home Regulations encouraged nursing homes to employ specially trained gerontological nurses. *The committee supports the recommendation of the IOM Committee on the Adequacy of Nurse Staffing in hospitals and nursing homes that nursing facilities use geriatric nurse specialists and geriatric nurse practitioners in both leadership and direct care positions (IOM, 1996a).* Most nursing homes, however, do not employ nurse practitioners in direct care positions.

In summary, the research evidence suggests that both nursing-to-resident staffing levels and the ratio of professional nurses to other nursing personnel are important predictors of high quality of care in nursing homes. Research provides abundant evidence that participation of RNs in direct caregiving and the provision of hands-on guidance to NAs in caring for residents is positively associated with quality of care. The research literature, however, does not answer the question of what particular skill mix is optimal (IOM, 1996a). Nor does it take into account possible substitutions for nursing staff and ways to best organize all staff. Moreover, as discussed later in this chapter, nurse staffing levels alone are a necessary, but not a sufficient, condition for positively affecting care in nursing homes. Training, supervision, environmental conditions, leadership and management, and organizational culture (or capacity) are essential elements in the provision of quality care to residents. Overall, there is a need for sufficient, well-trained, and motivated staff to provide consumer-centered care in nursing homes, as required in OBRA 87.

A few studies have examined the contributions to residents' well-being of other types of staff providing non-nursing services in nursing homes. One example is therapy. A study of physical and occupational therapy services in a clinical trial found therapy to have positive benefits for functional status and costs of care (Przybylski et al., 1996). Another clinical trial showed only modest benefits of physical therapy on mobility (Mulrow et al., 1994). A retrospective study of medical records reported that patients receiving high-intensity physical therapy had positive outcomes (Chiodo et al., 1992). A survey of nursing homes found that facility administrators perceived a positive relationship between the provision of daily rehabilitation therapy and the discharge of patients (Kochersberger et al., 1994). In a recent study, direct care staffing hours for these professional services (e.g., therapists and activity directors) had a consistent, significant negative relationship with deficiencies in nursing homes (Harrington et al., 2000h). In summary, the research reported has generally shown the importance of professionals providing therapy services in nursing homes. However, these studies offer little guidance on the appropriate level of nursing and medical care for different types of residents. *Overall, a strong need exists for research to examine the direct effects of health professionals (social workers, activities personnel, therapists, dietitians, dentists, pharmacists, and other personnel) on the quality of nursing home care.* Although it is obvious that these specialties are of critical importance, the amount and type of services delivered by such professionals have to be studied so that clear recommendations can be developed to improve quality of care.

Should Staffing Standards Be Increased?

Many clinicians, researchers, and consumer groups consider the current federal nursing home staffing standards to be inadequate to ensure quality of care in nursing homes. The National Citizens' Coalition for Nursing Home Reform (NCCNHR), a nonprofit organization formed in 1975 by a coalition of residents, advocates, ombudsmen, professionals, nursing home providers, and other groups, has criticized federal standards and recommended minimum federal staffing ratios (Burger et al., 1996). Based on expert opinion, NCCNHR (1995) adopted a recommended minimum staffing standard of 4.42 hours of total nursing time, adjusted for each nursing facility's casemix. These recommendations were endorsed by the National Committee to Preserve Social Security and Medicare and by the National Association of Directors of Nursing Administration in Long-Term Care (Mohler and Lessard, 1991; Mohler, 1993; NCCNHR, 1995).

An expert panel convened in 1998 at New York University for an invitational conference on nursing staff, casemix, and quality in nursing homes (Mezey and Kovner, 1998; Harrington et al., 2000c). This panel recommended an overall minimum nurse staffing level of 4.55 hours per resident day, including administrative staff [see Table 6.3]. It further recommended one full-time RN director of nursing and a full-time assistant director of nursing for facilities with 100 beds or more (proportionately adjusted for smaller facilities). In addition, it recommended that at least one RN nursing supervisor be on duty at all times (24 hours a day, 7 days a week) in each nursing home facility and that facilities of 100 beds or more have a full-time RN director for in-service education (proportionately adjusted for smaller facilities), who would be responsible for the administration and supervision of an ongoing training program for staff at all levels. The panel also recommended an increase in staffing levels at mealtimes, so that one staff member would be available for 30 to 60 minutes to assist each dependent individual with eating. Finally, it also recommended adjustments upward in staffing for increases in resident casemix.

The Omnibus Budget and Reconciliation Act, 1990 required the Secretary of Health and Human Services to conduct ". . . a study and report to Congress . . . on the appropriateness of establishing minimum caregiver to resident ratios and minimum supervisor to caregiver ratios for skilled nursing facilities." For a number of reasons, work on the study was delayed by HCFA. The due date for the report to Congress was extended to January 1, 1999. HCFA released the phase I report of the study in summer 2000. A range of problems have been noted among nursing home residents, including increased incidences of severe bed sores, malnutrition and dehydration, and abuse and neglect. The study found a strong relationship between staffing and quality and concluded that there may be critical ratios of nurses to residents below which nursing home residents are at substantially increased risk of quality problems (HCFA, 2000). No date is set yet for completion of phase 2 of the project. *The committee is pleased that HCFA has completed phase 1 of the study, and urges HCFA to expedite the completion and release of the full study.*

As discussed in Chapter 4, the committee found few studies of productivity and efficiency in nursing homes or of management practices that promote quality of care. The goal for nursing homes should be to have appropriate levels and mix of personnel who can organize the work to provide good care in an efficient manner.

In summary, the committee found a wide range of staffing levels in nursing facilities. Many facilities have adequate staffing levels and provide high quality of care to residents. However current staffing levels in some facilities are not sufficient to meet the minimum needs of residents for provision of quality of care, quality of life, and rehabilitation. As shown above, research provides abundant evidence of quality-of-care problems in some nursing homes and such problems are related at least in part to inadequate staffing levels.

The IOM (1996a) study, requested by Congress to examine the adequacy of nurse staffing in hospitals and nursing homes, found that a positive relationship exists between nursing staffing and quality of care, and that trends in resident characteristics suggest an increasing need for professional nursing presence. It further concluded that there was abundant evidence that participation of RNs in direct caregiving and provision of hands-on guidance to NAs in caring for residents is positively associated with quality of care. The IOM (1996a) report therefore recommended that more registered nurses be added to the staff in nursing homes and that by year 2000 a 24-hour presence of registered nurse coverage in nursing facilities be required as an enhancement to the current 8-hour requirement specified under OBRA 87. That committee recognized that its recommendation entails additional costs and, therefore, recommended that Medicare and Medicaid reimbursements be adjusted accordingly. *This committee endorses the recommendations of the 1996 IOM report* (IOM, 1996a). It regrets, however, that no directive or initiative is in place yet to implement these recommendations.

The committee concludes that in view of the increased acuity of nursing home residents, federal staffing levels must be made more specific and that the minimum level of staffing has to be raised and adjusted in accord with the casemix of residents. The objective should be to bring those facilities with low staffing levels up to an acceptable level and to have all facilities adjust staffing levels appropriately to meet the needs of their residents, by taking casemix into account. To ensure that the needs of residents for quality care are met, the committee recommends the following:

Recommendation 6.1: The committee recommends that HCFA implement the IOM 1996 recommendation to require RN presence 24 hours per day. It further recommends that HCFA develop minimum staffing levels (number and skill mix) for direct care based on casemix-adjusted standards.

Since July 1998, Medicare has been paying skilled nursing facilities based on the casemix of residents and HCFA's time study estimates of staff required to provide care for each RUG category. The Medicare rate calculation includes the amount of time for each type of nursing staff (RNs, LPNs, and NAs) that provides care for each RUG category. Therefore, increasing the minimum standards to those already paid for in Medicare PPS rates, in theory, would not increase Medicare costs. Although the Balanced Budget Act of 1997 cut Medicare nursing home reimbursement rates, some funds were restored by Congress in a budget passed in the fall of 1999. For a full discussion of reimbursement issues, see Chapter 8.

Twenty-six state Medicaid agencies also paid for nursing home care based on the casemix of residents in 1998 (Harrington et al., 2000g). Thus, there is a precedent for tying Medicaid reimbursement to the amount of staff time required to provide care for different types of residents. Analyses reviewed in Chapter 8 suggest that some state Medicaid reimbursement rates for nursing homes are extremely low and may not be sufficient to cover the cost of meeting minimum federal standards for quality of care. Low Medicaid reimbursement formulas and methods may discourage nursing homes from increasing staffing levels. Any increase in minimum staffing requirements should be related to reasonable adjustments in Medicaid reimbursement rates that pay for increased staff.

> **Recommendation 6.2: The committee recommends that Congress and state Medicaid agencies adjust their Medicaid reimbursement formulas for nursing homes to take into account any increases in the requirements of nursing time to meet the casemix-adjusted needs of residents.**

The cost of the additional staffing can be estimated by examining the differential time between the current staffing levels and the average facility staffing level needed, multiplied by the average wages of nursing home staff. Medicaid costs estimates would depend on the minimum requirements established by HCFA and the current staffing levels that are built into state Medicaid rates. Some states have rate methods that would allow increased staffing costs to be passed through in their rates. Other states would have to increase reimbursement rates to take into account the staff increases in cases where the states' rates did not cover the increased requirements. Facilities already meeting the proposed staffing standards would have no new costs, but facilities operating below the minimum would be required to increase their staffing levels (see Table 6.3 for facilities with the lowest staffing). Depending on the staffing standards adopted, the increased costs could range from $1.5 billion to $3.7 billion. Of this total, Medicaid would pay 67 percent (because it pays for 67 percent of residents), and these costs would be split approximately in half between the federal and state governments. Although the cost increases for staff would be substantial, they would represent only about a 4 percent increase in the total $87.5 billion spent on nursing homes in 1998 (Levit et al., 2000).

The American Health Care Association (AHCA, 1999) reported that the average RN wages per hour were $16.88, LPN wages were $12.88, and the NA wages were $7.44 in 1997. Since RNs represent 20.6 percent, LPNs 19.5 percent, and NAs 59.9 percent of the total nursing staff, the average nursing home wage per hour for nurses was about $10.43 in 1998. If the minimum requirements were set at the median of 3.21 hours per resident-day, the 1,343 facilities with the lowest staffing levels would have to increase staffing by 1.67 hours; 1,358 facilities would have staffing increased by 0.625 hour; 1,320 facilities would have to increase staffing by 0.415 hour; 1,397 would have to increase it by 0.245 hour; and 1,347 would have to increase it by 0.085 hour. The total increase in staffing would be about 409,600 hours per day in these facilities, if each facility is assumed to average 100 residents. At $10.43 per hour for 365 days, the total costs of the increase in staffing for a full year would be about $1.55 billion dollars. Another approach is to estimate the cost of increasing the average nursing hours reported on OSCAR (3.5 hours per resident-day) to the average hours reported on the HCFA time study (4.17 hours per resident-day) for all nursing facilities. This would result in a 0.67-hour increase per resident-day multiplied by $10.43 per hour for 1.5 million residents, times 365 days per year. The total cost of this increase would be about $3.3 billion.

Although difficult to estimate, increased professional nurse staffing levels might—under certain circumstances—produce some savings for the Medicare and Medicaid programs. For example, if an increased presence of professional nursing reduced the incidence of medical problems requiring hospitalization, some savings would accrue to offset higher staffing costs (Kayser-Jones et al., 1989; Kayser-Jones and Schell, 1997). If better staffing improved staff morale, the results might include higher worker productivity, lower turnover, and reduced on-the-job injuries, which are very common in nursing homes (IOM, 1996a). High personnel turnover is expensive. For example, replacement costs of staff are estimated at four times the employee's monthly salary when the costs of recruiting and training are included (Pillemer, 1996). Better staffing might even reduce the costs of supplies and drugs. For example, Phillips et al. (1993a) estimated that a reduction in the use of restraints actually saves facilities money by improving resident outcomes.

Reporting and Research Requirements

Effective monitoring of staffing levels depends on accurate, timely reporting by facilities. HCFA already requires facilities to report on their resident characteristics on a quarterly basis. *The committee believes that HCFA should require nursing facilities to provide quarterly reports on number and type of staff and staff stability.* Facilities should certify the accuracy of these data, and HCFA should review and audit the data regularly. HCFA should consult with consumer groups and with the nursing home industry in designing staffing report forms. By comparing staffing data with resident characteristics, HCFA will be better able to monitor compliance with staffing requirements and quality standards. To promote accountability to consumers and the public, HCFA should make these data available to the public on the Internet along with information on how to use and interpret the data as indicators of quality of care.

Furthermore, *the committee believes that HCFA should give high priority for research on staffing in nursing homes, and seek research funds to examine the actual time and the staff mix required to provide adequate processes and outcomes of care to nursing home residents. As new data become available about the appropriate staffing levels to meet the needs of residents, federal staffing standards and facility staffing practices should be modified appropriately.*

EDUCATION AND TRAINING OF STAFF IN NURSING HOMES

Registered and Licensed Practical Nurses

The issues of education and training are important to quality of care in nursing facilities (Maas et al., 1996). Registered nurses in nursing homes have substantially lower levels of education (74 percent with an associate or diploma degree) than nurses in hospitals (59 percent with associate or diploma degrees) (Maas et al., 1996; Moses, 1997). Many nurses in nursing homes have had no training in gerontology or chronic disease management (Bahr, 1991; Maas et al., 1996). Yet studies suggest the importance of nursing management by professional nursing staff and gerontology specialists in making improvements in quality of care (Schnelle, 1990; Schnelle et al., 1990; Hawkins et al., 1992; Anderson and McDaniel, 1998). All nursing homes should have a commitment to ongoing continuing education in the care of the chronically ill and disabled and to gerontological nursing. Training in resident assessment and care planning is also very important for nurses, particularly since some nursing schools do not provide training in the basic assessment of patients or in the supervision and management of ancillary personnel. Some states have recommended that each licensed nurse have at least 30 hours of training every two years, but few states have specified the particular areas of training needed.

Nursing management and leadership are central to providing high quality of care in nursing facilities, especially given the complex needs of residents. At present, there are no specific federal requirements for directors of nursing in nursing homes other than that they be RNs. Unlike hospitals, where only rarely do directors of nursing (DONs) have less than a bachelor's degree and often have graduate education, in nursing homes they often are graduates of either a diploma program or an associate degree program at a two-year college (Bahr, 1991; Moses, 1997), and rarely have advanced clinical training in gerontology. A bachelor's degree is considered the basic qualification for entry into professional practice by the American Academy of Nursing and the American Nurses' Association. Leadership and management are not part of the basic preparation in the diploma and associate degree programs. Furthermore, turnover among DONs is high, their salaries are relatively low, and they have limited opportunities for advancement—factors not conducive to strong leadership. Given the number of employees, budgets, and complexity of care provided in nursing facilities today, strong leadership from the DON is a prerequisite for provision of high-quality and cost-effective care (IOM, 1996a).

One of the problems with establishing training standards is that little research has been conducted to determine what would be a desirable standard for training. The amount and frequency of training, the nature and scope of training, and special needs for training (e.g., new technologies) should be examined by researchers to provide guidance in setting professional standards. Nonetheless, *nursing facilities should place greater emphasis on educational preparation in the employment of new DONs and licensed professionals.*

Nursing Assistants

Nursing assistants make up the largest proportion of caregiving personnel in nursing homes. They provide most of the direct care and spend the most time with residents, but they receive little training for provision of care in a nursing facility. The organization, use, and education of NAs make a substantial difference in the care, comfort, and health of nursing home residents, and also in the morale and health of the NAs. OBRA 87 required NAs in nursing homes to have a minimum of 75 hours of training and 12 hours of in-service training per year, and they must pass a competency test within four months of employment (see OBRA 87, sec.1819(b)(5)). Once the nursing assistants pass the competency examination, they are considered "certified nursing assistants." The training is specified in the legislation (the training for home health aides is the same as that for nursing assistants in nursing homes), but the exact nature of the training, certification, and requirements varies by states. Some states have gone beyond the minimum federal training requirements for nursing assistants. For example, California requires 150 hours of training before the NAs can take their competency test and work in facilities beyond the first four months of employment (Harrington et al., 2000c).

Medicare conditions of participation for nursing homes specify the training of nursing assistants required to provide personal care services. The training content must address each of the following subject areas through classroom and supervised practical training totaling at least 75 hours, with at least 16 hours devoted to supervised practical training. The training generally includes communication skills; observation, reporting, and documentation of patient status and the care or service furnished; reading and recording temperature, pulse, and respiration; basic infection control procedures; basic elements of body functioning; maintenance of a clean, safe, and healthy environment; recognition of emergencies and knowledge of emergency procedures; understanding of physical, emo-

tional, and developmental needs of, and ways to work with, the populations served, including the need for respect, privacy, and property; and
appropriate and safe techniques in personal hygiene and grooming
including adequate nutrition and fluid intake.

Supervised practical training means training in a laboratory or other
setting in which the trainee demonstrates knowledge while performing
tasks on an individual under the direct supervision of a registered nurse
or a licensed professional nurse. Each nursing assistant must pass a competency evaluation that addresses each of the subjects in the training
program, and each NA must complete a performance review at least every
12 months. The quality of training varies substantially across facilities and
states. Although states set some standards for training and competency
exams, these are minimal and not closely enforced. Some are concerned
that on-the-job training by nursing homes is weak and recommend that
such training be provided by community colleges or adult education programs, which would ensure that minimum standards for training are met
by all. However, research has not addressed these issues surrounding
training.

With the increased acuity of nursing home residents and the consequent complexity of care needed today, some argue that training should
be significantly increased and, especially, tied to the clinical problems
identified in nursing homes (Burgio and Burgio, 1990). Training for NAs
in nursing homes should include clinical care of the aged and disabled,
occupational health, and safety measures. NAs themselves are reported
to say they need more training and experience, particularly in the management of residents with dementia, depression, and aggression, and in
effective communication (Mercer et al., 1993). Ideally, training programs
should be structured to build-in career development for NAs. Increased
levels of training are expected to increase the quality of care in nursing
facilities. Unfortunately, research is lacking on the effect of different levels
and types of training on the quality of care provided in nursing homes.
There is some agreement among experts, however, that there is a relationship between the level and type of training and the quality of care that
nursing assistants provide.

Nursing Home Administrators

Probably no position in a nursing home is as central as that of the
administrator. Currently, federal Medicare and Medicaid requirements
do not set any standards for administrators. Some states have established
their own nursing home administration boards and requirements, but
these vary across states.

Christensen and Beaver (1996) and Singh (1997) have argued that the employment stability of nursing home administrators is a significant factor influencing the quality of care provided to residents in nursing homes. Singh and Schwab (1998) examined factors that cause the high turnover of nursing homes administrators (41 percent or higher annually). They found higher retention when administrators are involved in decision making, treated fairly, and given reasonable goals to achieve. They also found that turnover was lower in independently-owned facilities, nonprofit facilities, and larger-sized facilities than in chains, for-profit, and small facilities.

Singh and Schwab (1998) found that opportunities for educational and professional development were important factors in the retention of nursing home administrators. Castle and colleagues (1996) found a relationship between the number of hours worked by nursing home administrators, controlling for other factors, and the prevalence of pressure ulcers and the use of psychotropic medications. Castle and Banaszak-Holl (1997) showed that administrator's education, job tenure, and professional involvement were positive predictors of innovations in nursing homes.

Medical Directors and Practitioners in Nursing Homes

Medical services are relatively unavailable in day-to-day nursing home care. Medical practitioners have less of a presence except in rehabilitation and other facilities that provide more intensive medical services and supervision. Most nursing home residents, for whom scheduled physician visits are required, rarely leave the nursing facility to visit a primary care physician. Nonetheless, nursing home services must be provided in accord with care plans authorized and periodically reviewed by physicians. The attentiveness and leadership of the medical community are important in efforts to improve the quality of long-term care.

Medicare certification regulations promulgated in 1976 made medical directors responsible for quality oversight in nursing homes. OBRA 87 further strengthened the role of medical directors by defining their role. Medical directors are to provide oversight and participate in drug utilization review and quality assurance programs and to work with attending physicians on appropriate drug therapies and medical care issues.

The American Medical Directors Association has encouraged professional interaction and assisted in providing training programs for medical directors (Fortinsky and Raff, 1996). This effort appears to be leading to a greater level of interest by, and involvement of, physicians. Medical directors are reported to be spending more time in facilities to address quality issues (Fortinsky and Raff, 1996), but their overall time in facilities is less than 1.5 minutes per resident-day (see Figure 6.1). Zimmer et al.

(1993) pointed out that the average medical director spends little more than three hours a week in a facility. Many medical directors agree that such time is not sufficient and that more involvement by medical directors is essential (Levenson, 1993; Tangalos, 1993).

Few nursing homes have staff physicians; rather, they rely on community-based attending physicians to provide medical care to nursing home residents. Reports suggest that medical care in nursing homes tends to be provided by a small group of physicians, suggesting there may be problems accessing medical care for some nursing home residents (Fortinsky and Raff, 1996). Little research has focused on the role of physicians and the relationship of physician services to nursing home quality. Karuza and Katz (1994) studied physician staffing patterns in nursing homes in New York and found different organizational and practice patterns ranging from attending physicians in the community to in-house physicians and closed staff models. They argued that the lack of in-house physicians in many facilities was a problem for handling emergencies, diagnosing and treating acute medical problems, and managing infection control. Nurse practitioners can also play an important role in nursing home care by acting as substitutes for physicians or by working with physicians. Research studies on the value of nurse practitioners are discussed earlier under nursing home staffing.

Physician responsibility and liability for long-term care problems have emerged as new issues in nursing homes. Although medical directors are accountable for quality of care in nursing facilities, they generally have little authority within facilities (e.g., in terms of hiring and firing staff and in setting administrative policies) and little authority over attending physicians (Levenson, 1993). Attending physicians' actions, especially in drug selection and rehabilitation orders, may affect the financial operations of facilities, although the physicians themselves are paid for their medical services under Medicare Part B (i.e., they are not covered by PPS).

The growth of managed care also has important implications for physician services in nursing homes, especially as more acutely ill patients are being referred for posthospital care. Managed care plans and their physicians provide medical care to their members in nursing facilities. Reuben and colleagues (1999) described the approaches that three health maintenance organizations (HMOs) have taken to providing primary care for long-stay nursing home residents. HMOs that provided more visits to members in nursing homes had significantly fewer emergency room visits and hospitalizations compared with HMOs that provided fewer visits. These managed care programs performed significantly better on more than half of the process quality measures (e.g., response to falls and fevers), but no differences were observed in mortality. This study showed the value of a strong physician component devoted to nursing facility care and meticulous maintenance of the program.

One approach to improving the quality of nursing home care would be for facilities to vest greater authority and responsibility in medical directors for medical care services and require attending physicians and nurse practitioners to follow facility medical policies and procedures. Few facilities have established such requirements. A more stringent approach would be to develop closed panel staff to provide medical services within facilities so that attending physicians would have to meet certain education and credentialing standards before they could provide care to residents within the facility. *The committee believes that nursing homes should develop structures and processes that enable and require a more focused and dedicated medical staff responsible for patient care.* These organizational structures should include credentialing, peer review, and accountability to the medical director. Physicians should participate in the development of, and be responsive to, facility policies and procedures and regulatory requirements.

Physicians, nurse practitioners, and other primary care providers in long-term care need to have expertise relevant to the populations they are serving and the settings in which they are providing care. Those providing care to children, developmentally disabled, mentally disabled, chronically ill, or other special populations require expertise specific to each of these groups. In providing nursing home care to older populations, geriatric training is especially important, including training in multidisciplinary approaches to care, teamwork, and supervision of diverse professional and paraprofessional caregivers.

Medicare reimbursement policies could also help strengthen the quality of medical services provided to nursing home residents. In 1991, significant changes were made in physician reimbursement for nursing facility visits (Tangalos and Stone, 1993). Although the American Medical Directors Association supports the minimum visit requirements for residents to prevent resident abandonment by physicians, it argues that the appropriate number of physician visits should be based on patient acuity and medical necessity and not on arbitrary limits. The committee is concerned that HCFA rules do not adequately recognize the need for medical judgments that take into account the multiple complex medical problems that many nursing home residents have. Arbitrary limits set by fiscal intermediaries on the number of visits should be removed. *The committee believes that HCFA should make clear Medicare and Medicaid regulations for physician services in nursing homes and allow the number and type of services provided to be based on residents' medical needs and the severity of their illness.*

RESIDENTIAL CARE SETTINGS

Relationship Between Staffing and Quality

The committee found very little research examining the relationship between quality of care and the work force in residential care settings or even documenting the structure, process, or outcomes of care in these settings. Some researchers have expressed concerns about the quality of the personnel working in residential care settings (see Hawes et al., 1999), and periodic newspaper stories on assisted living provide case reports of problems. Also, a General Accounting Office (GAO, 1999a) study of assisted living facilities in four states found that more than one-fourth had been cited by state licensing, ombudsman, or other agencies. Frequent problems include poor care to residents and insufficient, unqualified, and untrained staff.

Based on participants' judgments, the Consumer Consortium on Assisted Living (CCAL, 1996) raised questions about the appropriate resident-to-staff ratio (taking casemix into account); management's understanding of the value of staff; ongoing training and staff development; supervisory systems to coordinate and oversee care delivery; and staff burnout. This group called for the development of standards or criteria for residential care staffing and staff training (CCAL, 1996).

Since residential care services are not provided under the Medicare and Medicaid programs (except under some state Medicaid waivers), there are no federal requirements for residential care personnel. States have the primary responsibility for regulating residential care facilities, and some do have staffing requirements. States vary considerably in their requirements for the work force, and some states have no educational requirements beyond a high school diploma for administrators. More than three-quarters of the work force in residential care settings, such as board and care homes and assisted living facilities, are unlicensed personal care workers and home health aides, while RNs and LPNs constitute less than 3 percent of the positions in these settings (Feldman, 1998).

The survey of board and care facilities in ten states, described in previous chapters, found 92 percent of the licensed homes and 62 percent of unlicensed homes provided personal care, such as assistance with activities of daily living (Hawes et al., 1995a). Most facilities were providing supervision or administration of medications, but only 21 percent had any licensed nursing staff (RNs or LPNs). Some states have passed nurse delegation acts that allow RNs to delegate medication administration to nursing assistants or personal care workers. Of staff giving injections, 28 percent were unlicensed with no formal training or expertise in giving injections. Only one state (Oregon) reported a program for training and certifying nursing assistants who pass medications. When staff were tested on their knowledge of aging and care practices or medications, only 14 percent of operators and staff scored at an acceptable level. Many of the professional nursing services provided in residential care facilities were arranged through home health care agencies. Since the conduct of that survey, however, licensing requirements in only 24 states and the District of Columbia allow nonnurses to administer medications—all of them include in-house medication training requirements. Five states require staff to be certified, 12 states require staff to complete a state- or Nursing Board-approved training course, nurse delegation protocols apply in 7 states, and physicians may authorize administration of medication in 1 state (Keren Brown-Wilson, personal communication, May 9, 2000).

Staffing requirements varied across states, but in general did not seem to address the individual needs of the residents. Ten agencies permitted admission or retention of bedfast residents, and 54 permit the retention of chairfast residents. However not all of those states impose staffing requirements. As an increasing number of frail and disabled people are admitted, this staffing situation becomes a health and safety issue (Hawes et al., 1993).

Hawes and colleagues (1999), in a national probability survey of assisted living facilities for the frail elderly, found that nearly all of the 2,945 facilities in the study reported that they provided or arranged for 24-hour staff, housekeeping, and three meals a day. Of the total in the study, 52 percent provided RN or LPN care on a part-time or full-time basis, 27 percent arranged or provided the care, and 21 percent did not provide the care. Facilities with higher nurse staffing were more likely to admit and retain residents with more care needs.

Staffing Standards

As stated earlier, a large body of research comparable to that for nursing facilities does not exist on work force issues in residential care settings. The Assisted Living Quality Coalition (ALQC, 1998) has recommended some minimum standards for staffing. It recommended that the administrator of assisted living facilities should be at least 21 years of age with at least a high school diploma and have adequate education, experience, and ongoing training to meet the needs of residents. In addition, the ALQC recommended a demonstrated management or administrative ability to maintain the overall operations of the setting.

The ALQC (1998) further recommended that staff numbers and qualifications should be sufficient to meet the scheduled and unscheduled needs of residents for services on a 24-hour basis and to monitor changes in residents' physical, cognitive, and psychosocial status. A minimum of one staff person should be awake and on-site at all times when one or more persons with cognitive impairments are present. More generally, staff should have "adequate skills, education, experience and ongoing training to serve the resident population in a manner consistent with the philosophy of assisted living" (ALQC, 1998, p. 84).

The coalition's recommendations have highlighted the need for states to develop more specific personnel standards and guidelines. The kinds of intensive time and resource-use studies described earlier for nursing homes have not been conducted in residential care settings. In part, this gap in information reflects variability of models, definitions, populations served, and state regulations. It also reflects the lack of Medicare and Medicaid funding for these services and the corresponding lack of incentive for policy makers to support even descriptive studies of resources associated with providing different types and amounts of care. Time and resource-use studies of the various types of personnel providing care are needed for residential care arrangements so that appropriate staffing standards can be developed. As Medicaid programs, in particular, begin to pay for more residential care services, federal and state governments have a greater interest in ensuring that these settings meet minimum standards of care and staffing.

Education and Training in Residential Care

In general, training requirements for staff in residential care facilities are set by states, not the federal government; and state policies vary. Hawes and colleagues (1995a) found that 20 percent of licensed board and care homes and 33 percent of unlicensed homes did not require any staff training. Of the facilities that required training, most did not require the training to be completed before staff began providing care.

The Consumer Consortium on Assisted Living (CCAL, 1996) reported concerns about the lack of regulated training requirements and ongoing programs for training and staff development. It recommended training staff in (1) better communication techniques with residents and with families; (2) respect for resident rights and ways to maximize resident autonomy; and (3) resident assessment and care planning activities for individualized resident care.

More generally, the Assisted Living Quality Coalition (1998) recommended that staff should have ongoing training to serve the resident population in a manner consistent with the philosophy of assisted living. It also recommended that such training be required for all staff that have contact with residents to ensure the skills necessary for providing high quality of care and monitoring changes in residents' conditions. It further recommended that in settings where residents have dementia, staff should "have a minimum of 12 hours of dementia-specific training per conducted by a qualified trainer (or facilitated by a trained staff member) to meet the needs/preferences of cognitively impaired residents effectively and to gain an understanding of the current standards of care for people with dementia" (ALQC, 1998, p. 84). ALQC further recommended that in settings where some skilled nursing services are delegated to paraprofessional staff, that staff should meet a documented protocol for supervision, training, and education requirements.

In summary, with regard to both staffing standards and education and training requirements, states should work to bring about more standardization and consistency in staffing standards across states. Providers should take the lead in ensuring the competence of, and provision of, appropriate training to all direct care personnel employed by residential care facilities. The committee does not believe that the first course of action should be enforcement by law or regulation at the federal level. It does caution, however, that if real quality-of-care problems were to emerge that could be related to inadequate staffing or training, then external regulations may be required to protect the health and safety of the residents.

HOME HEALTH AGENCY STAFF

Relationship Between Home Health Care Personnel and Quality

Research on the linkage between personnel and quality of care provided in a person's home is difficult to undertake because of the barriers to observing the care and identifying appropriate process and outcome measures. Most studies of home health care have examined predictors of use and expenditures rather than quality of care. R.A. Kane and colleagues (1994) described the problems of measuring home-based care quality because of the multiple goals for care, limited provider control, and unique family roles. The most highly rated outcomes were freedom from exploitation, satisfaction with care, physical safety, affordability, and physical functioning (R.A. Kane et al., 1994). Kane and Blewett (1993) developed measures that could be used to study problem-specific and patient-focused elements for older people in an ambulatory care setting. Kramer and colleagues (1990) developed quality indicator groups to classify clients into groups with similar needs and quality challenges. Although few studies have assessed quality of care, there are many complaints about home health aides and personal care workers (Harrington and Grant, 1990; Eustis et al., 1993). The key to high-quality care services is worker performance, knowledge, and skills (Eustis et al., 1993).

Home Health Agency Standards for Staff

Under Medicare, home health care services mean those services provided to individuals under the care of a physician by a home health agency, under a plan established and periodically reviewed by a physician, on a visiting basis in a place of residence such as the individual's home (Section 1861(m) of the Social Security Act [42 U.S.C. 1395x]). These services include:

- part-time or intermittent nursing care provided by or under the supervision of a registered professional nurse;
- physical or occupational therapy or speech-language pathology services;
- medical social services under the direction of a physician; and
- to the extent permitted in regulations, part-time or intermittent services of a home health aide who has successfully completed a training program approved by the Secretary.

To be eligible for Medicare home health benefits, a beneficiary must be homebound, under the care of a physician, and in need of skilled care—defined as intermittent skilled nursing services, physical therapy, speech therapy, and continuous occupational therapy. Once these conditions have been met, an individual may also receive medical social services, durable medical equipment (subject to a 20 percent copayment), and home health aide services. As long as the services are medically reasonable and necessary for the treatment of an illness or injury and certified by a physician (every 60 days), none of these services are limited to a specific time period or a specific number of visits (Vladeck and Miller, 1994).

Medicare will not pay for home health aide services unless the beneficiary also requires intermittent skilled nursing or therapy services. As a result of a court case (*Duggan v. Bowen*) settled in 1988, HCFA enlarged the definition of skilled care beyond the hands-on procedures (e.g., wound care, tube feeding) that had traditionally comprised skilled nursing care, to include certain services requiring skilled nursing judgment. Under this enlarged definition, individuals could receive home health aide coverage (Bishop and Skwara, 1993; Cohen and Tumlinson, 1997).

When Congress enacted OBRA 87, it included new legislative requirements for certified home health agencies similar to those for nursing homes. Certified home health agencies had to meet minimum requirements for nursing and training standards for home health aides.

The regulations require on-site supervision of the home health aide by a registered nurse every two weeks if the patient is receiving skilled nursing care (42 C.F.R. 484.36(d)). If another skilled service is being provided, an appropriate professional must make the supervisory visit. If the patient is not receiving skilled nursing services, physical or occupational therapy, or speech–language pathology services, the RN must make a supervisory visit at least every 62 days at a time when the aide is providing patient care.

Home health agency certification for Medicaid payment is linked to Medicare certification. Most states further link Medicaid with Medicare home health agency services through their state licensing statutes and regulations. A survey of states found that 10 states did not license home health agencies but used Medicare certification in 1999. Forty states and the District of Columbia have their own licensing laws for home health agencies (Harrington et al., 2000e) and their own regulations.

According to the Social Security Act (42 U.S.C. 1396d, Section 1905(a)(24)), personal care services (e.g., assisting people with activities of daily living such as eating and bathing) are those services "provided by an individual who is qualified to provide such services." States are allowed to designate qualified organizational providers which may include certified home health agencies or agencies that are neither licensed nor certified. Certified Medicare and Medicaid home health agencies are not required to provide personal care services, but they may choose to do so. Independent workers, usually known as personal care attendants, may also provide personal care services. The duties of home health aides and personal care attendants overlap in that both are allowed to provide direct care to clients, such as help with bathing, dressing, toileting, and eating (Harrington et al., 2000d,e).

Home Health Agency Staffing Levels

The Bureau of Labor Statistics estimated that there were 745,600 home health care employees in 1998. There were also about 130,000 RNs working in home health care or about 6 percent of the national pool of RNs (BLS, 2000). Skilled nursing, home health assistance, and therapy services are the major home health services provided, but little is known about the amount and type of services provided by certified and uncertified home health agencies. Likewise, little is known about the contribution of medical directors, physicians, and nurse practitioners in home health agencies.

Home health agency personnel are critical, yet little is known about the quality of care they provide. The monitoring of personnel by HCFA has been limited because overall enforcement of quality standards in home health agencies has been extremely limited (GAO, 1997b). *The committee believes that HCFA should increase its monitoring of home health staff including their education, knowledge, and competency, particularly for diverse population groups such as ventilator-dependent individuals and children with severe disabilities.* At the same time, *new research efforts are needed to develop uniform standards for the qualifications of home health care personnel and ways to improve quality of care for nursing, therapy, and medical services.*

Home health agencies are not required to appoint a medical director, although many have established formal and informal relationships with the medical community. No required visit schedule exists, but patients receiving home health services usually are seen by their physicians in an office setting.

Education and Training of Home Health Agency Staff

Certified agencies must have a qualified administrator who is either a physician, a registered nurse, or a health administrator with education and training and at least one year of supervisory experience. The Medicare conditions of participation for home health agencies (42 C.F.R. 484.36) also specify the training of home health aides to provide personal care services. The training generally covers the same areas described above for nursing assistants in nursing homes. The training must be provided through classroom and supervised practical training totaling at least 75 hours, with at least 16 hours devoted to supervised practical training (42 C.F.R. 484.36(a)). The person being trained must complete at least 16 hours of classroom training before beginning the supervised practical training.

Supervised practical training means training in a laboratory or other setting in which the trainee demonstrates knowledge while performing tasks on an individual under the direct supervision of a registered nurse or licensed professional nurse. The regulations also require 12 hours of in-service training for home health aides during each 12-month period (42 C.F.R. 484.36(b)(2)). The competency evaluation must address each of the subjects listed in the training program, and every home health agency must complete a performance review of each home health aide no less frequently than every 12 months.

Medicare specifies that the initial training of home health aides must be performed by or under the general supervision of a registered nurse who possesses a minimum of two years of nursing experience, at least one year of which must be in the provision of home health care. Other individuals may provide instruction under the supervision of such a nurse. The regulations also specify that the competency evaluation must be performed by a registered nurse (42 C.F.R. 484.36(b)(3)). The in-service training generally must be supervised by an RN who possesses a minimum of two years of nursing experience, at least one year of which must be in the provision of home health care.

States may have additional training requirements for home health workers, and the extent of these requirements varies considerably (Scala and Mayberry, 1997). A recent study found that California and Illinois both required 120 hours of home health aide training, New Hampshire required 100 hours, Kansas and New Jersey required 90 hours, and Texas required 80 hours (Harrington et al., 2000e). The United Hospital Fund of New York (1994) suggested increased training to improve the quality of home healthcare. It recommended three weeks of training at a minimum for home health aides after two weeks of classroom work and demonstration of competence in required skills. In addition, it recommended special training and support for home health aides who manage difficult-to-serve clients, such as those with Alzheimer's disease or AIDS.

The federal training requirements may also need updating. The training should ensure the skills necessary to provide high quality of care, promote autonomy, and monitor changes in patients' conditions. In addition to general competencies, home health aides should be trained and tested to ensure they can provide appropriate care when they are working with special populations such as demented clients, children, individuals with AIDS, and other groups.

Concern has been expressed by the community of people with disabilities needing long-term personal attendant services that Federal Medicare and Medicaid training requirements do not include instruction for providing consumer-directed services. For example, Scala and Mayberry (1997) have argued that the lack of adequate training and information for both consumers and staff is a major barrier to consumer-directed programs. A study of consumer-directed home and community-based services conducted by the National Council on the Aging also identified such training as a major issue (Cameron, 1996)

HOME CARE

As noted in the previous sections, the home care work force includes workers in home health and home care agencies, including personal care agencies, and those workers who are independent care providers. All of the problems with the home health care work force are also seen in home care, but very few studies have examined home care personnel issues and their relationship to quality. Most of the literature is on access to, and satisfaction with, consumer-directed models of personal care service discussed in earlier chapters. In these models, consumers select, train, and supervise personal care workers (DeJong et al., 1992; Fenton et al., 1997; Scala and Mayberry, 1997).

Benjamin (1998) conducted a study of California's personal care services program and examined the differences between agency model services and independent providers with client-directed care. The study found benefits and negative features of both models. The independent provider model provided more paid and unpaid hours to clients, but the worker compensation was much lower than in the agency model. Overall, clients were satisfied with both models. Clients receiving care from independent providers, however, reported more positive outcomes about how they felt in the service relationship and in their satisfaction with the technical and interpersonal aspects of care (Benjamin, 1998).

In states that have licensing requirements for personal care attendants, many require attendants to be supervised by an RN who visits the client every 60 to 180 days. Beyond these requirements, most states have few specific regulations regarding personnel in home care agencies or independent providers (Harrington et al., 2000e). It is unknown to what extent states monitor personnel requirements and the extent to which personnel issues are of concern.

As indicated in Chapter 3, although professionals involved with families in home care must meet basic standards of professional accreditation and licensure, demonstrate special expertise in the area of children's care, and have explicit training in areas related to the specific child in home care, families face particular problems in the long-term care of children. Many children receive needed care without difficulties, but many home care providers may not have the training or experience in the care of children. Instead, they come from a background of providing care for elderly patients (Feinberg, 1985). Moreover, agencies or programs may lack personnel equipped to supervise home and community-based care for children.

EDUCATION AND TRAINING RECOMMENDATIONS

As the discussion above indicates, the education and training requirements for formal long-term care providers and informal care providers are clearly important for ensuring high quality of care. The training should be directed to all professionals, not only nurses but also therapists, respiratory care providers, social workers, as well as other caregiving personnel. Although some minimum standards have been set for Medicare- and Medicaid-certified providers, these are generally weak, especially in light of the changing characteristics of those receiving care. Overall, the federal education and training requirements may not be adequate to ensure high quality of long-term care. Providers themselves are principally responsible for ensuring adequate training and competency of their work force. As a general principle, the work force must have the education, training, and commitment to provide care that is consistent with the needs of the individuals being served. The problem is that little research is available for many long-term care settings and services to show what appropriate amounts and types of education are necessary to achieve this.

Emphasis in the future should be placed not only on the content of training programs but more importantly on competency testing of skills for both formal and informal care providers. Training programs should be tailored to provide appropriate care to special population groups such as individuals with developmental disabilities or AIDS, children, and other groups. Providers also have to be trained and be competent in providing care that uses the most current clinical practice standards for different conditions such as dementia, diabetes, traumatic brain injury, and others. Professionals have to be competent in care assessment and planning, supervision of care workers, coordination of care services, and client- and family-centered care. Increased attention to the education and training of the long-term care work force is needed to ensure that staff has both the knowledge and the skills to provide high quality of care, with particular attention to client-directed care and the needs of special population groups.

> **Recommendation 6.3: The committee recommends that for all long-term care settings, federal and state governments, and providers, in consultation with consumers develop training, education, and competency standards and training programs for staff based on better knowledge of the time, skills, education, and competency levels needed to provide acceptable consumer-centered long-term care.**

For such education and training programs to work, strict policies for certification will be needed to establish improved standards for this work force. Both basic and ongoing training should promote the development of observational skills to monitor changes in resident or client conditions (including physical, cognitive, social, and psychological status) and to adjust care accordingly.

LABOR FORCE ISSUES

As stated earlier in this chapter, in addition to staffing levels and staff characteristics, the education and training of staff, job satisfaction, turnover, and salaries and benefits also affect the quality of care provided. The 1996 IOM report on the adequacy of nurse staffing included a review of the literature on labor shortages and the unstable labor pool for the nursing home market and the factors contributing to these problems (IOM, 1996a).

A serious shortage exists in the long-term care work force. The boom-ing economy is worsening the shortage of nurses, home health aides, certified nursing assistants, and personal care workers (Ryan, 1999; Rimer, 2000). As higher-paying jobs with better working conditions have opened up for the women who have typically held these jobs, workers are hard to find. With the national unemployment rate falling to 3.9 percent in April 2000 (3.5 percent for adult women), it is likely to remain difficult to attract staff into the long-term care industry (BLS, 2000). Shortage of home care workers is the subject of state task forces in Florida, Pennsylvania, and Maryland (Rimer, 2000).

The problem of recruiting workers is likely to worsen over time as the number of people needing long-term care increases relative to the popu-lation 20–64 years old, which makes up the work force (Lewin Group, 1999). The Bureau of Labor Statistics projects that jobs in the long-term care sector will increase by 1.64 million, or 53 percent, between 1996 and 2006 (BLS, 1998). Reflecting the growing emphasis on the provision of long-term care at home or in alternative residential settings rather than in institutions, total employment in nursing facilities is projected to grow less quickly than in other long-term care settings. BLS estimated that jobs in nursing and personal care facilities would increase by about 37 percent over 1996–2006 compared to increases of 59 percent in residential care facilities and 90 percent in home health. The vast majority of these addi-tional jobs will be for low-paid, low-benefit, low-skill home health aides, personal care workers, and certified nursing assistants. Obviously, an economic downturn could end the current shortage, but the long-run demographic imbalance between the demand for and supply of workers can only worsen over time, making it difficult to recruit the staff needed to achieve higher staffing levels.

Personnel Turnover

The American Health Care Association (1999) reported that in 1997 the turnover rate in nursing homes was 93 percent for NAs and 51 percent for RNs and LPNs. The turnover rate for directors of nursing was 32.5 percent, and for administrators was 22 percent (AHCA, 1999). Relatively high turnover rates of administrators and key supervisory personnel are worrisome for the operation of facilities, given the concerns about the caregiving work force and the vulnerability of many of those receiving long-term care. Although little research has been conducted in this area, it is widely recognized that administrative leadership is a crucial factor in improving the quality of care.

Turnover rates were also high in the home health care sector (Burbridge, 1993; MacAdam, 1993; Close et al., 1994; Crown et al., 1995).

Feldman et al. (1994) reported that turnover rates for home health care workers were much higher in private than in public agencies. The United Hospital Fund (1994) reported a 40 percent turnover rate of home health care workers; while Crown et al. (1992) reported 40–60 percent.

High turnover rates are not the only important factor in current labor force problems in long-term care. The length of employment is also important. A high turnover rate among a small percentage of employees in a facility is less likely to have an adverse impact on the quality of care, although it may affect certain care users and certain services. However, a high turnover rate for a large percentage of employees in a facility is likely to have a more widespread effect on quality of care. Data on tenure of leadership positions, turnover rates, and work force stability at the facility level are not available from any public source at this time. Yet in other businesses, such changes in leadership are reported in the press, and the Securities and Exchange Commission asks for this information from all publicly traded corporations so that stockholders have this information when making investment decisions. Such information is equally important for long-term care organizations.

Periodic shortages of personnel in long-term care can be attributed to cyclical economic conditions that increase the competition for unskilled workers and to structural features of the industry (Feldman et al., 1994; Feldman, 1996). Although cyclical economic conditions significantly affect the demand for unskilled workers, low wages and benefits along with difficult working conditions and heavy workloads also make recruitment difficult, even when unemployment rates are relatively high.

Wages and benefits for home and home health care workers, and for those in nursing homes, are significantly lower than for those in acute care settings (Crown et al., 1995; Feldman, 1996; Leavitt, 1998). For example, in 1996, RN wages in nursing homes were almost 19.7 percent lower than RN wages in hospitals. Wages of long-term care nursing assistants were 21 percent lower than hospital NA wages, although LPN wages were about the same as hospital LPNs (AHCA, 1997; Moses, 1997). Wages of RNs in home health and public health nursing were reported to be nearly 10 percent lower than those of RNs in hospitals in 1996 (Moses, 1997). Compared to hospital and nursing home workers, home care aides tended to work fewer weeks per year and were less likely to work full-time (Crown et al., 1995). Until wages and benefits in the long-term care sector are brought closer to parity with those of hospital workers, hospitals will continue to be the sought-after place of employment.

Restrictions related to the level of payment and benefits for independent care providers raise significant concerns (Litvak et al., 1987; Tilly and Bectel, 1999). Many consumer-directed long-term care programs base their service payments on assumptions of low hourly rates for caregivers and prohibit consumers from paying higher rates. To the extent that these prohibitions limit consumers' ability to pay competitive wages and benefits, they are likely to limit the ability of consumers to attract and retain more capable and skilled caregivers. If the current tight labor market persists and if recommendations for better pay for caregivers in nursing homes are adopted, restrictions on consumer-directed payments are likely to have an even greater impact on the availability of skilled caregivers.

Wages in other industries such as the fast food industry are sometimes higher than those of nursing assistants and home care aides in long-term care settings, and working conditions of the former may also be viewed as better. Even small differences in wages at that level influence where people are willing to work. Many paraprofessionals working in long-term care services earn, on average, only the minimum wage, which puts their income at less than the federal poverty level, and most have no benefits such as health insurance. Since many paraprofessionals are women and minorities who are supporting families, the low wages are a serious problem. Some workers take on two jobs or work extensive overtime to increase their income. Such conditions lead to fatigue and inefficiency, and could have a detrimental effect on the quality of care provided.

Factors contributing to low wages and benefits in long-term care include the limitations of Medicare and Medicaid reimbursements, high reliance on self-paying patients with limited financial resources, the profit orientation of many providers, and barriers to unionization (Burbridge, 1993; Close et al., 1994; Feldman, 1998). The low rates built into Medicare and Medicaid reimbursement rates are particularly important because these programs are the major payers for both nursing home and home health care services. Unless wages and benefits are set at levels that allow the long-term care industry to be competitive in the labor market, the work force is structured for instability. On the other hand, raising reimbursement rates will not by itself ensure that providers pass these increases on to workers unless accountability is built into the payment system.

Moving toward parity would undoubtedly be expensive for Medicare and Medicaid. Nonetheless, if improvement is to be made in the quality of nursing home care, a stable and well-motivated work force is needed. Government payers and providers of care must focus on improving compensation and working conditions.

Recommendation 6.4: For all long-term care service workers and settings, the committee recommends that federal and state governments, as appropriate, undertake measures to improve work environments including competitive wages, career devel-

opment opportunities, work rules, job design, and supervision that will attract and retain a capable, committed work force.

Important as wages and benefits are, Feldman (1998) and Close et al. (1994) found that work settings and management are critical in mediating the impact of compensation on turnover rates for paraprofessionals. Cohen-Mansfield (1997) and Blegen (1993) found that employee turnover rates are related to the adequacy of training, methods for managing workload and schedules, opportunities for career advancement, respect from administrators, organizational recognition, social climate and work level, staffing levels, clarity of roles, and participation in decision making. Much can be done to improve the working environment and the design of jobs for long-term care workers as part of a strategy to reduce turnover rates (Feldman et al., 1990; Feldman, 1993; Banaszak-Holl and Hines, 1996; Wilner, 1999).

Criminal Background Checks

Nursing homes and home health agencies are required under Medicare and Medicaid regulations to maintain written personnel policies and procedures. Federal regulations specify that nursing home residents and home health agency clients have the right to be free from abuse and neglect and to be in a safe and secure environment (OIG, 1998). To help facility managers screen out personnel with a record of abuse, each state under federal law is required to establish and maintain a registry of nursing aides that includes information on any finding by the state survey and certification agency of abuse, neglect, or misappropriation of property involving the elderly. Federal law does not require registries for registered nurses or licensed practical nurses, but state regulatory agencies monitor professional licenses, which may be suspended or revoked for breaches of conduct such as abuse of patients. There is no national system in place by which states can share information about known abusers, so workers can now evade state registries by moving from state to state. Moreover, current federal law does not require national criminal background checks of those working in long-term care.

The Office of the Inspector General (OIG, 1998) conducted a survey of states to determine their requirements for background checks of current and prospective employees of long-term care facilities and to see if states were maintaining registries on health workers. OIG found that 33 states required criminal background checks, but the coverage of such checks varied widely and not all facilities serving the elderly were included. They also found that a majority of states required checks of nurses aides seeking employment, but did not require checks of already employed aides or other personnel such as nurses. The sources for the criminal checks also varied.

The same study found that all 37 states contacted maintained registries for NAs, LPNs, RNs, and medical practitioners. Yet, 94 percent of the states did not initiate criminal background checks of personnel when they applied for certification or licensing, 29 percent did not require prior arrest or conviction information on renewal applications, and 13 percent did not have any provision for penalties for false statements on licensing or certification applications. OIG (1998) collected criminal records at eight randomly selected nursing homes and found that 5 percent of employees had been convicted of a variety of crimes including many serious offenses such as assault, robbery, and theft. OIG recommended federal requirements for criminal background checks of all workers in nursing homes and other long-term care facilities, and assistance in the development and expansion of a national abuse registry and state registries. It also recommend requiring states to improve reporting of abuse (OIG, 1998).

At the present time, certified nursing homes and home health agencies are not required by Medicare or Medicaid to conduct a criminal record check before hiring personnel. The American Health Care Association has also recommended the development of a national abuse registry and criminal background checks for workers. The Assisted Living Quality Coalition (1998) likewise recommended that a criminal record check and a check of any aide registry that is available should be conducted three days prior to employment for all new staff. It further recommended that staff not be retained if they have been convicted of a felony or any crime involving the abuse, neglect, or exploitation of others. HCFA recommended new legislation (HCFA, 1998a) to require criminal background checks for all nursing home personnel. This proposal is currently under study by members of the U.S. Senate Special Committee on Aging.

In 1999, Senators Kohl, Reed, and Byrd introduced legislation for the Patient Abuse Prevention Act (S. 1445) to require criminal background checks for personnel in nursing homes, intermediate care facilities for the mentally retarded, home health agencies, hospices, and other facilities that receive Medicare or Medicaid funds. The legislation would also require the creation of a national registry to list all long-term care employees including professional and non-professional staff who have been found to have abused, neglected, or mistreated residents. The registry would be incorporated into the existing provider database created by the Health Insurance Portability and Accountability Act of 1996. There are issues about where the national registry would be housed and who would pay for the background checks.

Because of the vulnerability of all individuals receiving long-term care services, the committee considers that measures are needed to protect clients.

> **Recommendation 6.5: The committee recommends federal legislation requiring timely performance of criminal background checks before hiring for all personnel in all long-term care settings.**

Long-term care providers should not hire or retain people convicted of a felony or misdemeanor that involves abuse or neglect of others. Federal support is needed to ensure that criminal background checks can be conducted in a timely fashion, especially because the high turnover of the work force demands quick responses in hiring.

Involvement of Informal Caregivers

Client and family involvement in the provision of long-term care services, generally on an unpaid basis, is of critical importance in the provision of long-term care. As indicated earlier in this report, family members provide an estimated 80 percent of the long-term care for elderly people (Barusch, 1991), and they provide homes and daily support for 90 percent of the people with developmental disabilities (Bass, 1990). Under some state programs and some federal demonstration projects, family members sometimes have been paid for such care.

The role of families in long-term care for children with special health care needs is given emphasis particularly in home and community-based services. Children generally do better, in terms of both physical growth and development and cognitive and educational development, in these settings than in institutional settings (Burr, 1985; Quint et al., 1990; Patterson et al., 1992; Perrin et al., 1997). However, data from a qualitative in-depth study of everyday family life experiences suggest that families of young children with severe disabilities continue to seek out-of-home placement. Without exception, the primary desire of all families was to care for their child at home. However when placement was considered, even if remote, the most frequently reported reasons were family "survival" and mitigating circumstances. The finding that one-quarter of the families had already sought or were considering placement for children in a young age range is provocative for policy and practice (Llewellyn et al., 1999).

The impact of chronic conditions on the family is one of the major problems confronting the health care system today (Coyne, 1997). Family care-giving is a critical but finite resource. Evidence, including results of randomized trials, suggests that supports for family caregivers can have positive effects on the health outcomes and well-being of those receiving care (e.g., Zimmerman, 1984; Meyers and Marcenko, 1989; Singer et al., 1989; Herman, 1991; Yoon et al., 1993; Agosta and Melda, 1995; McFarlane et al., 1995; Mittelman et al., 1996). These studies range from those in which the intervention consisted entirely of psychosocial support to family caregivers (e.g., Singer et al., 1989; McFarlane et al., 1995; Mittelman et al., 1996) to one study in which caregivers were part of a multi-element intervention (Yoon et al., 1993).

Some states are beginning to provide client and family training in caregiving activities for clients living at home so they can be involved in the hiring, supervision, and management of care at home. The benefits of client and family involvement in care are obvious in providing services beyond the formal caregiving services, but the major benefit may be in the involvement of client and family in monitoring the quality of care. *The committee believes that state and local government long-term care programs should make educational and ongoing support available to consumers and their families who are actively involved in the hiring, training, or supervision of caregiver-staff at home and encourage efforts to foster more interaction and cooperation between formal and informal caregivers.*

Another set of concerns expressed about informal caregivers involves liability for personal injuries. However, agencies that supply privately hired caregivers have faced little litigation charging negligence (Kapp, 1991). Perhaps more serious is the risk of liability for personal injury to independent care providers who are not covered by workers' compensation insurance. Scala and Mayberry (1997) have suggested that liability concerns for consumers and programs can be minimized by making the consumer the employer of record, delineating the responsibilities of the program and the consumer, educating and assisting consumers in the selection and supervision of care providers, encouraging consumers to require criminal history checks for their providers, and providing workers' compensation as a part of the benefits package.

CONCLUSION

To succeed, efforts to improve the quality of long-term care require a work force that is sufficient in size, with the necessary skills, competence, and commitment to provide the needed health and personal care services and to manage the delivery of this care in a supportive environment. This committee has serious concerns about each of these requirements and believes that numbers, skills, training, assessment, and positive management of frontline caregivers must become a higher priority for policy makers, managers, advocacy groups, health professionals, and researchers.

The committee recognizes that the recommendations presented in this chapter would entail additional costs for providers of care. Substantial improvements in the long-term care work force are not possible without increased resources for providers of care. Government policies of reimbursing for long-term care have an important influence in improving quality of care. Reimbursement issues are discussed further in Chapter 8.

7

Building Organizational Capacity

I n the past decade, much time, money, and effort has been spent on improving care in nursing homes, with less than adequate results. Measurement tools, quality standards, and external oversight mechanisms all are important for providing quality care, but they do not ensure a capacity to use the measures correctly, implement the standards effectively, or respond to oversight as intended.

This chapter discusses the organizational capacity of a provider to manage information and personnel, the technology and resources needed to translate knowledge into improved long-term care, and the management needed for meeting policy makers' demands for accountability. Specifically, it discusses the needed technology and resources that are generally not present in long-term care settings, ways to improve organizational capacity, and the effectiveness of the guidelines and quality management initiatives in long-term care. Although this chapter focuses mostly on nursing homes, many of the issues discussed are applicable directly or with some adaptation to those providing services in other long-term care settings, such as residential care facilities and home health care.

RECENT INITIATIVES TO IMPROVE CAREGIVING CAPACITY IN LONG-TERM CARE

A number of initiatives have been put in place in recent years to facilitate the ability of nursing homes to produce better outcomes for people using long-term care. These initiatives include the following:

- *Omnibus Budget Reconciliation Act of 1987 (OBRA 87) Regulations.* Regulatory standards articulated in OBRA 87 have provided nursing homes with a specific definition of quality (e.g., considering quality of life as well as quality of care). One effect was to focus nursing homes on their residents and on achievable quality.
- *Minimum Data Set (MDS).* Standardized clinical information systems have been developed in the form of the MDS. This data set is designed to help nursing homes organize their clinical activities to meet regulatory expectations for quality of care.
- *Practice Guidelines.* Evidence-based practice guidelines, which provide the best scientific advice available on how to treat common health problems, have been developed for some long-term care settings and common geriatric conditions (e.g., incontinence, behavioral agitation, depression, and pain). These guidelines bridge the gap between the clinical research literature and the providers, often in algorithms or steps to guide assessment and treatment and thus lead to better outcomes.
- *Quality Improvement Systems.* Some nursing homes have embraced improvement philosophies and methods that have primarily been successful in settings outside of health care. These quality improvement systems focus on consumer perspectives and preferences, organize staff efforts and care processes, and guide management activities.

Taken together, these four initiatives logically begin with policies to define goals for better nursing home care and they help providers meet these goals. The logic of this approach tempts a generalization to other long-term care settings. However, there is no strong evidence that these approaches have solved major quality problems in nursing home care.

FROM RULES, DATA, AND GUIDELINES TO EFFECTIVE PRACTICE

A review of the research literature and testimony presented to the committee generated insufficient evidence to conclude that the four initiatives to improve nursing home care have improved quality to the levels expected. Previous chapters have addressed issues related to OBRA 87 and MDS initiatives. This chapter focuses on the evidence about the effectiveness of practice guidelines, initiatives in quality management systems in long-term care, and the limitations of organizational capacity to translate knowledge into improved care.

Practice guidelines were developed with the hope that they would improve health outcomes and, often more importantly, contain costs (see, e.g., PPRC, 1988, 1989; IOM, 1990, 1992). They try to make user-friendly synthesis of evidence available to providers who are unable to evaluate broad scientific and clinical literature. Over time, despite charges about "cookbook medicine" and controversy over government-sponsored guidelines, the practice guidelines fulfill a need. Accordingly, health care organizations are using careful evidence-based processes to develop guidelines. In the long-term care area, both the American Medical Directors Association and the American Geriatrics Society support practice guidelines (AMDA, 1996; AGS, 1997, 1998).

Unfortunately, studies of acute and primary care report limited implementation of guidelines, although they have also begun to identify barriers to their use and propose ways of overcoming them (see, e.g., Chassin, 1993; James, 1993; Pestornik et al., 1996; Davis and Taylor-Vaisey, 1997; Cameron and Naylor, 1999; Guyatt et al., 1999; Katz, 1999). Although long-term care is less studied than acute care, guidelines appear neither routinely nor effectively implemented by nursing home providers, nor widely known by direct care nursing home staff.

QUALITY MANAGEMENT SYSTEMS

Many nursing homes report that they have made significant investments and progress in the quality improvement area. However, like practice guidelines, it is difficult to demonstrate objectively that quality management systems have significantly improved nursing home care. Even though originally developed for the industrial sector, they are being increasingly adopted by health care organizations (Berwick, 1989; Laffel and Blumenthal, 1989; IOM, 1990; Blumenthal and Kilo, 1998; Shortell et al., 1998). Quality management principles include the following:

- a focus on consumer needs and consumers' perceptions of how well their needs are met;
- an understanding that a system is composed of processes, all of which must work together to meet consumers' needs;
- a management responsible for process design and quality management;
- a focus on those processes needed to meet consumers' needs;
- a focus primarily on how the processes work, not on individual performance;
- a data-driven quality management system that is based on objective measurements, not on guesses, intuition, or anecdotes;
- quality management measures of consumers' values and perceptions, consumers' health and well-being, and resource use and costs, as they actually occur, not as they are intended to occur; and
- measures to identify improvement opportunities, set priorities, reduce

variation in processes (including errors) and outcomes (including adverse events) such as improved health and resource efficiency.

Two major nursing home provider organizations—the American Health Care Association and the American Association for Homes and Services for the Aging—and the Joint Commission on Accreditation of Healthcare Organizations (JCAHO) support the quality management systems approach. However, there are only anecdotal reports by nursing home providers that quality improvement systems have been implemented or that implementation has resulted in improved outcomes. Moreover, this anecdotal evidence is contradicted by two studies that used controlled designs to evaluate the effectiveness of continuous quality improvement interventions (McKenna et al., 1998; Schnelle et al., 1998). The Ohio pressure ulcer project reported no improvement in pressure ulcers (McKenna et al., 1998). The incontinence study (Schnelle et al., 1998) showed improved outcomes, but only while incontinence care was provided or monitored by research staff. The researchers concluded that although practice guidelines could be implemented to improve outcomes, such improved outcomes did not in themselves provide sufficient incentive for nursing homes to maintain the program without the external monitoring and consultation provided by research staff. Limited trained staff time and organizational capacity are a barrier to improved performance in nursing homes. The improvement principles mentioned above are demanding to implement, even in organizations that are relatively rich in resources and expertise, which most long-term care organizations are not.

Most applications and most research on quality management have focused on hospitals. A recent review of the literature by Shortell and colleagues (1998) revealed some evidence of improved outcomes and reduced costs in clinical care from quality improvement techniques. It did not find evidence of organization-wide improvements in clinical performance. Another recent review suggested that in studied hospitals, the techniques had little impact on organizational culture (Gerowitz, 1998).

ORGANIZATIONAL CAPACITY TO TRANSLATE KNOWLEDGE INTO PRACTICE

Defining expectations for quality care and extending the knowledge base needed to meet these expectations will lead to improvement only if nursing homes have the capacity to translate this knowledge into practice. Unfortunately, a large gap exists between current knowledge and the industry's capacity to implement that knowledge. The missing components are the number and competence of staff and the amount and type of needed resources.

OBRA 87 regulations, practice guidelines, and quality management systems fail to emphasize these critical capacity issues, perhaps because the technical expertise of long-term care providers and the necessary tangible resources are assumed. Practice guidelines, for example, provide specific recommendations about how to treat nursing home residents based on the best knowledge available in the clinical research literature. None of the guidelines, however, include a description either of the personnel necessary to implement recommended treatment steps or of the implementation costs (Schnelle et al., 1998).

Moreover, because implementation issues are not a major focus of controlled clinical trials, they also are not a major focus of the practice guidelines. Schnelle and colleagues (1998) recommended that guidelines should be evaluated to show how they apply to long-term care settings. The lack of emphasis on such basic implementation barriers as staffing adequacy and cost is common in efforts to improve long-term care.

Long-term care providers have deemphasized the importance of organizational capacity by failing to document systematically the costs or problems associated with delivering care consistent with OBRA 87 or other regulations. Instead, these providers suggest that existing resources are adequate not only to provide care consistent with regulations, but also to implement sophisticated improvement programs—all this without a significant increase in the direct care nursing home work force since OBRA 87 was enacted. Furthermore, most nursing homes, even highly motivated ones, lack the technical expertise and tangible resource capacity necessary to translate OBRA 87 regulations, practice guidelines, and quality improvement systems into practice. The rest of this chapter discusses two broad issues relevant to improving quality of care: (1) collecting and analyzing information and (2) translating this information into care processes that address quality problems.

Collecting and Analyzing Information

Regulations, data, guidelines, and quality improvement initiatives identified above all include information collection requirements. As Johnson and Kramer (1998) point out, improving quality requires identifying problems accurately. But an information system to measure the broad array of problems experienced by nursing home residents is difficult to design and even more difficult to implement. Nursing home residents suffer from multiple clinical and functional disabilities as well as quality-of-life problems.

Unfortunately, nursing homes have little experience using information either to evaluate the quality of care or to manage staff activities; they traditionally have not employed floor supervisors with training or expertise in information management. Even today, computers typically are not found at nurses' stations or otherwise accessible to direct care staff.

Some of the issues relevant to collecting the clinical information involved in the MDS and information on quality of life or satisfaction through resident or family interviews are discussed in Chapter 4. One of the primary barriers to accurate data collection in nursing homes is the absence of standardized clinical or life quality assessment protocols. Without standardized protocols nursing homes cannot plan or budget accurate quality assessments.

The MDS is generated from the perception of a nursing home workforce that is largely paraprofessional, temporary, and in need of more professional supervision. Such staff is not competent to provide the precise ratings in multiple areas of the MDS. Furthermore, accurately completing the annual or quarterly MDS reports is only part of the challenge. There are 18 resident assessment protocols (RAPs), which are triggered by problems noted in the MDS items. For example, a series of additional assessments are recommended for residents rated on the MDS as showing low oral food intake. Two separate studies reported that over 60 percent of nursing home residents would be triggered for these follow-up assessments (Pokrywka et al., 1997; Simmons and Reuben, 2000). Given the number of residents who need to have MDS and RAP assessments completed, it is surprising that there is no information about what staff time, supervisory oversight, or training mechanisms are necessary to collect these data accurately. Apparently, nursing homes are assumed to have both the tangible resources and the technical expertise necessary for accurate MDS and RAP assessments. The assumption of "adequate resources" seems particularly tenuous when the additional resource requirements of assessing resident or family perceptions of quality are considered. The latter measures are not covered in the MDS and involve significant technical challenges and resources that are different from those involved in completing the MDS, and assessment is only the first step in improving quality and not even the most labor-intensive step.

Translating Information into Practice

Assuming that accurate information can be collected, the result is not quality improvement unless it is translated into practice. Two major aspects of translating clinical or quality-of-life information into practice require organizing information to identify quality problems; and implementing, managing, and evaluating care processes to resolve quality problems.

Automated information-processing technologies help providers use

MDS information to evaluate outcomes. The barriers to using this information to improve care are due primarily to obsolete information technologies and the ability of staff to interpret the information. Mechanisms exist to organize MDS information either at the resident or at the aggregated level (e.g., facility or region). The resident assessment protocol (RAP) is a brief version of a practice guideline that makes recommendations about further assessment and treatment after a problem or potential problem has been identified (e.g., How do you assess and treat a resident whom you suspect is dehydrated?). This triggering system can be managed manually or with specially designed software. This triggering software may automatically generate care plans that are not appropriately individualized, This problem suggests that nursing home staff will need education in how to use information-processing technologies (Harrington et al., 1996).

Recently, software has been designed that aggregates MDS data into risk-adjusted quality indicators (e.g., number of residents with pressure ulcers who have high or low risk factors for that condition) (Zimmerman et al., 1995). The primary purpose of this is to identify facilities with unusual quality indicator scores. Quality indicators are now also incorporated in the survey process. Presumably, state survey staff can target problem facilities and motivate nursing homes that score poorly to correct problems. Whether this approach will achieve its purposes is unclear because it is based on the following three untested assumptions:

1. survey staff will know which processes to assess in nursing homes that have scored poorly on quality indicators;
2. nursing homes that score poorly do, in fact, implement different care processes than nursing homes that score well; and
3. significant and stable variation in the quality indicator performance scores will allow identification of both "good" and "bad" nursing homes.

One study reported that stable differences between nursing homes in Massachusetts were not evident on nine different indicators monitored over a three-year period (Porell et al., 1998). The authors concluded that it might not be possible to identify "good" nursing homes using clinical quality indicator data. Other studies have concluded that indicators are stable over a short time (Karon et al., 1999). Clearly, further research is needed on all three assumptions. As mentioned, quality indicator software produces summary scores which do not provide caregivers with the specific information necessary to influence the care of an individual resident, even though it might allow nursing homes to identify groups of residents with a common problem and monitor their progress over a period of time. Effective clinical practice requires constant adjustments in the resident's treatment. With this in mind, and because the health of nursing home residents can generally be expected to decline, a technology is needed to track the expected rate of decline for both individuals and for groups of residents in the same risk-adjusted categories (Kane et al., 1998b).

Lack of such automated information organization systems is a resource barrier to organizing MDS information for better care and regulation. Labor resources are less of a barrier to data organization than they are to accurate data collection. However, the time and intellectual resources required to prepare primary MDS data collection forms for computer entry are significant. In summary, better automated information systems to organize MDS data are essential to improve care in nursing homes.

IDENTIFYING EFFECTIVE INTERVENTIONS

The initiatives for improving care processes and outcomes include recommendations for assessment and treatment. Although the costs of implementing the assessment recommendations are unknown, they are likely to exceed nursing home resources. If the resources needed to implement treatments are factored in, nursing home resources are likely to be overwhelmed.

As was discussed earlier in this chapter, practice guidelines and RAPs are two initiatives designed to help nursing home staff identify processes that will improve outcomes. Two contradictory criticisms have been made about these initiatives. First, guidelines are too "prescriptive" and the nursing home work force (presumably mostly nurse assistants) should be able to design their own interventions to improve quality. This position puts significant pressure on an overworked, underpaid, and unstable paraprofessional work force. It also contradicts the basic assumption underlying practice guidelines that even highly paid professionals need advice and assistance. In fact, most guideline recommendations are intended to influence physician practice. Furthermore, as one reads the guidelines or RAPs with an eye toward implementing them, the argument that they are overly prescriptive loses force. Indeed, the second criticism is that these initiatives lack sufficient specificity for providers who are not expert in any one particular content area (e.g., depression) and who are consumed with the simple demands of daily care (Schnelle et al., 1998). Clearly no guidelines have been tested under realistic field conditions for the purpose of answering the following questions:

1. Can the guideline recommendations be implemented by staff who are not specifically trained in the guideline content area?

2. How time-consuming is it to implement the guidelines? What skills are needed to do so? How do these time and skill requirements match those typically available in nursing homes?
3. What are the effects of implementing the guidelines?

A great deal of clinical expertise, creativity, and time is needed to fully implement the assessment and treatment recommendations contained in the 12 practice guidelines available pertaining to nursing home residents and the 18 RAPs. At present, there is little reason to believe that nursing home staff will have either the technical expertise or reimbursed time necessary to implement even the assessment recommendations in the RAPs and practice guidelines.

At the same time, many low-tech, common sense interventions can improve nursing home quality outcomes. For example, multiple controlled clinical trials have demonstrated that urinary incontinence in most nursing home residents can be improved with simple toileting assistance programs (Creason et al., 1989; Schnelle, 1990; Colling et al., 1992; Hu et al., 1995). Although simple, these interventions are often more time-consuming to implement than the usual care processes conducted in nursing homes. Also, the labor costs associated with implementing care processes may be even more than those associated with conducting assessments.

The above discussion shows that practice guidelines and RAPs rarely have been developed with an eye towards getting providers to understand what personnel would most appropriately implement them and what are the costs associated with them.

CARE PROCESS IMPLEMENTATION AND IMPROVEMENT

Simple (i.e., not technically complicated) interventions can improve nursing home resident outcomes, but it is doubtful that there is enough staff to implement these simple but time-intensive interventions. Furthermore, improvement management models designed to facilitate the implementation of validated care processes require a significant expenditure of time for measurement and analysis. These expenses increase the total cost of implementing the processes.

The care patterns of nursing home staff have been described in observational studies by multiple research teams starting with the classic study by Baltes and her colleagues in 1983. This study documented that caregivers were more likely to reinforce resident behaviors characterized as dependent as opposed to independent (e.g., providing excessive physical assistance with movement instead of reinforcing residents for independent efforts to move). Not much has changed in 20 years. More recent observational studies in the areas of incontinence, mobility and exercise, dressing, and nutrition show that caregivers still tend to provide care that is time-efficient but is inconsistent with maintaining residents' highest level of functioning. For example, nursing aides (NAs) prefer to change wet residents because this takes significantly less time than toileting, even though toileting promotes continence (Schnelle et al., 1988a).

Nursing assistants employ time-efficient care practices that incidentally reinforce dependence and functional decline. Their workloads are inconsistent with the labor-intensive care processes to promote independence. However, no study has yet documented how many residents a nurse assistant can effectively care for, suggesting a large gap in this area.

Multiple studies indicate that staffing in nursing homes is inadequate to provide care that meets consumer expectations or is consistent with maximizing residents' independence. For example, families and residents interviewed in three different projects consistently identified staffing as their primary problem with nursing home care (VA, 1994; Gustafson and Gustafson, 1996; Norton et al., 1996). Inadequate staffing also was repeatedly identified as a problem in testimony both before this committee and before the Senate committee that commissioned the General Accounting Office to report on nursing home care (U.S. Special Committee on Aging, 1998, 1999). In addition, nursing aides themselves have reported in three separate studies that they have insufficient time to implement toileting programs or interventions designed to improve food intake among residents, and to individualize care (Kayser-Jones and Schell, 1997; Lekan-Rutledge et al., 1998; Walker et al., 1999). Finally, observational studies contrast the actual time spent providing usual care to the increased time required to implement care processes that promote better outcomes.

Controlled intervention studies by different research teams show that incontinence can be improved within one to three days using a toileting assistance program (Creason et al., 1989; Schnelle, 1990; Colling et al., 1992; Hu et al., 1995); but perhaps because of the increased staff time costs involved with a continence program, nursing home staff did not maintain improved continence by consistently providing the requested toileting assistance in even the most responsive residents after research staff left the facility (Schnelle et al., 1990; Schnelle et al., 1993, 1995b).

Similarly, other studies of ambulatory residents with high risk of functional decline show that mobility declines with inactivity, use of restraints, and fear of falling (Schnelle, 1992a; Schnelle et al., 1995b; MacRae et al., 1996). These residents need guidance and physical assistance with walking, which requires time- and attention-consuming care. An integrated protocol, called Functional Incidental Training (FIT) combines continence care with ambulation exercise. FIT implemented every two hours, four times a day for eight weeks, significantly increases walking endurance, physical activity levels and standing ability (Schnelle et al., 1995b), while contributing to continence training. Time cost analysis shows that staff time and cost differentials are high, but there is no apparent way to reduce the time needed to implement the intervention protocols (Schnelle et al., 1995a). Supervised exercise is necessary to prevent mobility declines and physically dependent residents need labor-intensive toileting assistance to be continent. Also, the frequency of walking assistance and incontinence care in these studies are consistent with resident and family preferences for such assistance (Schnelle et al., 1988a, 1995b; Simmons and Schnelle, 1999).

As in continence and mobility, the activity of daily living of dressing can be improved with slower, but greater resident involvement. Excessive assistance in dressing saves staff time but produces dependence (Beck et al., 1997; Rogers et al., 1999). However, the time needed to promote independent dressing exceeds the time that staff usually devote to assistance with dressing. One dressing intervention study reported that nursing staff failed to maintain residents' independence levels once research staff stopped implementing the prompting protocol (Beck et al., 1997).

Similarly, nutrition may be enhanced with labor intensive prompting strategies. Nursing home staff do not spend sufficient time assisting residents at risk for under-nourishment (Backstrom et al., 1987; Kayser-Jones et al., 1997; Steele et al., 1997). In addition, staff often either provide excessive physical assistance with feeding or pressure residents to eat quickly, apparently because of work-related time pressures (Kayser-Jones et al., 1997). Even residents who are physically capable of feeding themselves are at-risk for under-nutrition if they are regarded as "slow eaters" by nursing home staff. Two sudies reported that increased staff attention may be effective with nutrition (Lange-Alberts and Shott, 1994; Van Ort and Phillips, 1995) and an expert consensus group has reported that a staffing level of two to three residents per one aide is needed at mealtimes (Harrington et al., 2000c); the usual ratios are 10 to 1 or higher.

In summary, the various intervention studies reviewed here pertaining to four different domains—continence training, mobility, dressing, and nutrition—have reported consistent results. They provide strong evidence that simple interventions that use prompting and graduated physical assistance will produce better outcomes in nursing home residents. The interventions produce comparatively better results during the research period, in part because usual care processes are done too infrequently to promote better outcomes, or provide excessive physical assistance, which undermines the resident's ability to perform independently. Unfortunately, usual care practices are less time-consuming and less costly than promoting strategies that lead to more independence and better outcomes. The available time-based estimates of the staffing needed to implement better care processes indicate that nursing homes are inadequately staffed to provide care that maximizes residents' independence and, by implication, their quality of life. These labor resource barriers become more daunting when requirements of improvement management models are added. Such improvement management models involve their own intellectual and labor resource costs, which go beyond those just discussed.

MEASUREMENT ISSUES

The core components of an improvement management model, described earlier in this chapter, have been embraced by both nursing home providers and others in the health care industry in part because the model is intuitively appealing and has worked well in other settings, primarily industrial settings. However, the model may be more difficult to replicate successfully in health care settings due in part to measurement costs and related issues, although there is some evidence that continuous improvement models have been implemented successfully in acute care settings (Berwick and Bisognano, 1998).[1]

An improvement model focuses on work processes that are both under the control of providers and causally related to outcomes. The strategy is to frequently monitor these processes so as to identify and control the factors that interfere with their successful implementation. This should lead to continuous process improvements and thus, to improved outcomes. With this strategy, it would be inefficient to wait until outcomes are reported to conclude that care is either good or bad. In most cases, care processes have to be conducted poorly for extended periods to produce bad outcomes. Instead, the improvement model continuously analyzes work processes to prevent bad outcomes from ever occurring.

Implementing an improvement model successfully entails adding further to the already high measurement burden incurred by nursing homes. In industrial and service settings, where the improvement management model is most successful, very frequent and even continuous records of work processes are available. For example, continuous measures of assembly-line work processes are generated with computerized measurement technologies.

In most health care settings there are few, if any, process-monitoring technologies analogous to those in industrial settings. In nursing homes, nursing staff record some data relevant to processes on work flow-sheets (e.g., reposition every two hours, ambulate one time). However, these

---

[1]A more complete discussion of the barriers to implementing improvement models in nursing homes (e.g., unstable staff) has been published (Schnelle et al., 1993).

self-reported data are of suspect accuracy and in some cases are too non-descriptive (e.g., change wet residents as needed) to be useful for improvement management purposes.

Cost-efficient methods for measuring work processes in health care settings are largely unavailable at this time, and considerable creativity is needed to develop such methods. Recent research, for example, shows that approximately 48 percent of nursing home residents can accurately describe the care they receive (Simmons et al., 1997). Thus, it is possible that accurate reporters could be targeted and systematically interviewed as a means of determining whether care processes are being implemented (e.g., "Were you given walking assistance today?"). This system *could* work, but whether it is affordable and whether nursing home residents will cooperate is unknown. Other innovative monitoring systems have used hand-held computers to facilitate frequent records of care activities and microchips to continuously record resident movements, wetness levels, and staff contact with residents (Holmes, 1996). The microchip technology potentially permits continuous monitoring, similar to the continuous process data collection that occurs in industrial improvement models.

These high-tech solutions to process-monitoring have been criticized by some as dehumanizing care. At the same time, a counter-argument has been made that these methods provide the missing information needed to effectively manage consumer-centered care, and that nursing aides need the feedback provided by such information to sustain high motivation for their job. Clearly, more research is needed in this area, including studies that assess resident, family, and staff perceptions of these new technologies. Given the potential of automated process-monitoring systems to resolve both accuracy problems that have been reported with nursing home data recording systems and given their obvious usefulness for improvement management purposes, these research programs should receive a high priority.

Nonetheless, long-term care is years away from having a cost-effective process and information monitoring technology that is acceptable to all stakeholders and is as useful as the systems used in industrial settings. In the absence of such a technology, it is not surprising that nursing homes and other healthcare settings have experienced difficulty in implementing successful improvement models. Research is needed to test feasibility and cost effectiveness of implementing clinical practice guidelines and proven care interventions in long-term care settings. As stated earlier, there is an increasing number of guidelines and interventions that require rigorous testing to determine the costs of training, implementation, and maintenance, as well as the impact on key resident outcomes.

IMPROVING ORGANIZATIONAL CAPACITY

The high expectations for improved care created by post-OBRA 87 requirements, such as the MDS, suggest objective analyses of the resources needed to operationalize and implement the initiatives. Pressuring nursing homes to document care consistent with the regulatory requirements may be counterproductive in the absence of sound estimates of resource requirements and the match between these requirements and those actually available (Schnelle et al., 1997).

Certainly, current nursing home resources can be used more effectively and efficiently to improve care. But lack of a more realistic analysis of the resources needed and currently available to fulfill the intent of OBRA 87 prevents more objective resolution of these financially focused arguments. In addition, simply spending more money on nursing home care without improvements in other factors associated with quality care will not result in significant improvement (see Chapter 8 for a review of evidence linking payment to quality). This report emphaizes the inadequacy of staffing levels in nursing homes and the consequent deficiency in long-term care services. However, increasing staffing levels without simultaneously improving their education and training, and management systems will most certainly result in less-than-expected improvement. The management problems related to accurate measurement of staff performance as well as numerous other management issues must be resolved to fully realize the benefits of increased staffing.

The committee has made several recommendations throughout the report that could resolve organizational capacity problems that have been raised in this chapter. For example, recommendations made in Chapter 6 regarding staffing are necessary ingredients for significantly improving organizational capacity (see Recommendations 6.1, 6.2, and 6.3). In addition, the committee offers the following recommendations to resolve the primary organizational capacity problems that have been discussed in this chapter related to both technical (e.g., how to manage staff) and tangible resources (e.g., how many staff and with what education and training levels are needed, and what are the costs associated with them?).

Recommendation 7.1: The committee recommends that the Department of Health and Human Services fund research to examine the actual time and staff mix required in different long-term care settings to provide adequate processes and outcomes of care consistent with the needs and variability of consumers in these settings, and the fit between these needs and other existing staffing patterns. The Committee further recommends

that the Department of Health and Human Services, by establishing Centers for the Advancement of Quality in Long-Term Care, initiate research, demonstration, and training programs for long-term care providers to redesign care processes consistent with best practices and improvements in quality of life.

The committee believes that the Centers for the Advancement of Quality in Long-Term Care could be research, development, and teaching sites. Their functions could be partially listed as follows:

- Implement and develop clinical or quality-of-life assessment protocols for all long-term care settings as described in Recommendation 4.1.
- Implement and evaluate care processes that are demonstrated to improve measures of clinical or life quality.
- Demonstrate the resource requirements for implementing all assessment and care processes including the costs of training and managing staff in the provision of care.
- Serve as training sites for long-term care providers who are willing to invest in improving capacity.
- Serve as test sites for policy makers who need a realistic appraisal of the cost and feasibility of implementing regulatory standards being considered for legislative approval.

CONCLUSION

This chapter argues that most nursing homes, even highly motivated ones, may lack the technical expertise and resources—including but not limited to staffing levels—necessary to translate OBRA 87 regulations, practice guidelines, and quality improvement systems into practice. A strong case is made in this and the previous chapter that nursing home staffing levels are inadequate and that there will be little improvement until this issue is addressed. However, increasing staffing without simultaneously improving management systems will most certainly result in less-than-expected improvement. The management problems related to accurate measurement described in this chapter, as well as numerous other management issues, will have to be addressed to realize fully the benefit of increased staffing. These problems should not be used by any stakeholders to justify abandoning efforts to improve care. The discussions in this chapter support realistic directions for improvement that should take long-term care to the next level of quality.

8

Reimbursing to Improve Quality of Care

Over the past ten years, quality assurance initiatives for long-term care have focused on regulatory programs, such as strengthening the survey and certification process for providers. In contrast, relatively few efforts have highlighted the role that reimbursement can play in promoting or inhibiting the quality of long-term care. Contributing to the lack of emphasis on reimbursement is the paucity of conclusive data on the topic, a situation that has changed little since the 1986 Institute of Medicine (IOM) report on nursing homes. Some studies have linked poor quality of care in nursing homes to low Medicaid payment rates, but others have posited that quality-of-care deficiencies should be attributed to factors such as excess demand (Nyman, 1993). Although relatively little is known about the effect of reimbursement on quality of care in nursing homes, virtually nothing is known about its impact on other settings or on home and community-based services.

Two recent developments have directed new attention to the relationship between reimbursement and the quality of long-term care. First, the federal Balanced Budget Act of 1997 repealed federal standards for reimbursing nursing home care under the Medicaid program (the Boren amendment), giving states virtually unlimited freedom in setting nursing home payment rates. For Medicaid home and community-based waiver

---

Much of the information in this chapter draws from the background paper commissioned from J.M. Wiener and D.G. Stevenson for use by the committee.

service states have always had complete freedom in determining reimbursement levels. The nursing home industry has warned that Medicaid reimbursement levels already are too low and that further reductions would adversely affect the quality of care. Second, the Balanced Budget Act of 1997 also dramatically altered Medicare reimbursement methods for nursing homes and home health agencies and combined these changes with large budget savings. In some cases the changes have been major. As states gain new freedom to set Medicaid nursing home reimbursement levels and the federal government reduces Medicare payments, it becomes increasingly important to understand whether and how these changes might affect access and quality in long-term care. As reported below, changes in payment policies are creating great turmoil in the long-term care sector. The withdrawal of substantial resources from long-term care providers is troubling, especially because many of the recommendations in this report require more, not less, funding.

REIMBURSEMENT AND QUALITY

Research on reimbursement and its potential impact on the quality of care generally focuses on two broad areas of concern. First, what is the relationship between the costs of long-term care and the quality of care? This policy question is important because like most other areas of Medicaid policy, nursing home reimbursement levels and methods vary dramatically by state. For example, average Medicaid nursing home reimbursement rates for 1998 varied from a low of $62.58 per day in Nebraska to a high of $329.62 per day in Alaska. Second, does the method of payment (e.g., flat rate, prospective payment, use or type of casemix adjustment), independent of its level, affect the quality of care? This is potentially very important since government policy makers have considerable control over these policy levers.

Level of Cost or Payment and Quality

Although measuring cost and payment levels is comparatively straightforward, measuring the quality of care is not, and the way quality is assessed can significantly affect the results of studies that examine the relationship between the two. All of the studies examined here focused on nursing homes.

Most studies have analyzed the relationship between cost or payment and quality by using some form of input (e.g., staffing levels) or process indicator as the measure of quality. For example, using 1995–1996 Online Survey and Certification Assessment Reporting (OSCAR) System data, Harrington and colleagues (1998b,c) found a small but positive relationship between the amount of Medicaid reimbursement and nurse staffing levels (except for nursing assistants) and reported fewer certification deficiencies in facilities with higher staffing levels.

Questions can be raised about the appropriateness of using structural measures of quality because increased inputs imply, almost by definition, higher costs. That is, input and cost are likely to be positively related regardless of whether there is a relationship between cost and "real" quality. Several studies have found that higher reimbursement is associated with higher staffing, but they failed to find a significant relationship to other measures of quality (Nyman, 1988b; Zinn, 1994; Cohen and Spector, 1996). For example, Zinn (1994) found that higher reimbursement was associated with higher registered nurse staffing but, surprisingly, also with more use of restraints and a greater proportion of residents who were not toileted.

Only a few limited studies have examined the relationship between facility costs and quality using outcomes-based quality measures. Using 1983 data from Iowa, Nyman (1988b) found that costs were not significantly greater in nursing homes with higher quality as measured by various outcomes (including wearing clean clothing, being fully dressed, and having clean hair). At the same time, these outcome measures of quality were found to be associated with nursing time per patient. Similarly, using 1987 National Medical Expenditure Survey data, Cohen and Spector (1996) did not find a statistically significant relationship between reimbursement level and outcomes-based quality measures (including mortality, change in functional status, and presence of decubitus ulcers), while at the same time they did find a positive relationship between reimbursement level and staffing intensity. It appears that many aspects of quality care (e.g., staff attitude or administrative philosophy) do not require large expenditures and are not significantly related to facility costs (Ullman, 1987; Nyman, 1988b). Thus, improved quality might not necessarily imply higher costs, and poor quality might not simply be a result of inadequate resources.

The results of the Nyman (1988b) and Cohen and Spector (1996) studies illustrate the complexity of the relationship among costs, inputs, and outcomes and the dilemma for states in trying to establish payment rates that are adequate to produce quality care. Both found a relationship between cost or reimbursement level and staffing intensity, and both analyses found that professional staffing had a positive and significant relationship to quality of care in terms of outcomes. However, the effects of higher cost or reimbursement levels on staffing and of staffing on outcomes were not large enough for cost or reimbursement to have a statistically significant impact on quality as measured by outcomes.

Although there does not appear to be a simple relationship between cost and quality, logic suggests that there is some minimal level of reimbursement below which it will be either difficult or impossible for nursing homes to provide an adequate level of care. Moreover, current quality-of-care problems in long-term care should make policy makers alert to the possible negative impact of reducing the resources available to long-term care providers.

> **Recommendation 8.1: The committee recommends that, before making decisions to reduce reimbursements, state officials carefully assess the impact on access to services and on quality of care of any proposed reductions in Medicaid reimbursements for nursing home, home health and other home and community-based services.**

> **Recommendation 8.2: The committee recommends that the Department of Health and Human Services fund and support research to better understand the effects of payment policies on accessibility and quality of long-term care services, including the following:**
>
> - **the effects of low reimbursement rates or changes in Medicare and Medicaid reimbursement policies on providers of nursing home, home health, or other long-term care services;**
> - **the effects of current payment systems, such as prospective payment for nursing facilities and interim payment systems for home health agencies, on the accessibility and quality of services; and**
> - **whether states with low Medicaid reimbursement rates (adjusted for geographic variation in prices and other state-specific requirements) have lower quality of nursing home care.**

Method of Reimbursement and Quality

Setting Medicaid reimbursement rates for long-term care is one way in which states control expenditures and shape the long-term care market. To achieve savings, states focus not only on the overall level of reimbursement but also on the payment methodology used to reimburse long-term care providers. These policies differ most fundamentally on two levels: (1) whether they base payment on facility-specific costs or on a set of flat rates (set independently of an individual facility's costs) and (2) whether rates are set retrospectively or prospectively.

Facility-specific rates (set either prospectively or retrospectively) are based on an individual facility's costs, usually up to some ceiling. Under this type of payment, higher-cost facilities receive higher payments than lower-cost facilities. Under flat rates, nursing homes are paid a rate that is not based on the individual facility's costs. Typically, flat rates are based on the cost experience of all facilities in an area (sometimes adjusted for facility or patient characteristics such as the casemix of a nursing home's residents).

Under retrospective cost-based payment, nursing homes receive a facility-specific interim payment rate based on costs for some base year, with adjustment for inflation. If the actual costs (usually up to some ceiling) are different from the interim rate, either the state pays the facility or the facility pays the state the difference. This methodology encourages facilities to spend more (perhaps improving quality) because they can be reimbursed for their expenses, although ceilings on allowable costs and lags in altering rates affect on the incentive for facilities to increase spending.

Almost all states use prospective payment systems to pay nursing homes. Under prospective payment, providers receive a rate set in advance for a bundle of services, without adjustment for actual costs. Like a capitated payment for managed care, providers are at financial risk if facility costs exceed payments; alternately, providers can keep the surplus as profits should payments exceed their costs. To the extent that facilities make money by curtailing services, quality may be adversely affected. In theory, this should be more of a problem for flat-rate systems because there is no relationship between an individual facility's costs and its reimbursement. In contrast, facility-specific prospective payment systems periodically recalculate a facility's base costs. Thus, if a facility dramatically reduced its expenses, its future rate would also be reduced, limiting the extent to which it is in the nursing home's interest to reduce costs.

Empirical studies tend to support these theoretical expectations. Using cost-reporting data from eight states from 1978 to 1980, Holahan and Cohen (1987) found strong evidence that the cost containment incentives in state reimbursement systems appeared to have a real impact on cost increases: prospective and flat-rate systems generally reduced cost growth more than retrospective payment. Aggressive cost control strategies were also found to have a constraining effect on spending for direct care services (and therefore might adversely affect patient care). Patient care-related costs were constrained more than non-patient care-related costs in reimbursement systems with stronger cost-controlling incentives. At least in the short term, cost containment measures did not negatively affect access for Medicaid recipients.

Using 1981 Medicare and Medicaid Automated Certification Survey files and Medicare cost reports, Cohen and Dubay (1990) found that as cost containment incentives became stronger (e.g., the use of flat-rate payments), nursing homes responded by decreasing the severity of their casemix (e.g., limiting access for heavy care residents) and decreasing staffing levels. Nursing homes in states that paid flat rates had fewer nurses per bed than similar homes in cost-based reimbursement states. In addition, access for Medicaid recipients was worse in states with flat-rate reimbursement and better in states with prospective reimbursement. Finally, prospectively paid nursing facilities did not have costs that differed significantly from retrospectively paid facilities. However, facilities that were paid flat rates under Medicaid had significantly lower costs.

Prospective payment also can affect patient care services differently, depending on the bundle of services included in the unit of payment. For example, prospective payment rates may or may not include ancillary services such as prescription drugs and therapy services. In a study of five states, Moore and White (1998) compared New York—which includes prescription drugs in its prospective payments for nursing homes—to four states that reimburse prescription drugs on a fee-for-service basis (i.e., separate from the prospective rate). Their study found that prescription drug utilization for the treatment of selected medical conditions was significantly lower in New York than in the comparison states, suggesting that nursing homes responded to financial incentives of fixed payment.

Casemix Reimbursement

One variation of flat-rate reimbursement that many states have adopted is casemix reimbursement. An undesirable incentive of pure flat-rate payments (and, to a lesser extent, facility-specific methodologies) is for nursing homes to avoid costly residents who are severely disabled, since reimbursement is no greater for residents with heavy care needs than for those with light care needs. Casemix reimbursement systems are designed to mitigate the effects of these perverse incentives by matching the payment level to an individual's care needs. Under casemix reimbursement, nursing homes receive higher reimbursement when individuals require more services. The major theoretical strength of casemix reimbursement is to make nursing homes indifferent to the relative care needs of the individuals they admit.

Despite these advantages, casemix reimbursement also creates disincentives for nursing homes to rehabilitate residents (since they are paid more for more disabled residents) or to provide services that diminish their profits (since profits represent the difference between reimbursement and expenditures). These systems also create incentives for nursing homes to misreport resident conditions or services received. In their analysis of 1987 data from six states, Butler and Schlenker (1989) found some evidence that these problems did in fact occur and concluded that casemix reimbursement systems must include explicit ways to measure and ensure quality of care. In their review of the casemix reimbursement literature, Weissert and Musliner (1992) concluded that casemix payment by itself generally did little to improve quality of care. Higher casemix payments were not necessarily used to increase nursing home staffing levels or expenditures (Davis et al., 1998). In contrast, research is more positive on the use of casemix systems to improve access to care, although improving access for residents who require heavy care can create access difficulties for those who require light care (and arguably should be served outside of nursing homes).

Prospective Payment for Medicare Post-Acute Care Services

The Balanced Budget Act of 1997 (BBA 97) mandated the establishment of casemix-adjusted prospective payment systems for various Medicare post-acute care services, including nursing facility and home health services. These changes were expected to result in substantial reductions in Medicare expenditures for home health agencies and nursing facilities compared to what expenditures would have been without the changes. Reflecting concerns about the potential impact of these changes on people who use nursing home and home health services, the Medicare Payment Advisory Commission (MedPAC) recommended that DHHS establish systems to monitor quality of care as prospective payment is implemented for nursing homes and home health agencies (MedPAC, 1999).

The BBA 97 also moved nursing facility services into a prospective payment system (PPS), transitioning over three cost-reporting periods starting in July 1998. The new payment system is supposed to pay appropriately for the level of care needed and to control costs. Nursing facilities receive a casemix-adjusted, per diem payment based on a blend of national and facility-specific payment amounts. The payment bundles nursing, therapy, and capital payments into a single per diem amount. This is expected to constrain the growth in therapy or ancillary service use, where much of the recent growth in expenditures has occurred. Many observers argue that the methodology does not adequately account for the costs of nontherapy ancillaries such as prescription drugs (GAO, 1999e). A major concern is that the methods and data for casemix-adjusted payments are inadequate to design incentives that discourage providers from skimping on care or from avoiding consumers who need greater amounts of care (MedPAC, 1998). MedPAC recommendations for refining the nursing facility prospective payment system include (1) improving the system's ability to predict resources associated with patient need for nontherapy ancillary services (e.g., respiratory therapy, drugs); (2) updating payment weights to reflect such factors as changing technology and care patterns; and (3) developing methods to review the accuracy of facility assessments and classification of residents for payment purposes (MedPAC, 1999). The committee did not investigate payment issues at this level of specificity, but these recommendations appear reasonable in light of the committee's concerns.

In addition, the BBA 97 requires that nursing facilities reimburse therapists directly for services delivered in the facility, regardless of whether the service was provided by in-house staff or external organizations. Independent therapists will no longer be able to bill Medicare directly. As part of the transition, the cost limits for fiscal year 1998 will be adjusted to incorporate the cost limits frozen in 1994 and 1995. Like all prospective payment systems, a risk is that facilities may reduce what they spend on care in order to increase profits.

Although the BBA 97 also requires the implementation of a prospective payment system for home health, it gives the Health Care Financing Administration (HCFA) great discretion in its design. A home health prospective payment system was originally scheduled to be implemented in October 2000, but has been postponed by subsequent legislation. Reflecting congressional belief that aggregate payments were too high, reimbursement rates are to be adjusted downward by 15 percent when the prospective payment system is implemented.

In the meantime, an interim payment system based on modified cost limits is in place for home health care. Agencies are paid the lowest of their costs, 106 percent of the median cost for freestanding agencies, or average per-beneficiary expenditures. This third ceiling, average per-beneficiary expenditures, which is 75 percent based on facility-specific experience and 25 percent based on regional average costs, makes it difficult for agencies to change their service mix to provide either more expensive nursing services or more home health aide visits per patient.

The interim payment system for home health care is very controversial. Some researchers have warned that the system could restrict access to care, especially for high-use consumers (Komisar and Feder, 1998; Lewin Group, 1998). In addition, as originally specified by BBA 97, the interim payment system could be particularly difficult for several types of providers including home health agencies in rural areas, small agencies that have a large number of high-use residents, agencies that serve a more disabled population than in 1994 (the base year for payment calculations), and agencies that have formed as a result of recent mergers or acquisitions.

Implementation of the provisions of BBA 97 created great turbulence in the nursing home and home health industries. Nursing homes have complained that the budget cuts are too large, that consolidated billing is administratively burdensome, and that nontherapy ancillaries are not adequately recognized in the payment rate. Stock prices for publicly traded nursing home chains have plummeted dramatically, and seven national nursing home chains have filed for Chapter 11 bankruptcy protection, accounting for nearly 10 percent of the nation's nursing home beds (Childs, 2000; Editor, 2000; Vickery, 2000). While the industry blames changes in Medicare reimbursement policy for these problems, the General Accounting Office (GAO, 1999e) largely attributes them to poor business decisions.

The impact of the reimbursement changes on home health agencies has been even more dramatic, with Medicare expenditures falling drastically. Medicare home health expenditures declined 45 percent between 1997 and 1999 (CBO, 2000). In addition, the number of Medicare-certified home health agencies dropped from 10,444 in 1997 to 7,747 in 1999, a figure that is still far above the number of agencies in the early 1990s (NAHC, 2000). A GAO study of early implementation of the interim payment system found that it had not caused significant access problems for beneficiaries (GAO, 1998c). In part, this reflects the fact that the number of agencies nearly doubled between 1989 and 1997. The GAO did note the possibility of access problems for high-cost beneficiaries, but characterized them as relatively few and possibly related to other characteristics of the Medicare program. The 1999 MedPAC report noted concerns about the interim payment system but did not recommend further changes. The report noted the difficulties of designing a prospective payment system for home health care that "appropriately classified patients who require both short- and longer-term home health services" (MedPAC, 1999, p. 92).

Responding to the uproar caused by the Balanced Budget Act, in 1999 Congress passed and President Clinton signed the Medicare, Medicaid, and the State Children's Health Insurance Program (SCHIP) Balanced Budget Refinement Act of 1999. This legislation provides modest financial relief to a variety of providers, including nursing facilities and home health agencies. For nursing facilities, the legislation temporarily would increase the federal per diem by 20 percent for 15 Resource Utilization Groups (RUGs) in the categories of "extensive services," "special care," "clinically complex," "high rehabilitation," and "medium rehabilitation." According to the BBA, increased payments are made starting April 1, 2000, or with the implementation of a refined RUG system. In fiscal years 2001 and 2002, the federal per diem rate will increase by 4 percent for each year. In addition, starting in April 2000, separate payments are made for certain ancillary services.

For home health agencies, the legislation will add $1.3 billion in home health reimbursement over five years by delaying the 15 percent reduction in payments until after the first year of the prospective payment system. The law also slightly increases per-beneficiary cost for some agencies, removes the consolidated billing requirement for durable medical equipment, provides a $10 payment for completing a patient assessment, and revises the surety bond requirements.

Given the repercussions of these reimbursement changes for the long-term care industry, it is critical that the HCFA and Congress have accurate, up-to-date information.

Reimbursement Incentives to Improve Quality of Care

Some researchers have proposed that reimbursement be linked directly to quality of care (Zinn, 1994). Pointing out that reimbursement and quality assurance are typically defined by independent systems with separate objectives, Shaughnessy and Kurowski (1982) detailed several areas of research that have to be addressed before this linkage is possible, including the development of better process and outcomes measures, identification of quality norms, and development of incentives to change provider behavior. Although their article was written 18 years ago, most of the same limitations in the research base remain today.

There have been some experiments with outcomes-based incentives. A demonstration in San Diego in the early 1980s tested the effectiveness of monetary incentives in improving the health of nursing home residents and reducing Medicaid expenditures. These incentives for improved outcomes were found to have beneficial effects on quality, access, and number of hospital transfers (Norton, 1992). Other initiatives in Illinois, Connecticut, and Michigan have not been evaluated.

LIMITED NURSING HOME BED SUPPLY AND QUALITY OF CARE

Several studies done in the 1970s and early 1980s found a strong relationship between poor quality and a high percentage of Medicaid residents in nursing homes (Anderson et al., 1968; Kosberg and Tobin, 1972; Gottesman, 1974; Fottler et al., 1981; Weissert and Scanlon, 1985). These results are often interpreted as evidence that Medicaid nursing home reimbursement rates were too low to provide good quality care. If this were the case, then the quality-of-care problem could be alleviated simply by raising Medicaid reimbursement rates.

An alternative explanation is that the relationship between homes that are heavily dependent on Medicaid and low quality is attributable to an insufficient supply of nursing home beds available for Medicaid residents (i.e., excess demand), which means that facilities need not compete by providing high-quality care (Nyman, 1993, 1988a,b,c). Excess demand exists when not enough beds are available for consumers demanding care at a given market price, a condition that may be optimal for both the state and the nursing homes if not for the residents. Nursing homes typically charge two different rates—one for Medicaid residents and a higher rate for private-pay residents (Minnesota and North Dakota require that nursing homes charge the same rate to private and Medicaid recipients). Since private-pay rates are always higher than Medicaid reimbursement levels, profit-maximizing nursing homes would rather admit a private-paying individual than an individual supported by Medicaid. In an analysis of data from 43 states for 1969–1973, Scanlon (1980) found that excess demand resulted in a segmented nursing home market, with private-paying residents obtaining all desired care and public-paying residents filling any remaining beds. If excess demand exists for nursing home beds, it is excess Medicaid demand. Studies of Wisconsin and the 10 national long-term care channeling demonstration sites in the early 1980s also found evidence of excess demand (Nyman, 1985, 1988a,c).

Under excess demand, nursing homes can attract as many Medicaid residents as they want, regardless of quality. Although Medicaid residents prefer a higher quality of care, they cannot exercise these preferences under excess demand and must instead choose among the limited number of available beds. Hence, high-quality care is necessary only to attract more private-pay nursing home residents. In a market with a surplus of nursing home beds, however, nursing homes cannot act on their preference to admit private-paying residents over Medicaid-subsidized residents—they will accept either type in order to fill their beds. In this environment, both private- and Medicaid-paying residents would be able to exercise their preference for high-quality care. Consequently, nursing homes should increase quality in an attempt to attract residents.

Using 1978–1979 and 1983 data from Wisconsin, Nyman (1985, 1988a,c) found evidence to support his theory that excess demand was responsible for lower-quality nursing home care. He found that the low-quality–high-Medicaid relationship was stronger under conditions of excess demand. In addition, Nyman found that nursing homes in counties with a surplus bed supply spent more on patient care per empty bed than counties with a tight bed supply. Nyman posited that this evidence cast doubt on the assumption that the relationship between high Medicaid and low quality was simply from lower Medicaid payments. Based on 1987 nursing home survey and certification data, Zinn (1994) reached similar conclusions.

In addition to quality, the presence of excess demand in the nursing home market creates concern about access to nursing home care, especially for Medicaid residents. Private demand should not be affected by Medicaid demand or bed supply since private-pay residents always have admission preference. Using 1982–1984 data from the National Long-Term Care Survey and Area Resource, Ettner (1993) found that Medicaid residents had poorer access to nursing homes on average and that these differences seemed to exist mainly in areas in which bed supply was low or private competition for beds was greater. In addition, some nursing homes (e.g., Vencor, Inc.) have begun to focus on the private-pay and Medicare markets to the exclusion of the Medicaid market (Moss and Adams, 1998). Few facilities, however, can afford to exclude Medicaid residents completely since Medicaid pays for the large majority of nursing home residents.

There is some evidence that excess demand has declined in more recent years. In an evaluation of 1988 data from Wisconsin, Minnesota, and Oregon, Nyman (1993) found no evidence of excess demand (for Wisconsin, this finding contrasted with his analysis of 1983 data). In addition, national nursing home occupancy rates declined from 92 percent in 1985 to 88 percent in 1995 (NCHS, 1997). The number of nursing home beds also decreased substantially in a similar time period (Harrington et al., 1998a). However, there remains an extremely strong relationship between nursing home bed supply and use, leading most states to fear that a greater number of nursing home beds will result in higher Medicaid expenditures (Wiener et al., 1999). As a result, most states control the supply of nursing homes through certificate-of-need programs or moratoriums on new construction or certification for Medicaid.

State efforts to shift the balance of the long-term care system from institutional-based to home and community-based care by expanding home care services and using case management and preadmission screening efforts to encourage placement in settings other than nursing homes may also reduce excess demand. In all but a few states, however, home and community-based services are only a small proportion of Medicaid long-term care expenditures for the elderly. In addition, Medicare home health expenditures have skyrocketed since 1989 and the program has become more long-term care oriented. As the availability of home and community-based services increases, nursing homes will have to compete more actively with other types of long-term care providers (e.g., assisted living facilities and home health agencies) as well as with other nursing homes.

CONCLUSION

The impact of changes in reimbursement on the quality of long-term care is difficult to assess. Almost all of the research literature on the relationship between financing and quality is limited to nursing homes, is based on very old data, and does not reflect the regulatory changes required by the Omnibus Budget Reconciliation Act of 1987. Most studies on this topic were published in the mid- to late 1980s and relied on data from the late 1970s and early 1980s. Moreover, several studies focused on data from one or a few states, making it hard to generalize to the nation as a whole. In addition, the measures of quality in most of these studies were quite rudimentary, especially in terms of outcomes. Again, even less is known about reimbursement for nonmedical home care services and its effect on quality of care. The additional research recommended here is important to help policy makers make better-informed decisions about payment for long-term care.

In the meantime, because the quality of long-term care is already problematic, states and the federal government should be cautious in their quest for Medicare and Medicaid savings. Because many of the recommendations proposed in this report will likely mean additional costs for providers, (e.g., for additional staff), the withdrawal of substantial resources from long-term care providers is a matter of concern.

Although research on nursing homes suggests that higher rates are not necessarily used to improve resident care and that many elements of quality care do not require spending more money, direct resident care expenditures are particularly vulnerable to rate reduction initiatives. Lowering Medicaid nursing home reimbursement rates may be especially problematic in states with high levels of excess demand, since nursing homes in these states do not have to compete for consumers on the basis of quality. Reducing excess demand would lower the quality risks of reducing nursing home rates, but probably would result in higher Medicaid expenditures overall.

9

Closing Remarks

During the three years this committee met, it reviewed much of the available data and research, and learned a lot about the various issues surrounding long-term care. This chapter highlights just some of the conclusions the committee reached. As is clear from the discussions in the preceding chapters, it is easier to propose a comprehensive examination of long-term care than to identify, collect, and analyze relevant data sufficient to support comparable descriptions and assessments across the diverse settings, services, and populations.

Throughout the study the committee's work was impeded by the lack of common definitions across and within states to describe many of the providers of long-term care; and a lack of comprehensive, timely, and reliable information on the quality of care received from the various long-term care sources. Although steps are being taken in that direction, no core set of quality measures are available with common elements and data collection protocols that apply across long-term care settings and services—to nursing homes, home care, and supportive services, the great variety of congregate residences, and other settings or services. The result is that very little is known about the quality of care and outcomes in settings other than nursing homes. What information is available often is not comparable, and does not take into account how people perceive their experience of long-term care.

The committee believes that long-term care should be consumer-centered focusing on the needs, circumstances, and preferences of people using care and involving them, to the extent possible, in planning, delivering, and evaluating care. The notion of consumer-centered care is not new, but there is now tangible evidence, at least in the acute and primary care encounters, of consumer-centered care in many facets of health care delivery and financing. The committee finds guarded optimism in the increased acceptance of consumer-centered service as a core principle for assessing and improving long-term care. However, moving toward meaningful consumer-centered services in long-term care settings would require a mix of changes in consumer and provider attitudes, business practices, public policies, care processes, and management structures. Achieving such changes requires research, and time and effort to integrate the elements of consumer-centered care into the training and attitude of the full range of paid caregivers. A prerequisite to such care is an adequate supply of caregivers who are appropriately trained and sensitive to provide such care.

Broadly speaking, consumers and their families should have access to information, training, and resources necessary for them to participate in self-care and in the direction of their care providers at the level they choose. A recent General Accounting Office report (GAO, 1999a) on assisted living singled out inadequate contracts as a major problem in that sector. People receiving formal long-term care in any setting should have a care contract or admission agreement that is clear, understandable, and enforceable to ensure that long-term care users (or their representatives) have access to accurate, complete, and understandable information about the services that individual caregivers and provider organizations offer. For children receiving long-term care, family members have central roles in a child's care team including approval of care plans for the child and participation in updating the objectives and services set forth in the care plan, but are not always aware of their role. When care providers change their policies or practices, they should present information or, if appropriate, create training programs for consumers and directly related parties.

Public information and reporting to the community and to consumers should be required of providers annually, and should include financial and quality information, results of consumer surveys, and findings of regulatory and accrediting bodies. Federal and state laws should include specific provisions regarding consumer protections for nursing homes, residential care, and home care, and should provide specific mechanisms in addition to existing regulatory bodies to oversee the rights of consumers.

Supportive public policies are essential for the expansion of consumer-centered care because those using long-term care often rely heavily on public programs to help pay for care over long periods of time. Ideally, the policies governing such programs should permit various levels of participant involvement and direction, offer consumers access to a flexible array of benefits, and make available the assistance and resources people need to successfully determine and direct their services. No one approach is sufficient for the diverse groups using long-term care.

The range of benefits, risks, and resources associated with different approaches to consumer-directed personal care services for people with disabilities is only beginning to be identified. Before these principles could be translated into workable and cost effective programs, developmental and feasibility research and evaluation is needed in several areas.

Regardless of the approach to long-term care adopted, the committee emphasizes the importance of reliable and timely data on which to base decisions. The committee's work on several of the issues it was asked to examine was impeded by the lack of availability of timely, reliable, and valid data across states and settings. Very little is known about the quality of care and outcomes in settings other than nursing homes. Most information still focuses on nursing homes; consequently, this report devotes disproportionate attention to them. This emphasis reflects, to a large extent, the concentration of public expenditures in the nursing home setting and the monitoring of that spending to ensure accountability.

An increasing number of elderly people are living in settings that are neither homes nor nursing homes. Some with disabilities who previously would have resided in nursing homes are seeking alternative settings. Lack of data, however, makes it difficult to assess the nature and extent of this shift. Alternatives to nursing home care are found in a variety of residential settings, but they are not systematically and frequently enumerated with uniform and meaningful definitions. The Bureau of the Census, for instance, classifies people as residing either in households or in group quarters, which include both institutions, such as nursing homes, and other non-institutional group quarters, such as rooming and boarding houses, group foster care, and board and care homes. Furthermore, Census classifies both small board and care arrangements and apartments in assisted living facilities as households, not institutions. Assisted living facilities are growing rapidly. In the absence of clear and uniform definitions of these and other residential arrangements we have no way of measuring the growth of these settings nationally or how many and what type of clients they serve.

Despite periodic reports about poor conditions in some residential care settings and fraud in sectors of the home health care industry, comprehensive information about quality of care is scarce for the home and community-based services which are preferred by many users of long-term care and their families and advocates. Informed choices about long-term care alternatives depend on better information.

The evidence reviewed by the committee indicates that the quality of care in nursing homes may have improved in some areas during the past decade, to a large extent due to provider response to the 1987 Nursing

Home Reform Act and the forces that gave rise to this legislation. Improvements are best documented for the use of physical and chemical restraints in nursing homes. The evidence also suggests that serious quality problems appear to continue to affect residents of this country's nursing homes, with persistently poor providers of care remaining in operation. Taken together, government databases and investigative reports, research studies, legislative hearings, and similar sources point in this direction. Serious deficiencies remain in the implementation of government programs to assess and enforce basic standards of quality in long-term care. The information base available for nursing homes suggests a number of problems including variation in state survey and enforcement processes, restricted federal funding for state programs, and inadequate attention to home and community-based services. Particularly worrisome is the continued participation in Medicare and Medicaid of persistently poor-performing providers, especially those who have been repeatedly dropped from the program and reinstated. A number of federal initiatives to improve the regulation of nursing homes have been announced, but it is important for Congress and advocacy groups to continue the monitoring of their implementation and consequences. Their effectiveness cannot be assumed.

The committee acknowledges that issues surrounding the quality of long-term care are closely intertwined with the broader issues of access, work force, and costs. Over the course of this study, the committee became increasingly persuaded that the amounts and ways we pay for long-term care are probably inadequate to support a work force sufficient in numbers, skills, stability, and commitment to provide adequate clinical and personal services for the increasingly frail or complex populations using long-term care. Adequate funding is necessary but not sufficient for good-quality care. For some policy makers and consumer advocates, the combination of poor care and high shareholder profits and corporate executive pay for some long-term care providers undermines arguments for higher provider payments. Nonetheless, the information available to the committee on staffing levels and skills, management, training, wage levels, working conditions, and turnover suggests that resource constraints are a serious problem. This situation has important implications because the long-term care work force is the essential pathway to many improvements in processes of care based on better understanding of care processes and outcomes, internal quality improvement strategies, and more effective regulation. Efforts to identify effective care processes often point to technically simple but time-consuming interventions that, especially when combined with increasing care measurement and analysis requirements, imply a need for additional resources.

The committee, in closing, hopes that its findings and conclusions will provide some insights for the current discussions on policies for meeting the care needs of long-term care users. Hopefully it will lead to the needed research and data collection for obtaining a comprehensive and reliable description of the various long-term care arrangements throughout the country, their size, services provided and staffing levels and training, the characteristics of those receiving care, and the staffing and quality of care provided in the different settings and services. Such information is essential for policy development and evaluation of long term care in the United States.

The committee's assessment about the quality in long-term care is mixed. Important steps are being taken to develop long-term care services that are consumer-centered, and to provide alternatives that respond not only to people's differences but also to their usual preferences for options that provide more autonomy and privacy, and fewer disruptions in their lives. At the same time, consumer-centered care is not a simple concept that can be defined and interpreted in an identical fashion for all those using long-term care services under all circumstances.

On the other hand, the committee found it disappointing that less has been achieved than was hoped in the 1980s when many of the quality initiatives discussed were launched. In particular grave neglect and problems in care persist in some nursing homes, and few—despite some examples to the contrary—have physical environments or policies that promote the quality of life most people desire regardless of their functional limitations or settings in which they receive care. Although the nursing home reforms were enacted in 1987, the Health Care Financing Administration issued the implementing regulations in late 1990, and the enforcement regulations became effective in 1995. Change is a process that takes time to produce definitive results. As discussed earlier, beyond nursing homes, little is known about the quality of long-term care or its outcomes.

Although this report has discussed much that is disappointing or negative about long-term care in this country, it is not intended as a condemnation of those providing, managing, or regulating long-term care. Although some are guilty of inattention, neglect, incompetence, or even abuse, most are trying to do their work well and responsibly, often under difficult circumstances, and understaffed with low compensation.

References

AAHSA (American Association of Homes and Services for the Aging). *Improving Quality in Long-Term Care.* Statement Submitted to the IOM Committee on Improving Quality in Long-Term Care. Washington, DC: AAHSA, 1998.

Aaronson, W.E., Zinn, J.S., and Rosko, M.D. Do For-Profit and Not-for-Profit Nursing Homes Behave Differently? *The Gerontologist* 34(6):775–786, 1994.

Abt Associates. *Evaluation of the Long-Term Care Survey Process.* Cambridge, MA: Abt Associates, 1996.

Abt Associates and CHSRA (Center for Health System Research and Analysis). Analysis of the Validity of Quality of Care Determinations. Chapter 4 in *Evaluation of the Long Term Care Survey Process.* Bethesda, MD: Abt Associates, 1996.

ACHCA (American College of Health Care Administrators). "Testimony to the IOM Committee on Improving Long-Term Care." Presented to the Committee, March 13, 1998.

Adams, M., and Beatty, P. Consumer-Directed Personal Assistance Services: Independent Living, Community Integration and the Vocational Rehabilitation Process. *Journal of Vocational Rehabilitation* 10:93–101, 1998.

Adler, M. Population Estimates of Disability and Long-Term Care. *ASPE Research Notes.* [WWW document]. URL: http://aspe.hhs.gov/rn/rn11.htm (accessed on February 24, 1999), 1995.

Agosta, J., and Melda, K. *Supplemental Security Income for Children with Disabilities: An Exploration of Child and Family Needs and the Relative Merits of the Cash Benefit Program.* Salem, OR: Human Services Research Institute, 1995.

AGS (American Geriatrics Society). *Clinical Practice Guidelines: Guideline for Restraint Use.* New York: AGS, 1997.

AGS. *The Management of Chronic Pain in Older Persons.* New York: AGS, 1998.

Aharony, L., and Strasser, S. Patient Satisfaction: What We Know About and What We Still Need to Explore. *Medical Care Review* 50(1):49–79, 1993.

AHCA (American Health Care Association). *Facts and Trends 1997: The Nursing Facility Sourcebook.* Washington, DC: AHCA, 1997.

AHCA. *Facts and Trends 1998: The Nursing Facility Sourcebook.* Washington, DC: AHCA, 1998.

AHCA. *Facts and Trends 1999: The Nursing Facility Sourcebook.* Washington, DC: AHCA, 1999.

AHCPR. *Clinical Practice Guideline: Pressure Ulcers in Adults.* Rockville, MD: AHCPR, 1994.

Albert, S.M., and Logsdon, R.G. Assessing Quality of Life in Alzheimer's Disease. *Journal of Mental Health and Aging* 5(1):3–111, 1999.

Alecxih, L.M.B., Lutsky, L., Corea, J., and Coleman, B. *Estimated Cost Savings from the Use of Home and Community-Based Alternatives to Nursing Facility Care in Three States.* Washington, DC: American Association of Retired Persons, 1996.

Allen, S.M., and Mor, V. The Prevalence and Consequences of Unmet Need. *Medical Care* 35(11):1132–1148, 1997.

Aller, L.J., and Van Ess Coeling, H. Quality of Life: Its Meaning to the Long-Term Care Resident. *Journal of Gerontological Nursing* 21(2):20–25, 1995.

ALQC (Assisted Living Quality Coalition). *Assisted Living Quality Initiative: Building a Structure That Promotes Quality.* Washington, DC: ALQC, 1998.

AMDA (American Medical Directors Association). *Depression: Clinical Practice Guideline; Heart Failure: Clinical Practice Guideline; Pressure Ulcers: Clinical Practice Guideline; Urinary Incontinence: Clinical Practice Guideline.* Columbia, MD: AMDA, 1996.

Americans with Disabilities Act of 1990. 42 U.S.C. 12101 et seq. (28 C.F.R. § 41.51).

Amerman, E., Schneider, B., and Frnak, M. *Clinical Protocol Series in Community-Based Long-Term Care: Overview and Trainer's Guide.* Philadelphia, PA: Philadelphia Corporation on Aging, 1995.

Anderson, N., Holmberg, R.H., Schneider, R.E., and Stone, L.B. *Nursing Home Care: A Minnesota Analysis.* Minneapolis: American Rehabilitation Foundation, 1968.

Anderson, R.A., and McDaniel, R.R. RN Participation in Organizational Decision Making and Improvements in Resident Outcomes. *Health Care Management Review* 24(1):7–16, 1998.

AOA (Administration on Aging). *1998 Long-Term Care Ombudsman Program Report.* Washington, DC: AOA, 1998.

Applebaum, R.A., and Austin, C. *Long-Term Care Case Management: Design and Evaluation.* New York: Springer Publishing, 1990.

Applebaum, R.A., Harrigan, M., and Kemper, P. *Evaluation of the National Long-Term Care Demonstration: Tables Comparing Channeling to Other Community Care Demonstrations.* Princeton, NJ: Mathematica Policy Research, 1986.

Applebaum, R.A., Straker, J.K., and Geron, S.M. *Assessing Satisfaction in Health and Long-Term Care: Practical Approaches to Hearing the Voice of the Consumer.* New York: Springer, 1999.

Arling, G., Nordquist, R.H., Brant, B.A., and Capitman, J.A. Nursing Home Case Mix. *Medical Care* 25:9–19, 1987.

Arling, G., Karon, S., Sainfort, F., Zimmerman, D.R., and Ross, R. Risk Adjustment of Nursing Home Quality Indicators. *The Gerontologist* 37(6):757–766, 1997.

Arno, P.S., Levine, C., and Memmott, M.M. The Economic Value of Informal Caregiving. *Health Affairs* 18(2):182–188, 1999.

Avorn, J., Dreyer, P., Connely, K., and Soumerai, S.B. Use of Psychoactive Medication and the Quality of Care in Rest Homes. *New England Journal of Medicine* 320(4):227–232, 1989.

Backstrom, A., Norberg, A., and Norberg, B. Feeding Difficulties in Long-Stay Patients at Nursing Homes. Caregiver Turnover and Caregivers' Assessments of Duration and Difficulty of Assisted Feeding and Amount of Food Received by the Patient. *International Journal of Nursing Studies* 24(1):69–76, 1987.

Badelt, C., Holzmann-Jenkins, A., Matul, C., and Osterle, A. *Analyse der Auswirkungen des Pflegevorsorgesystems.* Translated by Hopperger, J.P. Venice, Austria: Bunderministeriums for Arbeit, Gesundh'eit, und Soziales, 1997.

Bahr, R.T. *Mechanisms of Quality in Long Term Care: Service and Clinical Outcomes.* New York: National League for Nursing Press, 1991.

Baltes, M.M., Honn, S., Barton, E.M., Orzech, M.J., and Lago, D. On the Social Ecology of Dependence and Independence in Elderly Nursing Home Residents: A Replication and Extension. *Journal of Gerontology* 38:556–564, 1983.

Banaszak-Holl, J., and Hines, M.A. Factors Associated with Nursing Home Staff Turnover. *The Gerontologist* 36(4):512–517, 1996.

Banaszak-Holl, J., Zinn, J., and Mor, V. The Impact of Market and Organizational Characteristics on Nursing Care Facility Service Innovation: A Resource Dependency Perspective. *Health Services Research* 31(1):97–117, 1996.

Barkan, B. The Regenerative Community: The Live Oak Living Center and the Quest for Autonomy, Self-Esteem, and Connection in Elder Care. In Gamroth, L.M., Semradek, J., and Tornquist, E.M., eds. *Enhancing Autonomy in Long-Term Care: Concepts and Strategies.* New York: Springer, 1995.

Barnes, L.E.A. Residential Care Operators: Perspectives on Mental Illness and Caregiving Roles. A Nursing Perspective on Severe Mental Illness. In Chafetz, L., ed. *New Directions for Mental Health Services* No. 58, Summer 1993.

Barney, J.L. Community Presence in Nursing Homes. *The Gerontologist* 27(3):367–369, 1987.

Barusch, A.S. *Elder Care: Family Training and Support.* Thousand Oaks, CA: Sage Publications, 1991.

Bass, D.S. *Caring Families: Supports and Interventions.* Silver Springs, MD: National Association of Social Workers Press, 1990.

Beatty, P., Adams, M., and O'Day, B. Virginia's Consumer-Directed Personal Assistance Services Program: A History and Valuation. *American Rehabilitation* 24(3):31–35, 1998a.

Beatty, P.W., Richmond, G.W., Tepper, S., and DeJong, G. Personal Assistance for People with Physical Disabilities: Consumer-Direction and Satisfaction with Services. *Archives of Physical Medicine and Rehabilitation* 79 (6), 674–677, 1998b.

Beck, C., Heacock, P., Mercer, S.O., Walls, R.C., Rapp, C.G., and Vogelpohl, T.S. Improving Dressing Behavior in Cognitively Impaired Nursing Home Residents. *Nursing Research* 46:126–132, 1997.

Benjamin, A.E. *Comparing Client-Directed and Agency Models for Providing Supportive Services at Home.* Los Angeles: University of California, 1998.

Bennett, C. *Nursing Home Life: What It Is and What It Could Be.* New York: Tiresias Press, 1980.

Bernabei, R., Murphy, K., Jrijters, D., DuPaquier, J.N., and Gardent, H. Variations in Training Programmes for Resident Assessment Instrument Implementation. *Age and Ageing* 26(Suppl 2):31–35, 1997.

Bernabei, R., Gambassi, G., and Mor, V. Introducing Functional Outcomes in Geriatric Pharmaco-epidemiology: The SAGE Database. *Journal of the American Geriatrics Society* 46:250–252, 1998.

Berwick, D.M. Continuous Improvement as an Ideal in Health Care. *New England Journal of Medicine* 320:53–56, 1989.

Berwick, D.M., and Bisognano, M. Health Care Services. In Juran, J.M., and Godfrey, A.B., eds. *Jurans Quality Handbook.* New York: McGraw-Hill, 1998.

Birren, J.E., Lubben, J.E., Rowe, J.C., and Deutchman, D.E. *The Concept and the Measurement of Quality of Life in the Frail Elderly.* San Diego, CA: Harcourt Brace, 1991.

Bishop, C., and Skwara, K.C. Recent Growth of Medicare Home Health. *Health Affairs* 12(3):95–110, 1993.

Blanchette, K. *A National Overview of Adult Foster Care for the Elderly.* Washington, DC: American Association of Retired Persons, 1996.

Blaum, C.S., Fries, B.E., and Fiatarone, M.A. Factors Associated with Low Body Mass Index and Weight Loss in Nursing Home Residents. *Journal of Gerontology: Series A, Biological Sciences and Medical Sciences* 50(3):M162–M168, 1995.

Blaum, C.S., O'Neill, E.F., Clements, K.M., Fries, B.E., and Fiatarone, M.A. Validity of the Minimum Data Set for Assessing Nutritional Status in Nursing Home Residents. *American Journal of Clinical Nutrition* 66(4):787–794, 1997.

Blegen, M.A. Nurses' Job Satisfaction: A Meta-Analysis of Related Variables. *Nursing Research* 42(1):36–41, 1993.

Bliesmer, M.M., Smayling, M., Kane, R., and Shannon, I. The Relationship Between Nursing Staffing Levels and Nursing Home Outcomes. *Journal of Aging and Health* 10(3):351–371, 1998.

BLS (Bureau of Labor Statistics). Employment Projections and Industry Occupation Matrix, U.S. Department of Labor, Washington, DC, 1998.

BLS (Bureau of Labor Statistics). *National Industry–Occupation Employment Matrix* [WWW document]. URL: http://stats.bls.gov/oep/nioem/ (accessed March 27–30, 2000), 2000.

Blumenthal, D., and Kilo, C.M. A Report Card on Continuous Quality Improvement. *The Milbank Quarterly* 76(4):625–648, 1998.

Bowers, B., and Becker, M. Nurse's Aides in Nursing Homes: The Relationship Between Organization and Quality. *The Gerontologist* 32(3):360–366, 1992.

Braddock, D., Hemp, R., Parish, S., and Westridge, J. *The State of the States in Developmental Disabilities: Fifth Edition.* Washington, DC: American Association on Mental Retardation, 1998.

Braden, B.R., Cowan, C.A., Lazenby, H.C., Martin, A.B., McDonnell, P.A., Sensenig, A.L., Stiller, J.M., Whittle, L.S., Donham, C.S., Long, A.M., and Stewart, M.W. National Health Expenditures, 1997. *Health Care Financing Review* 20(1):83–126, 1998.

Braun, B.I. The Effect of Nursing Home Quality on Patient Outcome. *Journal of the American Geriatrics Society* 39(4):329–338, 1991.

Brod, M., Stewart, A.L., and Sands, L. Conceptualization of Quality of Life in Dementia. *Journal of Mental Health and Aging* 5(1):7–19, 1999.

Buchanan, J.L., Bell, R.M., Arnold, S.B., Witsberger, C., Kane R.L., and Garrard, J. Assessing Cost Effects of Nursing-Home-Based Geriatric Nurse Practitioners. *Health Care Financing Review* 11(3):67–78, 1990.

Burbridge, L. The Labor Market for Home Care Workers: Demand, Supply, and Institutional Barriers. *The Gerontologist* 33(1):41–46, 1993.

Burger, S.G. Individualized care: The key to quality of life. Speech delivered at the Minnesota Department of Health, Facility and Provider Compliance Staff In-Service, Minneapolis, April 22, 1999.

Burger, S.G., Frazer, V., Hunt, S., and Frank, B. National Citizens' Coalition for Nursing Home Reform. In *Nursing Homes: Getting Good Care There.* San Luis Obispo, CA: American Source Books, 1996.

Burgio, L.D., and Burgio, K.L. Institutional Staff Training and Management: A Review of the Literature and a Model for Geriatric, Long-Term Care Facilities. *International Journal of Geriatric Psychiatry* 30(4):287–302, 1990.

Burke, B., and Cornelius, B. *Analysis of Staff Time Based on HCFA's Multistate Case-Mix and Quality Demonstration and HCFA's Staff Time Measurement Study for National SNF System.* Baltimore, MD: Health Care Financing Administration, 1998.

Burr, C.K. Impact on the Family of a Chronically Ill Child. Pp. 24–40 in Hobbs, N., and Perrin, J.M., eds. *Issues in the Care of Children with Chronic Illness.* San Francisco: Jossey-Bass, 1985.

Burton, L.C., German, P.S., Rovner, B.W., Brant, L.J., and Clark, R.D. Mental Illness and the Use of Restraints in Nursing Homes. *The Gerontologist* 32(2):164–170, 1992.

Butler, P.A., and Schlenker, R.E. Case-Mix Reimbursement for Nursing Homes: Objectives and Achievements. *The Milbank Quarterly* 67(1):103–136, 1989.

Burwell, B. *Medicaid Long Term Care Expenditures in FY 1998*. Boston: The Medstat Group, 1999.

Callahan, E.J., Bertakis, K.D., Azari, R., Robbins, J.A., Helms, L.J., and Chang, D.W. The Influence of Patient Age on Primary Care Resident Physician–Patient Interaction. *Journal of the American Geriatrics Society* 48:30–35, 2000.

Cameron, C., and Naylor, C.D. No Impact from Active Dissemination of the Ottawa Ankle Rules: Further Evidence of the Need for Local Implementation of Practice Guidelines. *Canadian Medical Association Journal* 160(8):1165–1168, 1999.

Cameron, K.A. *International and Domestic Programs Using "Cash and Counseling" Strategies to Pay for Long-Term Care*. Washington, DC: United Seniors Health Cooperative, 1993.

Cameron, K.A. State Demonstrations and Initiatives in Consumer Choice and Direction. Findings from the National Survey of States. In *Consumer-Directed, Long-Term Care Services*. Symposium conducted at the annual meeting of the Gerontological Society of America, Washington, DC, November 1996.

Capezuti, E., Evans, L., Strumpf, N., and Maislin, G. Physical Restraint Use and Falls in Nursing Home Residents. *Journal of the American Geriatrics Society* 44:627–633, 1996.

Capitman, J., Abrahams, R., and Ritter, G. Measuring the Adequacy of Home Care for Frail Elders. *The Gerontologist* 37(3):303–313, 1997.

Cassell, E.J. *The Nature of Suffering and the Goals of Medicine*. New York: Oxford University Press, 1991.

Castle, N.G. The Use of Physical Restraints in Nursing Homes: Pre- and Post-Nursing Home Reform Act. *Journal of Health and Social Policy* 9(3):71–89, 1998a.

Castle, N.G. Variation in Psychotropic Drug Use in Nursing Homes. *Journal of Health and Social Policy* 10(3):13–36, 1998b.

Castle, N.G., and Banaszak-Holl, J. Top Management Team Characteristics and Innovation in Nursing Homes. *The Gerontologist* 37 (5):572–580, 1997.

Castle, N.G., and Mor, V. Hospitalization of Nursing Home Residents: A Review of the Literature, 1980–1995. *Medical Care Research and Review* 53:123–148, 1996.

Castle, N.G., and Mor, V. Physical Restraints in Nursing Homes: A Review of the Literature Since the Nursing Home Reform Act of 1987. *Medical Care Research and Review* 55(2):139–170, 1998.

Castle, N.G., Fogel, B., and Mor, V. Quality of Care in Nursing Homes Administered by Members of the American College of Health Care Administrators. *Journal of Long Term Care Administration* 24(2):11–16, 1996.

Census (Bureau of the Census). *65+ in the United States. Current Population Reports, Special Studies*. Washington, DC: Government Printing Office, 1996.

CBO (Congressional Budget Office). *An Analysis of the President's Budgetary Proposals for Fiscal Year 2001*. Washington, DC: Government Printing Office, 2000.

CCAL (Consumer Consortium on Assisted Living). *What Do Consumers Want in Assisted Living? A Conference Report*. Falls Church, VA: CCAL, 1996.

Chassin, M.R. Improving Quality of Care with Practice Guidelines. *Frontiers of Health Services Management* 10(1):40–44, 1993.

Chassin, M.R., and Galvin, R.W. The Urgent Need to Improve Health Care Quality. Institute of Medicine National Roundtable on Health Care Quality. *Journal of the American Medical Association* 280(11):1000–1005, 1998.

Cherry, R.L. Agents of Nursing Home Quality of Care: Ombudsmen and Staff Ratios Revisited. *The Gerontologist* 21(2):302–308, 1991.

Cherry, R.L. Community Presence and Nursing Home Quality of Care: The Ombudsman as a Complementary Role. *Journal of Health and Social Behavior* 34(4):336–345, 1993.

Childs, N. Nursing Facility Bankruptcies Top 10 Percent in 21 States. *Provider* 26(4):13, 2000.

Chiodo, L.K., Gerety, M.B., Mulrow, C.D., Rhodes, M.C., and Tuley, M.R. The Impact of Physical Therapy on Nursing Home Patient Outcomes. *Physical Therapy* 72(2):168–173, 1992.

Christensen, C., and Beaver, S. Correlation Between Administrator Turnover and Survey Results. *Journal of Long-Term Care Administration* 24(2):4–7, 1996.

CHSRA (Center for Health Systems Research and Analysis). *Summary of Insights from Survey Studies. Report Completed for the Health Care Financing Administration.* Madison, WI: CHSRA, October 1997.

Clark, D., and Brown, M. *How to Organize and Direct an Effective Resident Council.* Jefferson, MO: Missouri Long-Term Care Ombudsman Office and the Missouri Division on Aging, 1998.

Clark, R. and Turek-Brezina, J. Licensed Board and Care Homes: Preliminary Findings from the 1991 National Health Provider Inventory. *ASPE Research Notes* March, 1993.

Clark, R.E., Turek-Brezina, J., Chu, C.W., and Hawes, C. *Licensed Board and Care Homes: Preliminary Findings from the 1991 National Health Provider Inventory.* Washington, D.C.: U.S. Department of Commerce, 1994.

Cleary, P.D., and McNeil, B.J. Patient Satisfaction as an Indicator of Quality Care. *Inquiry* 25:25–36, 1988.

Cleary, P.D., Edgman-Levitan, S., Roberts, M., Moloney, T.W., McMullen, W., Walker, J.D., and Delbanco, T.L. Patients Evaluate Their Hospital Care: A National Survey. *Health Affairs* 10(4):254–267, 1991.

Close, L., Estes, C.L., Linkins, K., and Binney, E. A Political Economy Perspective on Front-Line Workers in Long-Term Care. *Generations* 18(3):23–27, 1994.

Cohen, J.W., and Dubay, L.C. The Effect of Medicaid Reimbursement Method and Ownership on Nursing Home Costs, Case Mix and Staffing. *Inquiry* 27:183–200, 1990.

Cohen, J.W., and Spector, W.D. The Effect of Medicaid Reimbursement on Quality of Care in Nursing Homes. *Journal of Health Economics* 15:23–28, 1996.

Cohen, M.A., and Tumlinson, A. Understanding the State Variation in Medicare Home Health Care. The Impact of Medicaid Program Characteristics, State Policy, and Provider Attributes. *Medical Care* 35(6):618–633, 1997.

Cohen-Mansfield, J. Turnover Among Nursing Home Staff. A Review. *Nursing Management* 28(5):59–64, 1997.

Cohen-Mansfield, J., Werner, P. and Marx, M.S. An Observational Study of Agitation in Agitated Nursing Home Residents. *International Psychogeriatrics* 1:153–165, 1989.

Colling, J., Ouslander, J., Hadley, B.J., Eisch, J., and Campbell, E. The Effects of Patterned Urge Response Toileting (PURT) on Urinary Incontinence Among Nursing Home Residents. *Journal of the American Geriatrics Society* 40(2):135–141, 1992.

Conroy, J. *The Hissom Outcome Study: A Report on 6 Years of Movement into Supportive Living: The People Who Once Lived at Hissom Memorial Center: Are They Better Off?* Report Number I of a Series on Well-Being of People with Developmental Disabilities in Oklahoma. Submitted jointly to Oklahoma Department of Human Services and U.S. District Court, Northern District of Oklahoma. Ardmore, PA: Center for Outcome Analysis, 1996.

Covert, S.B., Macintosh, J.D., and Shumway, D.L. Closing the Laconia State School and Training Center: A Case Study in Systems Change. Pp. 197–212 in Bradley, V.J., Ashbaugh, J.W., and Blaney, B.C., eds. *Creating Individual Supports for People with Developmental Disabilities: A Mandate for Change at Many Levels.* Baltimore, MD: Paul H. Brookes, 1994.

Coyne, I.T. Chronic Illness: The Importance of Support for Families Caring for a Child with Cystic Fibrosis. *Journal of Clinical Nursing* 6(2):121–129, 1997.

Creason, N.S., Grybowski, J.A., Burgener, S., Whippo, C., Yeo, S.A., and Richardson, B. Prompted Voiding Therapy for Urinary Incontinence in Aged Female Nursing Home Residents. *Journal of Advanced Nursing* 14:120–126, 1989.

Crooks, V.C., Schnelle, J.F., Ouslander, J.P., and McNees, M.P. Use of the Minimum Data Set to Rate Incontinence Severity. *Journal of the American Geriatrics Society* 43(12):1363–1369, 1995.

Crown, W., MacAdam, M., and Sadowsky, E. *Health Aides: Characteristics and Working Conditions of Aides Employed in Hospitals, Nursing Homes and Home Care.* Waltham, MA: Brandeis University, 1992.

Crown, W., Ahlburg, D.A., and MacAdam, M. The Demographic and Employment Characteristics of Home Care Aides: A Comparison with Nursing Home Aides, Hospital Aides, and Other Workers. *The Gerontologist* 35(2):162–170, 1995.

Davidson, G., Penrod, J., Kane, R.A., Moscovice, I., and Rich, E. Modeling the Costs of Case Management in Long-Term Care. *Health Care Financing Review* 13(1):73–81, 1991.

Davis, D.A., and Taylor-Vaisey, A. Translating Guidelines into Practice. A Systematic Review of Theoretic Concepts, Practical Experience and Research Evidence in the Adoption of Clinical Practice Guidelines. *Canadian Medical Association Journal* 157(4):408–416, 1997.

Davis, M.A., Freeman, J.W., and Kirby, E.C. Nursing Home Performance Under Case-Mix Reimbursement Responding to Heavy Care Incentives and Market Changes. *Health Services Research* 33(4):815–834, 1998.

DeJong, G., Batavia, A.I., and McKnew, L.B. The Independent Living Model of Personal Assistance in National Long-Term-Care Policy. *Aging and Disability* 89–95, 1992.

DeParle, N. The Health Care Financing Administration on Medicare Payment Reforms. Testimony before the U.S. Senate Finance Committee, March 17, 1999.

DHHS (Department of Health and Human Services). *Informal Caregiving: Compassion in Action.* Washington, DC: DHHS, 1998.

Desbiens, N., Wu, A.W., Broste, S.K., Wenger, N.S., Conners, Jr., A.F., Lynn, J., Yasui, Y., Phillips, R.S., and Fulkerson, W. Pain and Satisfaction with Pain Control in Seriously Ill Hospitalized Adults: Findings from the SUPPORT Research Investigations. For the SUPPORT Investigators: Study to Understand Prognosis and Preferences for Outcomes and Risks of Treatment. *Critical Care and Medicine* 24:1953–1961, 1996.

Diamond, T. *Making Gray Gold: Narratives of Nursing Home Care.* Chicago: University of Chicago Press, 1992.

Donabedian, A. Evaluating the Quality of Medical Care. *Milbank Quarterly* 44:166–203, 1966.

Doty, P., Kasper, J., and Litvak, S. Consumer-Directed Models of Personal Care: Lessons from Medicaid. *Milbank Quarterly* 74(3):377–409, 1996.

Dywbad, G., and Bersani, H. *New Voices: Self-Advocacy by People with Disabilities.* Cambridge, MA: Brookline Books, 1996.

Edelman T. An Unpromising Picture: Implementation of Reform Law's Enforcement Provisions Troubles Advocates. *Quality Care Advocate* March 1997.

Edelman, T. Improving the Quality of Care in Long-Term Care. Testimony of the National Senior Citizens Law Center prepared for the Institute of Medicine Committee on Improving Quality in Long-Term Care. Washington, DC, 1998a.

Edelman, T. What Happened to Enforcement? *Nursing Home Law Letter* 1–2:1–46, 1998b.

Edelman, T. What Happened to Enforcement? Part 2: The Experiences of Five States. Study Funded by the Commonwealth Foundation. Washington, DC: National Senior Citizens Law Center, 1998c.

Editor. Stock Checks. *Provider* 26(4):18, 2000.

Ejaz, F.K., Jones, J.A., and Rose, M.S. Falls Among Nursing Home Residents: An Examination of Incident Reports Before and After Restraint Reduction Programs. *Journal of the American Geriatrics Society* 42:960–964, 1994.

Emanuel, E.J., and Emanuel, L.L. Four Models of the Doctor–Patient Relationship. *Journal of the American Medical Association* 267:2221–2226, 1992.

Emanuel, E.J., Weinberg, D.S., Gonin, R., Hummel, L.R., and Emanuel, L.L. How Well Is the Patient Self-Determination Act Working: An Early Assessment. *American Journal of Medicine* 95:619–628, 1993.

Estes, C.L., and Swan, J.H. *The Long-Term Care Crisis: Elders Trapped in the No-Care Zone.* Beverly Hills, CA: Sage Publications, 1993.

Ettner S.L. Do Elderly Medicaid Patients Experience Reduced Access to Nursing Home Care? *Journal of Health Economics* 11:259–280, 1993.

Eustis, N.N., Kane, R.A., and Fischer, L.R. Home Care Quality and Home Care Workers: Beyond Quality Assurance as Usual. *The Gerontologist* 33(1):47–54, 1993.

Evans, L., and Strumpf, N. Tying Down the Elderly. A Review of the Literature on Physical Restraint. *Journal of the American Geriatrics Society* 37:65–74, 1989.

Evashwick, C.J. *The Continuum of Long-Term Care: An Integrated Systems Approach.* Albany, NY: Delmar Publishing, 1996.

Fagin, R.M., Williams, C.C., and Burger, S.G. *Meeting of Pioneers in Nursing Home Culture Change.* Rochester, NY: Lifespan of Greater Rochester, 1997.

Feder, J., Edwards, J., and Kidder, S. *The Long-Term Care Ombudsman Program: Efforts and Limitations in Quality Assurance.* Washington, DC: Center for Health Policy Studies, Georgetown University, 1988.

Feinberg, E.A. Family Stress in Pediatric Home Care. *Caring* IV(5):38–44, 1985.

Feldman, P.H. Work Life Improvements for the Home Aide Work Force: Impact and Feasibility. *The Gerontologist* 33(1):47–54, 1993.

Feldman, P.H. Labor Market Issues in Home-Based Care. In Fox, D., and Raphael, C., eds. *Home-Based Care for a New Century.* Malden, MA: Blackwell Publishers, 1996.

Feldman, P.H., Work Force Issues and Quality of Long-Term Care. Background paper prepared for the Institute of Medicine, Committee on Improving Quality in Long Term Care, 1998.

Feldman, P.H., Sapienza, A., and Kane, N. *Who Cares for Them? Workers in the U.S. Home Care Industry.* Westport, CT: Greenwood-Praeger Press, 1990.

Feldman, P.H., Sapienza, A., and Kane, N. On the Home Front: The Job of the Home Aide. *Generations* 18(3):16–19, 1994.

Fenton, M., Entrikin, T., Morrill, S., Marburg, G., Shumway, D., and Nerney, T. *Beyond Managed Care: An Owner's Manual for Self-Determination.* Concord, NH: Self-Determination for Persons with Developmental Disabilities, 1997.

Ferrell, B.A. Pain Evaluation and Management in the Nursing Home. *Annals of Internal Medicine* 123:681–687, 1995.

Flanagan, S.A., and Green, P.S. *Consumer-Directed Personal Assistance Service: Key Operational Issues for State CD-PAS Programs Using Intermediary Services Organizations.* Cambridge, MA: The Medstat Group, 1997.

Folkemer, D., Jensen, A., Lipson, L., Stauffer, M., and Fox-Grange, W. Adult Foster Care for the Elderly: A Review of State Regulatory and Funding Strategies. Washington, DC: American Association of Retired Persons, 1996.

Foner, N. Nursing Home Aides: Saints or Monsters? *The Gerontologist* 34(2):245–250, 1994.

Fortinsky, R.H., and Raff, L. Physicians in Nursing Homes: Challenges and Opportunities. *Nursing Home Medicine* 4(1):8–13, 1996.

Fottler, M.D., Smith, H.L., and James, W.L. Profits and Patient Care Quality in Nursing Homes: Are They Compatible? *The Gerontologist* 21(5):532–538, 1981.

Fowler, F.J., Barry, M.J., Lu-Yao, G., Wasson, J.H., and Bin, L. Outcomes of External Beam Radiation Therapy for Prostate Cancer: A Study of Medicare Beneficiaries in Three Surveillance, Epidemiology, and End Results Areas. *Journal of Clinical Oncology.* 14(8):2258–2265, 1996.

Freedman, J.A., Cook, C.A., Robinson, T., and Kinney, E.D. Collaborative QI in Community-Based Long-Term Care. *Joint Commission Journal on Quality Improvement* 21(12):701–710, 1995.

Friedland, R.B., and Summer, L. *Demography Is Not Destiny.* Washington, DC: National Academy on Aging Society, 1999.

Fries, B.E., Schneider, D., Foley, W., Gavazzi, M., Burke, R., and Cornelius, E. Refining a Case-Mix Measure for Nursing Homes: Resources Utilization Groups (RUGS-III). *Medical Care* 32(7):668–685, 1994.

Fries, B.E., Hawes, C., Morris, J.N., Phillips, C.D., Mor, V., and Park, P.S. Effect of the National Resident Assessment Instrument on Selected Health Conditions and Problems. *Journal of the American Geriatrics Society* 45:994–1001, 1997.

Frisoni, G.B., Franzoni, S., Rozzini, R., Ferucci, L., Boffelli, S., and Trabucchi, M. Food Intake and Mortality in the Frail Elderly. *Journal of Gerontology: Medical Sciences* 50A(4):M203–M210, 1995.

Frytak, J. Quality of Life. In: Kane, R.L., and Kane, R.A., eds. *Assessing Older People: Measures, Meaning, and Practical Applications.* New York: Oxford University Press, 2000.

Frytak, J.R., Kane, R.A., Finch, M.D., Jane, R.L., and Maude-Griffin, R. Outcome Trajectories for Assisted Living and Nursing Facility Residents in Oregon. *Health Services Research,* in press.

GAO. *Board and Care: Insufficient Assurances That Residents' Needs Are Identified and Met.* GAO/HRD-89-50. Washington, DC: GAO, 1989.

GAO. *Home Health Care: HCFA Evaluation of Community Health Accreditation Program Inadequate.* GAO-HRD-92-93. Washington, DC: GAO, 1992a.

GAO. *Home Health Care: HCFA Properly Evaluated JCAHO's Ability to Survey Home Health Agencies.* GAO-HRD-93-33. Washington, DC: GAO, 1992b.

GAO. *Medicaid Long-Term Care: Successful State Efforts to Expand Home Services while Limiting Costs.* GAO-HEHS-94-167. Washington, DC: GAO, 1994.

GAO. *Medicare Allegations Against ABC Home Health Care.* GAO-OSI-95-17. Washington, DC: GAO, 1995.

GAO. *Medicare Home Health Utilization Expands While Program Controls Deteriorate.* GAO-HEHS-96-16. Washington, DC: GAO, 1996a.

GAO. *Medicaid Long-Term Care: State Use of Assessment Instruments in Care Planning.* GAO-PEMD-96-4. Washington, DC: GAO, 1996b.

GAO. *Long-Term Care: Consumer Protection and Quality of Care Issues in Assisted Living.* GAO-HEHS-97-93. Washington, DC: GAO, 1997a.

GAO. *Medicare Home Health Agencies: Certification Process Ineffective in Excluding Problem Agencies.* GAO-HEHS-98-29. Washington, DC: GAO, 1997b.

GAO. *California Nursing Homes: Care Problems Persist Despite Federal and State Oversight.* GAO-HEHS-98-202. Washington, DC: GAO, 1998a.

GAO. *Medicare: Improper Activities by Mid-Delta Home Health.* GAO-OSI-98-5. Washington, DC: GAO, 1998b.

GAO. *Medicare Home Health Benefit: Impact of Interim Payment System and Agency Closures on Access to Services.* GAO-HEHS-98-238. Washington, DC: GAO, 1998c.

GAO. *Assisted Living: Quality of Care and Consumer Protection Issues in Four States.* GAO-HEHS-99-27. Washington, DC: GAO, 1999a.

GAO. *Nursing Homes: Additional Steps Needed to Strengthen Enforcement of Federal Standards.* GAO-HEHS-99-46. Washington, DC: GAO, 1999b.

GAO. *Nursing Homes: Complaint Investigation Processes Often Inadequate to Protect Residents.* GAO-HEHS-99-80. Washington, DC: GAO, 1999c.

GAO. *Nursing Home Care: Enhanced HCFA Oversight of State Programs Would Better Ensure Quality.* GAO-HEHS-00-6. Washington, DC: GAO, 1999d.

GAO. *Skilled Nursing Facilities: Medicare Payment Changes Require Provider Adjustments But Maintain Access.* GAO/HEHS-00-23. Washington, DC: GAO, 1999e.

Garrard, J., Chen, V., and Dowd, B. The Impact of the 1987 Federal Regulations on the Use of Psychotropic Drugs in Minnesota Nursing Homes. *American Journal of Public Health* 85(6):771–776, 1995.

Garrard, J., Cooper, S.L., and Goertz, C. Drug Use Management in Board and Care Facilities. *The Gerontologist* 37(6):748–756, 1997.

Geron, S.M. Using Measures of Subjective Well-Being and Client Satisfaction in Health Assessment of Older People. *Health Care in Later Life* 1(3):185–196, 1996.

Geron, S.M. *The Home Care Satisfaction Measures (HCSM): Study Design and Initial Results of Item Analyses.* Boston: Boston University School of Social Work, 1997.

Gerowitz, M.B. Do TQM Interventions Change Management Culture? *Quality Management in Health Care* 6(3):6–11, 1998.

Gerteis, M., Edgman-Levitan, S., Daley, J., and Delbanco, T.L., eds. *Through the Patient's Eyes: Understanding and Promoting Patient-Centered Care.* San Francisco: Jossey-Bass, 1993.

Gilles, M.O., Groc, I., and Legros, M. *La Prestation Depedance: Experimentations Resultats des Phases 1 et 2 du Programme d'Evaluation de l'Expetrimentation d'une Prestation Dependance.* Translated by Tilly, J. Paris, France: Centre de Recherche pour l'Etude et l'Observation des Conditions de Vie, 1995.

Glass, A.P. Improving Quality of Care and Life in Nursing Homes. *Journal of Applied Gerontology* 7:406–423, 1988.

Gold, M.R., Siegel, J.E., Russell, L.B., and Weinstein, M.C., eds. *Cost-Effectiveness in Health and Medicine.* New York: Oxford University Press, 1996.

Goldberg, H.B., Burstein, N.R., Moore, T., and Schmitz, R.J. *Case-Mix Adjustment for a National Home Health Prospective Payment System: Interim Report.* Cambridge, MA: Abt Associates, 1998.

Goodwin, J.S. Geriatrics and the Limits of Modern Medicine. *New England Journal of Medicine* 340(16):1283–1285, 1999.

Gottesman, L.E. Nursing Home Performance as Related to Resident Traits, Ownership, Size, and Source of Payment. *American Journal of Public Health* 64(3):269–276, 1974.

Graber, D.R., and Sloane, P.D. Nursing Home Survey Deficiencies for Physical Restraint Use. *Medical Care* 33(10):1051–1063, 1995.

Grana, J.M., and Yamashiro, S.M. *An Evaluation of the Veterans Administration Housebound and Aid and Attendant Allowance Program.* Prepared for the Office of the Assistant Secretary for Policy and Evaluation, Department of Health and Human Services. Washington, DC: Project HOPE, 1987.

Gubrium, J.F. *Speaking of Life: Horizons of Meaning for Nursing Home Residents.* Hawthorne, NY: Aldine de Gruyeter, 1993.

Gustafson, D.H., and Gustafson, R. Re-Engineering Long-Term Care Quality of Life Improvement. Paper presented at the symposium on: *Improving the Quality of Life for Nursing Home Residents: The Challenges and the Opportunities.* Baltimore, MD, July 11–12, 1996.

Guyatt, G.H., Sinclair, J., Cook, D.J., and Glasziou, P. Users' Guides to the Medical Literature: XVI. How to Use a Treatment Recommendation. Evidence-Based Medicine Working Group and the Cochrane Applicability Methods Working Group. *Journal of the American Medical Association* 281(19):1836–1843, 1999.

Harrington, C. The Federal Nursing Home Survey and Regulation Process. Testimony to the U.S. Senate Special Committee on Aging. Washington, DC: U.S. Senate, July 28, 1998.

Harrington, C., and Carrillo, H. The Regulation and Enforcement of Federal Nursing Home Standards. *Medical Care Research and Review* 56(4):471–494, 1999.

Harrington, C., and Carrillo, H. *Analysis of HCFA's On-Line Survey Certification and Reporting (OSCAR) System Data.* San Francisco: University of California, 2000.

Harrington, C., and Grant, L.A. The Delivery, Regulation and Politics of Home Care: A California Case Study. *The Gerontologist* 30(4):451–461, 1990.

Harrington, C., Summers, P.R., Curtis, M., and Maynard, R. *Study of the Resident Assessment Information System.* San Francisco: University of California, Department of Social and Behavioral Sciences, 1996.

Harrington, C., Carrillo, H., Mullan, J., and Swan, J.S. Nursing Home Staffing in the States: The 1991–1995 Period. *Medical Care Research and Review* 55(3):334–363, 1998a.

Harrington, C., Swan, J.H., Griffin, C., and Clemena, W. *1996 State Data Book on Long Term Care Program and Market Characteristics.* San Francisco: University of California, Department of Social and Behavioral Sciences, 1998b.

Harrington, C., Zimmerman, D., Karon, S.L., Robinson, J., and Beutel, P. *Nursing Home Staffing and its Relationship to Deficiencies.* San Francisco: University of California, Department of Social and Behavioral Sciences, 1998c.

Harrington, C., Carrillo, H., Thollaug, S.C., and Summers, P.R. Nursing Facilities, Staffing, Residents, and Facility Deficiencies, 1991 through 1997. San Francisco: Univeristy of California, 1999.

Harrington, C., LeBlanc, A.J., Wood, J., Satten, N., and Tonner, M.C. *Medicaid Home and Community Based Services in the States: Policy Issues and Future Directions.* San Francisco: University of California, Department of Social and Behavioral Sciences, 2000a.

Harrington, C., Carrillo, H., Thollaug, S.C., Summers, P.R., and Wellin, V. *Nursing Facilities, Staffing, Residents, and Facility Deficiencies, 1992 Through 1998.* Report prepared for the U.S. Health Care Financing Administration and the Agency for Health Care Policy and Research. San Francisco: University of California, Department of Social and Behavioral Sciences, 2000b.

Harrington, C., Kovner, C., Mezey, M., Kayser-Jones, J., Burger, S., Mohler, M., Burke, R., and Zimmerman, D. Experts Recommend Minimum Nurse Staffing Standards for Nursing Facilities in the United States. *The Gerontologist* 40(1):5–16, 2000c.

Harrington, C., LaPlante, M., Newcomer, R.J., Bedney, B., Shostak, S., Summers, P., Weinberg, J., and Basnett, I. *A Review of Federal Statutes and Regulations for Personal Care and Home and Community-Based Services: A Final Report.* San Francisco: University of California, Department of Social and Behavioral Sciences, 2000d.

Harrington, C., Summers, P.R., and Wellin, V. *State Medicaid Home Health Licensing and Certification.* Prepared for the Health Care Financing Administration. San Francisco: University of California, Department of Social and Behavioral Sciences, 2000e.

Harrington, C., Carrillo, H., Wellin, V., Norwood, F., and Miller, N. 1915(c) Medicaid Home and Community-Based Waiver Participants, Services, and Expenditures, 1992–1997. San Francisco: University of California, Department of Social and Behavioral Sciences, 2000f.

Harrington, C., Swan, J.H., Wellin, V., Clemena, W. and Carrillo, H. *1998 State Data Book on Long Term Care Program and Market Characteristics.* San Francisco: University of California, Department of Social and Behavioral Sciences, 2000g.

Harrington, C., Zimmerman, D., Karon, S.L., Robinson, J., and Beutel, P. Nursing Home Staffing and its Relationship to Deficiencies. *Journal of Gerontology* forthcoming 2000h.

Harrington, C., Carrillo, H., Wellin, V., Miller, N., and LeBlanc, A.J. Predicting State Medicaid Home and Community-Based Waiver Participants and Expenditures, 1992–1997. *The Gerontologist* forthcoming 2000i.

Harris, L. and Associates. The ICD Survey of Disabled Americans: Bringing Disabled Americans into the Mainstream. *Incitement* 9:12, 1993.

Hawes, C. *Assuring Nursing Home Quality: The History and Impact of Federal Standards in OBRA 1987.* Paper prepared for the Commonwealth Fund. Research Triangle Park, NC: Research Triangle Institute, 1996.

Hawes, C., Wildfire, J.B., and Lux, L.J. *The Regulation of Board and Care Homes: Results of a 50-State Survey.* Washington, DC: American Association of Retired Persons, 1993.

Hawes, C., Mor, V., Wildfire, J., Iannacchione, V., Lux, L., Green, R., Greene, A., Wilcox, V., Spore, D., and Phillips, C.D. *Analysis of the Effect of Regulation on the Quality of Care in Board and Care Homes. Executive Summary.* Providence, RI: Brown University, 1995a.

Hawes, C., Morris, J.N., Phillips, C.D., Mor, V., Fries, B.E., and Nonemaker, S. Reliability Estimates for the Minimum Data Set for Nursing Home Resident Assessment and Care Screening (MDS): Results from the Final Field Testing. *The Gerontologist* 35(2):172–178, 1995b.

Hawes, C., Morris, J.N., Phillips, C.D., Fries, B.E., and Mor, V. Development of the Nursing Home Resident Assessment Instrument in the U.S. *Age and Ageing* 26(S2):19–26, 1997a.

Hawes, C., Mor, V., Phillips, C.D., Fries, B.E., Morris, J.N., Steele-Friedlob, E., Greene, A.M., and Nennstiel, M. The OBRA-87 Nursing Home Regulations and Implementation of the Resident Assessment Instrument: Effects on Process Quality. *Journal of the American Geriatrics Society* 45:977–985, 1997b.

Hawes, C., Rose, M., and Phillips, C.D. *A National Study of Assisted Living for the Frail Elderly: Results of a National Survey of Facilities.* Beachwood, OH: Myers Research Institute, Menorah Park Center on Aging, 1999.

Hawkins, A.M., Burgio, L.D., Langford, A., and Engel, B.T. The Effects of Verbal and Written Supervisory Feedback on Staff Compliance with Assigned Prompted Voiding in a Nursing Home. *Journal of Organizational Behavior Management* 13:137–150, 1992.

HCFA (Health Care Financing Administration). 42 CFR Parts 401–498. Medicare and Medicaid Programs: Survey, Certification and Enforcement of Skilled Nursing Facilities and Nursing Facilities: Final Rule. *Federal Register* 59(217), 1994.

HCFA. *State Operations Manual: Provider Certification.* Transmittal No. 272. Washington, DC: HCFA, 1995a.

HCFA. *State Operations Manual: Provider Certification.* Transmittal No. 273. Washington, DC: HCFA, 1995b.

HCFA. *State Operations Manual: Provider Certification.* Transmittal No. 274. Washington, DC: HCFA, 1995c.

HCFA. *Assuring the Quality of Nursing Home Care.* DHHS Fact Sheet. Washington, DC: HCFA Press Office, July 21, 1998a.

HCFA. *A Report to Congress: Study of Private Accreditation (Deeming) of Nursing Homes, Regulatory Incentives and Non-Regulatory Incentives, and Effectiveness of the Survey and Certification System.* Washington, DC: HCFA, 1998b.

HCFA. Letter to the Honorable Charles E. Grassley, Chairman, U.S. Senate Special Committee on Aging: Nursing Home Initiative Update #12. Washington, DC: HCFA, August 1999a.

HCFA. *Assuring Quality for Nursing Home Residents.* HCFA Fact Sheet Press Release. Washington, DC: HCFA Press Office, December 14, 1999b.

HCFA. *State Operations Manual. Survey and Enforcement Process for SNFs and NFs. Part 7.* Baltimore, MD: HCFA, 1999c.

HCFA. *Report to Congress: Appropriateness of Minimum Nurse Staffing Ratios in Nursing Homes, Phase 1.* Baltimore, MD: HCFA, 2000.

Health Care Financing Review. *Medicare and Medicaid Statistical Supplement, 1999.* Washington, DC: HCFA, 1999.

Heller, T. Residential Relocation and Reactions of Elderly Retarded Persons. In Janicki, M. and Wisniewski, H., eds. *Aging and Developmental Disabilities: Issues and Approaches.* Baltimore, MD: Brookes, 1985.

Heller, T., Hahn, J.E., and Factor, A. Nursing Home Reform: The Impact of Moving out of Nursing Homes on People with Developmental Disabilities. *Policy Research Brief* 7:1–7, 1995.

Heller, T., Miller, A.B., and Factor, A. Environmental Characteristics of Nursing Homes and Community-Based Settings, and the Well-Being of Adults with Intellectual Disabilities. *Journal of Intellectual Disabilities* 42(5):418–428, 1998.

Henderson, J.N., and Vespari, M.D., eds. *The Culture of Long Term Care: Nursing Home Ethnography.* Westport, CT: Bergin and Garvey, 1995.

Herman, S. Use and Impact of a Cash Subsidy Program. *Mental Retardation* 29(5):253–258, 1991.

Hobbs, N., and Perrin, J., eds. *Issues in the Care of Children with Chronic Illness.* San Francisco: Jossey-Bass, 1985.

Hobbs, N., Perrin, J.M., and Ireys, H.T. *Chronically Ill Children and Their Families.* San Francisco: Jossey-Bass, 1985.

Hoeffer, B., Rader, J., McKenzie, D., Lavelle, M., and Stewart, B. Reducing Aggressive Behavior during Bathing Cognitively Impaired Nursing Home Residents. *Journal of Gerontological Nursing* 23(5):16–23, 1997.

Hofland, B. Autonomy in Long-Term Care: Background Issues and a Programmatic Response. *The Gerontologist* 28:3–9, 1988.

Holahan, J.F., and Cohen, J.W. Nursing Home Reimbursement: Implications for Cost Containment, Access, and Quality. *Milbank Quarterly* 65(1):112–147, 1987.

Holmes, D. *Bar-Code Technology in Long-Term Care Operations and Research.* Paper presented at the Annual Meeting of the American Association of Homes and Services for the Aging, Philadelphia, 1996.

Horowitz, A.V., and Reinhard, S. Home Care for Persons with Serious Mental Illnesses. Pp. 269–292 in Fox, D.M., and Raphael, C., eds. *Home-Based Care for a New Century.* Malden, MA: Blackwell Publishers, 1997.

Hu, T.W., Igou, J.F., Kaltreider, D.L., Yu, L.C., Rohner, T.J., Dennis, P.J., Craighead, W.E., Hadley, E.D., and Ory, M.G. A Clinical Trial of a Behavioral Therapy to Reduce Urinary Incontinence in Nursing Homes. *Journal of the American Medical Association* 273(17):1366–1370, 1995.

Hughes, S.L., Conrad, K.J., Manheim, L.M., and Edelman, P.L. Impact of Long-Term Home Care on Mortality, Functional Status, and Unmet Needs. *Health Services Research* 23:269–294, 1988.

IOM (Institute of Medicine). Takeuchi, J., Burke, R., and McGeary, M., eds. *Improving the Quality of Care in Nursing Homes.* Washington, DC: National Academy Press, 1986.

IOM. Lohr, K.N., ed. *Medicare: A Strategy for Quality Assurance,* Vol. 1. Washington, DC: National Academy Press, 1990.

IOM. Field, M.J., and Lohr, K.N., eds. *Guidelines for Clinical Practice: From Development to Use.* Washington, DC: National Academy Press, 1992.

IOM. Wehling, J., Feasley, J., and Estes, C., eds. *Real People, Real Problems. Evaluation of the Long-Term Care Ombudsman Program of the Older Americans Act.* Washington, DC: National Academy Press, 1995.

IOM. Wunderlich, G., Sloan, F., and Davis, C., eds. *Nursing Staff in Hospitals and Nursing Homes: Is it Adequate?* Washington, DC: National Academy Press, 1996a.

IOM. *Best at Home: Assuring Quality Long-Term Care in Home and Community-Based Settings.* Washington, DC: National Academy Press, 1996b.

IOM. Field, M.J., and Cassel, C.K., eds. *Approaching Death: Improving Care at the End of Life.* Washington, DC: National Academy Press, 1997.

Jackson, J.L., and Kroenke, K. Patient Satisfaction and Quality of Care. *Military Medicine* 162(4):273–277, 1997.

James, B.C. Implementing Practice Guidelines through Clinical Quality Improvement. *Frontiers of Health Services Management* 10(1):3–37, 1993.

Jessop, D.J., and Stein, R.E.K. Providing Comprehensive Health Care to Children with Chronic Illness. *Pediatrics* 93:602–607, 1994.

Jette, A.M., Smith, K.W., and McDermott, S.M. Quality of Medicare-Reimbursed Home Health Care. *The Gerontologist* 36(4):492–501, 1996.

Johnson, M.F., and Kramer, A.M. *Quality of Care Problems Persist in Nursing Homes Despite Improvements Since the Nursing Home Reform Act.* Paper prepared for the Institute of Medicine Committee on Improving the Quality of Long-Term Care. Washington, DC, October 1998.

Justice, D, Folkemer, D., Donahoe, E., and Nelssen, H. *Integral Role of Case Management in Authorizing Services Under State Community Care Programs.* Washington, DC: National Association of State Units on Aging, 1991.

Kane, R.A. Goals of Home Care: Therapeutic, Compensatory, Either, or Both? *Journal on Aging and Health* 11(3):299–321, 1999.

Kane, R.A. Long-Term Case Management for Older Adults. In Kane, R.L., and Kane, R.A. eds. *Assessing Older People: Measures, Meaning, and Practical Applications.* New York: Oxford University Press, 2000.

Kane, R.A., and Degenholtz, H.D. Case Management as a Force for Quality Assurance and Quality Improvement in Home Care. *Journal of Aging and Social Policy* 9(4):5–28, 1997.

Kane, R.A., and Frytak, J. *Models for Case Management in Long-Term Care: Interactions of Case Managers and Home Care Providers.* Minneapolis, MN: University of Minnesota, National Long-Term Care Resource Center, 1994.

Kane, R.A., and Kane, R.L. *Long-Term Care: Principles, Policies, and Programs.* New York: Springer, 1987.

Kane, R.A., and Wilson, K.B. *Assisted Living in the United States: A New Paradigm for Residential Care for Frail Older Persons?* Washington, DC: American Association of Retired Persons, 1993.

Kane, R.A., Kane, R.L., Arnold, S., Garrard, J., McDermott, S., and Kepferle, L. Geriatric Nurse Practitioners as Nursing Home Employees: Implementing the Role. *The Gerontologist* 28(4):469–477, 1988.

Kane, R.A., Illston, L.H., Kane, R.L., Nyman, J.A., and Finch, M.D. Adult Foster Care for the Elderly in Oregon: A Mainstream Alternative to Nursing Homes. *American Journal of Public Health* 81:1113–1120, 1991a.

Kane, R.A., Finch, M., Geron, S.M., Skay, C., Stoner, T., and McGuire, D. *Development and Field Testing of a Uniform Long-Term Client Instrument for Florida.* Report prepared for the Florida Department of Health and Rehabilitative Services. Minneapolis, MN: University of Minnesota, National Long-Term Care Resource Center, 1991b.

Kane, R.A., Penrod, J., Davidson, G., Moscovice, I., and Rich, E. What Cost Case Management in Long-Term Care. *Social Services Research* 65(2):281–303, 1991c.

Kane, R.A., Kane, R.L., Illston, L.H., and Eustis, N.N. Perspectives on Home Care Quality. *Health Care Financing Review* 16(1):69–89, 1994.

Kane, R.A., O'Connor, C.M., and Baker, M.O. *Delegation of Nursing Activities: Implications for Patterns in Long-Term Care.* Washington, DC: American Association of Retired Persons, 1995.

Kane, R.A., Caplan, A.L., Urv-Wong, E.K., Freeman, I.C., Avoskar, M.A., and Finch, M. Everyday Matters in the Lives of Nursing Home Residents: Wish for and Perception of Choice and Control. *Journal of the American Geriatric Society* 45:1086–1093, 1997.

Kane, R.A., Baker, M.O., Salmon, J., and Veazie, W. *Consumer Perspectives on Private Versus Shared Accommodations in Assisted Living Settings.* Washington, DC: American Association of Retired Persons, 1998a.

Kane, R.A., Kane, R.L., Ladd, D. and Veazie, W. Variation in State Spending for Long-Term Care: Factors Associated with More Balanced Systems. *Journal of Health Policy, Politics and Law* 23(2):363–390, 1998b.

Kane, R.A., Kane, R.L., and Ladd, D. *The Heart of Long-Term Care.* New York: Oxford Press, 1998c.

Kane, R.A., Giles, K., Lawton, M.P., and Kane, R.L. Development of Measures and Indicators of Quality of Life in Nursing Homes: Wave I. Report submitted to Health Care Financing Administration. Minneapolis, MN: University of Minnesota School of Public Health, 1999.

Kane, R.L. Setting the PACE in Chronic Care. *Contemporary Gerontology* 6(12):47–50, 1999.

Kane, R.L., and Blewett, L.A. Quality Assurance for a Program of Comprehensive Care for Older Persons. *Health Care Financing Review* 14(4):89–110, 1993.

Kane, R.L., Bell, R.M., and Riegler, S.Z. Value Preferences for Nursing Home Outcomes. *The Gerontologist* 26:303–308, 1986.

Kane, R.L., Finch, M., Chen, Q., Blewett, L., Burns, R., and Moskowitz, M. Post-Hospital Care for Medicare Patients. *Health Care Financing Review* 16(1):131–154, 1994.

Kane, R.L., Kane, R.A., Finch, M., Harrington, C., Newcomer, R., Miller, N., and Hulbert, M. S/HMOs, The Second Generation: Building on the Experience of the First Social Health Maintenance Organization Demonstrations. *Journal of the American Geriatrics Society* 45:1010–1017, 1997.

Kane, R.L., Chen, Q., Finch, M., Blewett, L., Burns, R., and Moskowitz, M. Functional Outcomes of Post-Hospital Care for Stroke and Hip Fracture Patients Under Medicare. *Journal of the American Geriatrics Society* 46(12):1525–1533, 1998.

Kane, R.L., and Huck, S. The Implementation of the PACE Demonstration Project. *Journal of the American Geriatrics Society* 44:218–228, 2000.

Kapp, M.B. Improving Choices Regarding Home Care Services: Legal Impediments and Empowerments. *Saint Louis University Public Law Review* 10:441–484, 1991.

Karon, S.C., Sainfort, F., and Zimmerman, D.R. Stability of Nursing Home Quality Indicators Over Time. *Medical Care* 37(6):570–579, 1999.

Karuza, J., and Katz, P.R. Physician Staffing Patterns Correlates of Nursing Home Care: An Initial Inquiry and Consideration of Policy Implications. *Journal of the American Geriatrics Society* 42:787–793, 1994.

Kassirer, J.P. Adding Insult to Injury: Usurping Patients' Prerogatives. *New England Journal of Medicine* 308:898–901, 1983.

Katz, D.A. Barriers Between Guidelines and Improved Patient Care: An Analysis of AHCPR's Unstable Angina Clinical Practice Guideline. *Health Services Research* 34(1-2):377–389, 1999.

Kauffman, C. Abuse and Neglect: An Investigative Report on Quad-City Nursing Homes. *Quad-City Times.* Series. December 1–8, 1996.

Kayser-Jones, J. Mealtime in Nursing Homes. *Journal of Gerontological Nursing* 22(3):26–31, 1996.

Kayser-Jones, J. Inadequate Staffing at Mealtime. *Journal of Gerontological Nursing* 23(8):14–21, 1997.

Kayser-Jones, J., and Schell, E. The Effect of Staffing on the Quality of Care at Mealtime. *Nursing Outlook* 45(2):64–72, 1997.

Kayser-Jones, J., Wiener, C.L., and Barbaccia, J.C. Factors Contributing to the Hospitalization of Nursing Home Residents. *The Gerontologist* 29(4):1502–1510, 1989.

Kayser-Jones, J., Schell, E., Porter, C., and Paul, S. Reliability of Percentage Figures Used to Record the Dietary Intake of Nursing Home Residents. *Nursing Home Medicine* 5(3):69–76, 1997.

Kayser-Jones, J., Schell, E.S., Porter, C., Barbaccia, J.C., Steinbach, C., Bird, W.F., Redford, M., and Pengilly, K. A Prospective Study of the Use of Liquid Oral Dietary Supplements in Nursing Homes. *Journal of the American Geriatrics Society* 46(11):1378–1386, 1998.

Kayser-Jones, J., Schell, E.S., Porter, C., Barbaccia, J.C., and Shaw, H. Factors Contributing to Dehydration in Nursing Homes: Inadequate Staffing and Lack of Professional Supervision. *Journal of the American Geriatrics Society* 47(10):1187–1194, 1999.

Kinney, E.D., Freeman, J.A, and Cook, C.A. Quality Improvement in Community-Based Long-Term Care: Theory and Reality. *American Journal of Law and Medicine* 20(1-2):59–77, 1994.

Kochersberger, G., Hielema, F., and Westlund, R. Rehabilitation in the Nursing Home: How Much, Why, and With What Results. *Public Health Reports* 109(3):372–376, 1994.

Komisar, H.L., and Feder J. *The Balanced Budget Act of 1997: Effects on Medicare's Home Health Benefit and Beneficiaries Who Need Long-Term Care.* New York: Commonwealth Fund, 1998.

Kosberg, J., and Tobin, S.S. Variability Among Nursing Homes. *The Gerontologist* 12:214–219, 1972.

Kramer, A.M. *Betrayal: The Quality of Care in California Nursing Homes.* Testimony Before the U.S. Senate Special Committee on Aging. Washington, DC, July 28, 1998.

Kramer, A.M. *The Nursing Home Initiative: Results at Year One.* Testimony Before the U.S. Senate Special Committee on Aging. Washington, DC, June 30, 1999.

Kramer, A.M., Shaughnessy, P.W., Bauman, M.K., and Crisler, K.S. Assessing and Assuring the Quality of Home Health Care: A Conceptual Framework. *Milbank Quarterly* 68:413–443, 1990.

Krauss, N.A., and Altman, B.M. Characteristics of Nursing Home Residents—1996. *MEPS Research Findings No. 5.* Rockville, MD: Agency for Health Care Policy and Research, 1998.

Kravitz, R. Patient Satisfaction with Heath Care: Critical Outcome or Trivial Pursuit? *Journal of General Internal Medicine* 13:280–282, 1998.

Kruzich, J.M., Clinton, J.F., and Kelber, S.T. Personal and Environmental Influences on Nursing Home Satisfaction. *The Gerontologist* 32(3):342–350, 1992.

Kuhlthau, D., Walker, D.K., Perrin, J.M., Bauman, L., Gortmaker, S.L., Newacheck, P.W., and Stein, R.E. Assessing Managed Care for Children with Chronic Conditions. *Health Affairs* 17(4):42–52, 1998.

Kuntz, C. *Persons with Severe Mental Illness: How Do They Fit into Long-Term Care?* Report prepared by the Office of Disability, Aging, and Long-Term Care Policy. Washington, DC: Department of Health and Human Services, May 1995.

La Monica, E.L., Oberst, M.T., Madea, A.R., and Wolf, R.M. Development of a Patient Satisfaction Scale. *Research in Nursing and Health* 9:43–50, 1986.

Laffel, G., and Blumenthal, D. The Case for Using Industrial Quality Management Science in Health Care Organizations. *Journal of the American Medical Association* 262:2869–2872, 1989.

Laine, C., and Davidoff, F. Patient-Centered Medicine: A Professional Evolution. *Journal of the American Medical Association* 275(2):152–156, 1996.

Laird, C. *Limbo.* Novato, CA: Chandler and Sharp Publishers, 1985.

Laliberte, I., Mor, V., Berg, K., Intrator, O., Calore, K., and Hiris, J. Impact of the Medicare Catastrophic Coverage Act on Nursing Homes. *Milbank Quarterly* 75(2):203–233, 1997.

Landgraf, J.M., Abetz, L., and Ware, J.E. *Child Health Questionnaire: A User's Manual*, 1st Edition. Boston: The Health Institute, New England Medical Center, 1996.

Lange-Alberts, M., and Shott, S. Nutritional Intake. Use of Touch and Verbal Cueing. *Journal of Gerontological Nursing* 20(2):36–40, 1994.

Lasser, R.A., and Sunderland, T. Newer Psychotropic Medication Use in Nursing Home Residents. *Journal of the American Geriatrics Society* 46(2):202–207, 1998.

Lavizzo-Mourey, R.J., Zinn, J., and Taylor, L. Ability of Surrogates to Represent Satisfaction of Nursing Home Residents with Quality of Care. *Journal of the American Geriatrics Society* 40:39–47, 1992.

Lawton, M.P., and Bader, J. Wish for Privacy by Young and Old. *Journal of Gerontology* 25(1):48–54, 1970.

Lawton, M.P., Van Haitsma, K., and Klapper, J. Observed Affect in Nursing Home Residents with Alzheimer's Disease. *Journal of Gerontology—Psychological Sciences* 51B(1):3–14, 1996.

Lawton, M.P., Van Haitsma, K., Perkinson, M. and Ruckdeschel, K. Observed Affect and Quality of Life in Dementia: Further Affirmations and Problems. *Journal of Mental Health and Aging* 5(1): 69–81, 1999.

Leavitt, T. The Demographic and Employment Characteristics of Home Care Aides in the 1990s. Unpublished paper prepared for the Institute of Medicine Committee on Improving Quality in Long-Term Care, June 11–12, 1998.

LeBlanc, A.J., Tonner, M.L., and Harrington, C. *State Medicaid Programs Offering Personal Care Services.* San Francisco: University of California, 2000a.

LeBlanc, A.J., Tonner, M.L., and Harrington, C. *Medicaid 1915(c) Home and Community Based Services Waivers Across the States: Program Structure and Barriers to Growth.* San Francisco: University of California, 2000b.

Lekan-Rutledge, D., Palmer, M.H., and Belyea, M. In Their Own Words: Nursing Assistants' Perceptions of Barriers to Implementation of Prompted Voiding in Long-Term Care. *The Gerontologist* 38(3):370–378, 1998.

Levenson, S.A., ed. *Medical Direction in Long-Term Care.* Durham, NC: Carolina Academic Press, 1993.

Levin, B.L., and Petrila, J. *Mental Health Services: A Public Health Perspective.* New York: Oxford University Press, 1996.

Levine, J.M., Marchello, V., and Totolos, E. Progress Toward a Restraint-Free Environment in a Large Academic Nursing Facility. *Journal of the American Geriatrics Society* 43(8):914–918, 1995.

Levit, K.R., Lazenby, H.C., Braden, B.R., Cowan, C.A., Sensenig, A.L., McDonnell, P.A., Stiller, J.M., Won, D.K., Martin, A.B., Sivarajan, L., Donham, C.S., Long, A.M., and Stewart, M.W. National Health Expenditures, 1996. *Health Care Financing Review* 19(1):161–200, 1997.

Levit, K.R., Cowan, C., Lazenby, H., Sensenig, A., McDonnell, P., Stiller, J., Martin, A., and the Health Accountants Team. Health Spending in 1998: Signals of Changes. *Health Affairs* 19(1):124–132, 2000.

Lewin/ICF and James Bell Associates. *Descriptions of and Supplement Information on Board and Care Homes Included in the Update of the National Health Provider Inventory.* Washington, DC: Lewin/ICF, 1990.

Lewin Group. *Implications of the Medicare Home Health Interim Payment System of the 1997 Balanced Budget Act.* Washington, DC: National Association for Home Health Care, February 1998.

Lewin Group. Unpublished Analysis of U.S. Census Bureau Projections. Fairfax, VA: the Lewin Group, 1999.

Libow, L., and Starer, P. Care of the Nursing Home Patient. *New England Journal of Medicine* 321:93–96, 1989.

Lidz, C.W., Fischer, L., and Arnold, R.M. *The Erosion of Autonomy in Long-Term Care.* New York: Oxford University Press, 1992.

Life Services Network of Illinois. *Life Services Network's Nursing Facility Resident Satisfaction Questionnaire.* Presented at the American Association of Homes and Services for the Aging State Executive Forum Meeting, October 21, 1997.

Linn, M., Furel, L., and Linn, B.A. Patient Outcome as a Measure of Quality of Nursing Home Care. *American Journal of Public Health* 67(4):337–344, 1977.

Litvak, S., and Kennedy, J. *Policy Issues and Questions Affecting the Medicaid Personal Care Services Option Benefit.* Oakland, CA: World Institute on Disability, 1991.

Litvak, S., Zukas, H., and Heumann, J.E. *Attending to America—Personal Assistance for Independent Living: A Survey of Attendant Service Programs in the United States for People of All Ages with Disabilities.* Berkeley, CA: World Institute on Disability, 1987.

Llewellyn, G., Dunn, P., Fante, M., Turnbull, L., and Grace, R. Family Factors Influencing Out-of-Home Placement Decisions. *Journal of Intellectual Disabilities Research* 43(3):219–233, 1999.

Llorente, M.D., Olsen, E.J., Leyva, O., Silverman, M.A., Lewis, J.E., and Rivero, J. Use of Antipsychotic Drugs in Nursing Homes: Current Compliance with OBRA Regulations. *Journal of the American Gerontological Society* 46:198–201, 1998.

Locker, D., and Dunt, D. Theoretical and Methodological Issues in Sociological Studies of Consumer Satisfaction with Medical Care. *Social Science and Medicine* 12:283–292, 1978.

Logsdon, R., Gibbons, L., McMurry, S., and Teri, L. Quality of Life in Alzheimer's Disease: Patient and Caregiver Reports. *Journal of Mental Health and Aging* 5(1):21–32, 1999.

Lustbader, W. The Pioneer Challenge: A Radical Shift in the Culture of Nursing Homes. In Noelker, L.A. and Harel, Z., eds. *Linking Quality of Long Term Care and Quality of Life.* New York: Springer, 2000

Maas, M., Buckwalter, K., and Specht, J. Nursing Staff and Quality of Care in Nursing Homes Pp. 361–424 in *Nursing Staff in Hospitals and Nursing Homes: Is It Adequate?* Washington, DC: National Academy Press, 1996.

MacAdam, M. Home Care Reimbursement and Effects on Personnel. *The Gerontologist* 33(1):55–63, 1993.

MacRae, P.G., Schnelle, J.F., Simmons, S.F., and Ouslander, J.G. Physical Activity Levels of Ambulatory Nursing Home Residents. *Journal of Aging and Physical Activity* 4:264–278, 1996.

Manton, K.G. A Longitudinal Study of Sectional Change and Mortality in the United States. *Journal of Gerontology* 43(5):S153–S161, 1988.

Manton, K.G., Singer, B.H., and Suzman, R.M. *Forecasting the Health of Elderly Populations.* New York: Springer-Verlag, 1993.

Manton, K.G., Corder, L., and Stallard, E. Chronic Disability Trends in Elderly United States Populations: 1982–1994. *Proceedings of the National Academy of Sciences* 94(6):2593–2598, 1997.

Mattimore, T.J., Wenger, N.S., Desbiens, N.A., Teno, J.M., Hamel, M.B., Lit, H., Califf, R., Connors, A.F., Lynn, J., and Oye, R.K. Surrogate and Physician Understanding of Patients' Preferences for Living Permanently in a Nursing Home. *Journal of the American Geriatrics Society* 45(7):818–824, 1997.

McFarlane, W.R., Lukens, E., Link, B., Dushay, R., Deakins, S.A., Newmark, M., Dunne, E.J. Horen, B., and Toran, J. Multiple-Family Groups and Psychoeducation in the Treatment of Schizophrenia. *Archives of General Psychiatry* 52 (8):679–687, 1995.

McKenna, M., Moyers, J., and Feuerberg, M. Review of Non-Regulatory Quality Improvement Interventions. Pp. 339–384 in *HCFA Report to Congress: Study of Private Accreditation (Deeming) Nursing Homes, Regulatory Incentives and Non-Regulatory Initiatives, and Effectiveness of the Survey and Certification System*, Vol. II. Washington, DC: HCFA, 1998.

Mechanic, D. Emerging Trends in Mental Health Policy and Practice. *Health Affairs* 17(6):82–98, 1998.

Mechanic, D. *Mental Health and Social Policy: The Emergence of Managed Care.* Fourth Edition. Boston: Allyn and Bacon, 1999.

MedPAC (Medicare Payment Advisory Commission). *Health Care Spending and the Medicare Program: A Data Book.* Washington, DC: MedPAC, 1998.

MedPAC. *Report to the Congress: Medicare Payment Policy.* Washington, DC: MedPAC, 1999.

Mercer, S.O., Heacock, P., and Beck, C. Nurse's Aides in Nursing Homes: Perceptions of Training, Work Loads, Racism and Abuse Issues. *Journal of Gerontological Social Work* 21(1/2):95–112, 1993.

Meyers, J., and Marcenko, M. Impact of a Cash Subsidy Program for Families of Children with a Severe Developmental Disability. *Mental Retardation* 27:383–386, 1989.

Mezey, M., and Kovner, C. Expert Recommendations on Minimum Nurse Staffing Standards for Nursing Homes. Letter to the IOM Committee. New York: John A. Hartford Foundation Institute for Geriatric Nursing, November 16, 1998.

Mezey, M.D., and Lynaugh, J.E. The Teaching Nursing Home Program: Outcomes of Care. *Nursing Clinics of North America* 24(3):769–780, 1989.

Mezey, M.D., and Lynaugh, J.E. Teaching Nursing Home Program: A Lesson in Quality. *Geriatric Nursing* (Mar–Apr):76–77, 1991.

Miller, N.A. Medicaid 2176 Home and Community-Based Waivers: The First Ten Years. *Health Affairs* 11(4):162–171, 1992.

Miller, N.A. Patient-Centered Long-Term Care. *Health Care Financing Review* 19(2):1–10, 1997.

Miller, N.A., Ramsland, S., and Harrington, C. Trends and Issues in the Medicaid 1915(c) Waiver Program. *Health Care Financing Review* 20(4):139–160, 1999a.

Miller, N.A., Ramlsand, S., Goldstein, E., and Harrington, C. *States' Use of Medicaid Community-Based Long Term Care 1990–1997.* Baltimore, MD: University of Maryland, Baltimore County, 1999b.

Miltenburg, T., Ramakers, C., and Mensink, J. *A Personal Budget for Clients, Summary of an Experiment with Cash Benefits in Home Care in the Netherlands.* Nijmegen, Netherlands: Institute for Applied Social Sciences, 1996.

Mittelman, M.S., Ferris, S.H., Shulman, E., Steinberg, G., and Levin, B. A Family Intervention to Delay Nursing Home Placement of Patients with Alzheimer Disease. A Randomized Controlled Trial. *Journal of the American Medical Association* 276(21):1725–1731, 1996.

Mohler, M. *Combined Federal and State Nursing Services Staffing Standards.* Washington, DC: National Committee to Preserve Social Security and Medicare, 1993.

Mohler, M., and Lessard, W. *Nursing Staff in Nursing Homes: Additional Staff Needed and Cost to Meet Requirements and Quality of OBRA 87.* Testimony prepared for the U.S. House of Representatives Select Committee on Aging. Washington, DC, 1991.

Mollica, R.L. Assisted Living and State Policy. *Journal of Long-Term Care Administration* 24(3):11–14, 1996.

Mollica, R.L. State Assisted Living Policy: 1998 [WWW document]. URL http:// aspe.os.dhhs.gov/daltcp/reports.htm (accessed October 27, 1998), 1998.

Mollica, R., Reinardy, J., Kane, R.A., Fralich, J., Potthoff, S., Nyman, J., and Leone, A. *Preliminary Findings and Recommendations Concerning Kansas Long-Term Care System.* Minneapolis, MN: University of Minnesota, National Long-Term Care Resource Center, 1994.

Monk, A., Kaye, L.W., and Litwin, T. *Resolving Grievances in the Nursing Home: A Study of the Ombudsman Program.* New York: Columbia University Press, 1984.

Montogmery, R. and Kosloski, K. Respite Revisited: Re-Assessing the Impact. In Katz, P.R., Kane, R.L., and Mezey, N.D., eds. *Quality of Care in Geriatric Settings.* New York: Springer, 1995.

Moore, T., and White, A. *Drug Utilization and MDS-Based Outcomes for Elderly Nursing Home Residents.* Cambridge, MA: Abt Associates, 1998.

Mor, V. Hospitalization of Nursing Home Residents: A Review of Clinical, Organizational and Policy Determinants. Providence, RI: Brown University Gerontology Center, 1999.

Mor, V., Sherwood, S., and Gutkin, C. A National Study of Residential Care for the Aged. *The Gerontologist* 26(4):405–417, 1986.

Mor, V., Intrator, O., Fries, B., Phillips, C., Teno, J., Hiris, J., Hawes, C., and Morris, J. Changes in Hospitalization Associated with Introducing the Resident Assessment Instrument. *Journal of the American Geriatrics Society* 45(8):1002–1010, 1997.

Morris, J.N., Hawes, C., Fries, B.E., Phillips, C.D., Mor, V., Katz, S., Murphy, K., Drugovich, M.L., and Friedlob, A.S. Designing the National Resident Assessment Instrument for Nursing Homes. *The Gerontologist* 30(3):293–307, 1990.

Morris, J.N., Nonemaker, S., Murphy, K., Hawes, C., Fries, B.E., Mor, V., and Phillips, C. A Commitment to Change: Revision of HCFA's RAI. *Journal of the American Geriatrics Society* 45(8):1011–1016, 1997.

Mortimore, E., Miller, P., Santoro, V., and Feuerberg, M. Evidence on Processes: Problem Identification. In *A Report to Congress: Study of Private Accreditation (Deeming) of Nursing Homes, Regulatory Incentives and Non-Regulatory Incentives, and Effectiveness of the Survey and Certification System.* Washington, DC: HCFA, 1998.

Moseley, C. B. The Impact of Federal Regulations on Urethral Catheterization in Virginia Nursing Homes. *American Journal of Medical Quality* 11:222–226, 1996.

Moses, E.B. *The Registered Nurse Population: Findings from the National Sample Survey of Registered Nurses, March 1996.* Washington, DC: Department of Health and Human Services, 1997.

Moss, M., and Adams, C. Industry Focus. For Medicaid Patients: Doors Slam Closed—Citing Finances, Nursing Homes Evict the Needy. *Wall Street Journal* April 7, 1998.

Msall, M.E., DiGaudio, K., Rogers, B.T., LaForest, S, Catanzaro, N.L., Cambell, J., Wilczenski, F., and Duffy, L.C. Functional Independence Measure for Children (Wee-FIM). Conceptual Basis and Pilot Use in Children with Developmental Disabilities. *Clinical Pediatrics (Philadelphia)* Jul;33(7):421–430, 1994.

Mukamel, D.B., and Brower, C.A. The Influence of Risk Adjustment Methods on Conclusions About Quality of Care in Nursing Homes Based on Outcome Measures. *The Gerontologist* 38(6):695–703, 1998.

Mulrow, C.D., Gerety, M.B., Kanten, D., Cornell, J.E., DeNino, L.A., Chiodo, L., Aguilar, C., O'Neil, M.D., Rosenberg, J., and Solis, R.M. A Randomized Trial of Physical Rehabilitation for Very Frail Nursing Home Residents. *Journal of the American Medical Association* 271(7):519–524, 1994.

Munroe, D.J. The Influence of Registered Nursing Staffing on the Quality of Nursing Home Care. *Research in Nursing and Health* 13(4):263–270, 1990.

NAHC (National Association for Home Care). Basic Statistics About Home Care [WWW Document]. URL: http:www.nahc.org/Consumer/hcstats.html (accessed May 9, 2000), 2000

National Blue Ribbon Panel on Personal Assistance Services. Dautel, P., and Frieden, L., eds. *Consumer Choice and Control: Personal Attendant Services and Supports in America.* Houston, TX: Independent Living Research Utilization, 1999.

National Institute on Consumer-Directed Long-Term Services. *Principles of Consumer-Directed Home and Community-Based Services.* Washington, DC: National Council on the Aging, 1996.

NCCNHR (National Citizens' Coalition for Nursing Home Reform). *A Consumer Perceptive on Quality Care: The Residents' Point of View.* Washington, DC: NCCNHR, 1985.

NCCNHR. *Consumers' Minimum Standard for Nurse Staffing in Nursing Homes.* Washington, DC: NCCNHR, 1995.

NCCNHR and NCPSSM (National Committee to Preserve Social Security and Medicare). *Summary of Reported State Minimum Staffing Requirements.* Washington, DC: NCCNHR, 1998.

NCHS (National Center for Health Statistics). An Overview of Nursing Homes and Their Current Residents: Data from the 1995 National Nursing Home Survey. In Strahan, G.W., ed. *Advance Data from Vital and Health Statistics,* No. 280. Hyattsville, MD: NCHS/CDC Department of Health and Human Services, 1997.

NCHS. An Overview of Home Health and Hospice Care Patients: 1996 National Home and Hospice Care Survey. In Haupt, B.J., ed. *Advance Data from Vital and Health Statistics,* No. 297. Hyattsville, MD: NCHS/CDC Department of Health and Human Services, 1998.

NCHS. Characteristics of Elderly Home Health Users: Data from the 1996 National Home and Hospice Care Survey. In Munson, M.L., ed. *Advance Data from Vital and Health Statistics,* No. 309. Hyattsville, MD: NCHS/CDC Department of Health and Human Services, 1999a.

NCHS. *The National Home and Hospice Care Survey: 1996 Summary.* Hyattsville, MD: NCHS/CDC Department of Health and Human Services, 1999b.

NCHS. An Overview of Nursing Homes and their Current Residents: Data from the 1997 National Nursing Home Survey. In Gabrel, C.S., ed. *Advance Data from Vital and Health Statistics,* No. 311. Hyattsville, MD: NCHS/CDC Department of Health and Human Services, 2000.

Nelson, H.W. A Study of Oregon Volunteer Long-Term Care Ombudsman Organizational Commitment and Burnout as Related to Selected Variables. Ph.D. dissertation. Corvallis, OR: Oregon State University, 1993.

Neu, C.R., and Harrison, S.C. *Posthospital Care Before and After the Medicare Prospective Payment System.* RAND R-3590-HCFA. Santa Monica, CA: RAND, 1988.

Newacheck, P.W., Strickland, B., Shonkoff, J.P., Perrin, J.M., McPherson, M., McManus, M., Lauver, C., Fox, H., and Arango, P. An Epidemiologic Profile of Children with Special Health Care Needs. *Pediatrics* 102(1):117–123, 1998.

Newcomer, R.J., and Grant, L.A. Residential Care Facilities: Understanding Their Role and Improving Their Effectiveness. Pp. 101–124 in Tilson, D., ed. *Aging in Place: Supporting the Frail Elderly in Residential Environments.* Glenview IL: Scott, Foresman, and Co., 1990.

Norton, E. Incentive Regulation of Nursing Homes. *Journal of Health Economics* 11:105–128, 1992.

Norton, P.G., van Maris, B., Soberman, L., and Murray, M. Satisfaction and Residents and Families in Long-Term Care: Construction and Application of an Instrument. *Quality Management in Health Care* 4(3):38–46, 1996.

Nosek, M., Fuhre, M., and Potter, C. Life Satisfaction of People with Physical Disabilities: Relationship to Personal Assistance, Disability Status, and Handicap. *Rehabilitation Psychology* 40(3):192–202, 1995.

Nyman, J.A. Prospective and "Cost-Plus" Medicaid Reimbursement, Excess Medicaid Demand, and Quality of Nursing Home Care. *Journal of Health Economics* 4:237–259, 1985.

Nyman, J.A. The Effect of Competition on Nursing Home Expenditures Under Prospective Payment. *Journal of Health Economics* 4:237–259, 1988a.

Nyman, J.A. Improving the Quality of Nursing Home Outcomes: Are Adequacy- or Incentive-Oriented Policies More Effective. *Medical Care* 26(12):1158–1171, 1988b.

Nyman, J.A. Excess Demand, the Percentage of Medicaid Patients, and the Quality of Nursing Home Care. *Journal of Human Resources* 23(1):76–92, 1988c.

Nyman, J.A. Testing for Excess Demand for Nursing Homes. *Medical Care* 31:680–693, 1993.

OBRA (Omnibus Budget Reconciliation Act of 1987). Public Law 100-203. Subtitle C: Nursing Home Reform. Signed by President Reagan, Washington, DC, December 22, 1987.

OBRA (Omnibus Budget Reconciliation Act of 1990). Public Law 101-508, Section 4801(B)(e)(17)(B). Washington, DC, 1990.

OIG (Office of the Inspector General, Department of Health and Human Services). *Improving Safeguards in Long-Term Care.* Report to the U.S. Senate Special Committee on Aging. Washington, DC: OIG, 1998.

OIG. *Long-Term Care Ombudsman Program: Complaint Trends.* OEI-02-98-00350. Washington, DC: OIG, 1999a.

OIG. *Nursing Home Survey and Certification: Deficiency Trends.* OEI-02-98-00331. Washington, DC: OIG, 1999b.

OIG. *Quality of Care in Nursing Homes: An Overview.* OEI-02-99-00060. Washington, DC: OIG, 1999c.

O'Keefe, H. *Determining the Need for Long-Term Care Services: An Analysis of Health and Function Eligibility Criteria in Medicaid Home and Community-Based Waiver Programs.* Washington, DC: National Association of Retired Persons, 1996.

Ooi, W.L., Morris, J.N., Brandeis, G.H., Hossain, M., and Lipsita, L.A. Nursing Home Characteristics and the Development of Pressure Sores and Disruptive Behaviours. *Age and Ageing* 28(1):45–52, 1999.

Ouslander, J., and Kane, R. The Costs of Urinary Incontinence in Nursing Homes. *Medical Care* 22:69–79, 1984.

Ouslander, J.G., Osterweil, D., and Morley, J. *Medical Care in the Nursing Home.* Second Edition. New York: McGraw-Hill, 1997.

Palmer, M.H., German, P.S., and Ouslander, J.G. Risk Factors for Urinary Incontinence One Year After Nursing Home Admission. *Research in Nursing and Health* 14:405–412, 1991.

Palmer, M.H., Bennett, R.G., Marks, J., McCormick, K.A. and Engel, B.T. Urinary Incontinence: A Program That Works. *Journal of Long Term Care Administration* Summer:19–25, 1994.

Patterson, J.M., Leonard, J.J., and Titus, J.C. Home Care for Medically Fragile Children: Impact on Family Health and Well-Being. *Journal of Developmental and Behavioral Pediatrics* 13:248–255, 1992.

Pearson, A., Hocking, S., Mott, S., and Riggs, A. Quality of Care in Nursing Homes: From the Resident's Perspective. *Journal of Advanced Nursing* 18:20–24, 1993.

Perrin, J.M. Services for Children with Chronic Physical Disorders and their Families. Pp. 329–349 in Mor, V., and Allen, S.M., eds. *Living in the Community with Disability.* New York: Springer Publishing, 1998.

Perrin, J.M., and Bloom, S.R. Coordination of Care for Households with Children with Special Health Needs. Pp. 711–718 in Wallace, H.M., Nelson, R.P., and Sweeney, P.J., eds. *Maternal and Child Health Practices,* 4th Edition. Oakland, CA: Third Party Publishing, 1994.

Perrin, J.M., Shayne, M.W., and Bloom, S.R. *Home and Community Care for Chronically Ill Children.* New York: Oxford University Press, 1993.

Perrin, J.M., Thyen, U., and Bloom, S. Care at Home for Children with Chronic Illness: Program and Policy Implications. Pp. 219–244 in Fox, D.M. and Raphael, C., eds. *Home-Based Care for a New Century*. Malden, MA: Blackwell Publishers and Milbank Memorial Fund, 1997.

Perrin, J.M., Ettner, S.L., McLaughlin, T.J., Gortmaker, S.L., Bloom, S.R., and Kuhlthau, K. State Variations in Supplemental Security Income Enrollment for Children and Adolescents. *American Journal of Public Health* 88:928–931, 1998.

Perrin, J.M., Kuhlthau, K., McLaughlin, T.J., Ettner, S.L., and Gortmaker, S.L. Changing Patterns of Conditions among Children Receiving SSI Disability Benefits. *Archives of Pediatric and Adolescent Medicine* 153:80–84, 1999.

Pestotnik, S.L., Classen, D.C., Evans, R.S., and Burke, J.P. Implementing Antibiotic Practice Guidelines Through Computer-Assisted Decision Support: Clinical and Financial Outcomes. *Annals of Internal Medicine* 124(10):884–890, 1996.

Phillips, C.D., Hawes, C., and Fries, B.E. Reducing the Use of Physical Restraints in Nursing Homes: Will it Increase Costs? *American Journal of Public Health* 83(3):342–348, 1993a.

Phillips, C.D., Chu, C.W., Morris, J.N., and Hawes, C. Effects of Cognitive Impairments on the Reliability of Geriatric Assessments in Nursing Homes. *Journal of the American Geriatrics Society* 41(2):136–142, 1993b.

Phillips, B.R., Brown, R.S., Bishop, C.E., Klein, A.C., Ritter., G.A., Schore, J.L., Skavara K.C., and Thornton C.V. Do Preset Per Visit Payment Rates Affect Home Health Agency Behavior? *Health Care Financing Review* 16(1):91–107, 1994.

Phillips, C.D., Hawes, C., Mor, V., Fries, B.E., Morris, J., and Nennstiel, M. Facility and Area Variation Affecting the Use of Physical Restraints in Nursing Homes. *Medical Care* 34(11):1149–1162, 1996.

Phillips, C., Morris, J.N., Hawes, C., Fries, B.E., Mor, V., Nennstiel, M., and Iannacchione, V. Association of the Resident Assessment Instrument (RAI) with Changes in Function, Cognition and Psychosocial Status. *Journal of the American Geriatrics Association* 45(8):986–993, 1997.

Picker Institute. *Surveys of Rehabilitation Programs and Home Care Services*. Boston, MA: Picker Institute, 1995.

Pillemer, K. *Solving the Frontline Crisis in Long-Term Care: A Practical Guide to Finding and Keeping Quality Nursing Assistants*. Cambridge, MA: Frontline Publishing Company, 1996.

Pillemer, K., and Moore, D.W. Abuse of Patients in Nursing Homes: Findings from a Survey of Staff. *The Gerontologist* 29(3):314–320, 1989.

Pokrywka, H.S., Koffler, K.H., Remsburg, R., Bennett, R.G., Roth, J., Tayback, M., and Wright, J.E. Accuracy of Patient Care Staff in Estimating and Documenting Meal Intake of Nursing Home Residents. *Journal of the American Geriatrics Society* 45(10):1223–1227, 1997.

Porell, F., and Caro, F.G. Facility-Level Outcome Performance Measures for Nursing Homes. *The Gerontologist* 38(11):665–684, 1998.

Porell, F., Caro, F.G., Silva, A., and Monane, M. A Longitudinal Analysis of Nursing Home Outcomes. *Health Services Research* 33(4):835–865, 1998.

Portenoy, R.K. Opioid Therapy for Chronic Nonmalignant Pain Current Status. Pp. 247–288 in *Progress in Pain Research and Management*, Vol. 1. Seattle, WA: IASP Press, 1994.

Powers, L.E. Family and Consumer Activism in Disability Policy. Pp. 413–433 in Singer, G.H.S., Powers, L.E., and Olson, A.L., eds. *Redefining Family Support: Innovations in Public–Private Partnerships*. Baltimore, MD: Paul H. Brookes, 1996.

PPRC (Physician Payment Review Commission). Increasing Appropriate Use of Services: Practice Guidelines and Feedback of Practice Patterns. In *Annual Report to Congress*. Washington, DC: PPRC, 1988.

PPRC. Effectiveness Research and Practice Guidelines. In *Annual Report to Congress*. Washington, DC: PPRC, 1989.

ProPAC (Prospective Payment Assessment Commission). *Report and Recommendations to the Congress. Annual Report of the Commission*. Washington, DC: ProPAC, 1997.

Przybylski, B.R., Dumont, E.D., Watkins, M.E., Warren, S.A., Beaulne, A.P., and Lier, D.A. Outcomes of Enhanced Physical and Occupational Therapy Service in a Nursing Home Setting. *Archives of Physical Medicine and Rehabilitation* 77(6):554–561, 1996.

Quill, T.E. Partnerships in Patient Care: A Contractual Approach. *Annals of Internal Medicine* 98:228–234, 1983.

Quint, R., Chesterman, E., Crain, L.S., Winkleby, M., and Boyce, W.T. Home Care for Ventilator-Dependent Children: Psychosocial Impact on the Family. *American Journal of Diseases of Children* 144:1238–1241, 1990.

Rabins, P., Kasper, J., Leinman, L., Black, B., and Patrick, D. Concept and Methods in the Development of the ADRLQ: An Instrument for Assessing the Health-Related Quality of Life in Persons with Alzheimer's Disease. *Journal of Mental Health and Aging* 5(1):34–49, 1999.

Rader, J., Lavelle, M., Hoeffer, B., and McKenzie, D. Maintaining Cleanliness: An Individualized Approach. *Journal of Gerontological Nursing* 22(3):32–38, 1996.

Ragged Edge. How Kansas Got "Consumer Control" into the Law. *Ragged Edge* (July/August):21–25, 1997.

Reilly, K.E. Skilled Nursing Facility Prospective Case-Mix Payment and Nursing Time. Paper prepared for the John H. Hartford Institute for Gerontological Nursing. Boston, MA: Abt Associates, 1998.

Reinhardy, J., Kane, R.A., and Mollica, R. *CAILS Assessment Project*. Report Prepared for the Vermont Department of Aging and Disabilities. Minneapolis, MN: University of Minnesota, National Long-Term Care Resource Center, 1994.

Reuben, D.B., Schnelle, J.F., Buchanan, J.L, Kington, R.S., Zellman, G.C., Farley D.O., Hirsch, S.H., and Ouslander J.G. Primary Care of Long-Stay Nursing Home Residents: Approaches of Three Health Maintenance Organizations. *Journal of the American Geriatrics Society* 47:131–138, 1999.

Ribeiro, B., and Smith, S. Evaluation of Urinary Catheterization and Urinary Incontinence in a General Nursing Home Population. *Journal of the American Geriatrics Society* 33:479–481, 1985.

Richmond, G.W., Beatty, P., Tepper, S., and DeJong, G. The Effect of Consumer-Directed Personal Assistance Services on the Productivity Outcomes of People with Disabilities. *Journal of Rehabilitation Outcomes Measurement* 1(4):48–51, 1997.

Rimer, S. Nationwide, a Shortage of Home Health Aides [WWW document]. URL: http://www.nytimes.com/yr/mo/day/news/national/oldworkers.html, January 3, 2000.

Rodin, J. Aging and Health: Effects of the Sense of Control. *Science* 233:1271–1275, 1986.

Rogers, J.C., Holm, M.B., Burgio, L.D., Granieri, E., Hsu C., Hardin, J.M., and McDowell, B.J. Improving Morning Care Routines of Nursing Home Residents with Dementia. *Journal of the American Geriatrics Society* 47(9):1049–1057, 1999.

Rosenthal, G.E., and Shannon, S.E. The Use of Patient Perceptions in the Evaluation of Health-Care Delivery Systems. *Medical Care* 35(11):NS58–NS68, 1997.

Ross, C.K., Steward, C.A., and Sinacore, J.M. A Comparative Study of Seven Measures of Patient Satisfaction. *Medical Care* 33(4):392–406, 1995.

Rotegard, L.L., Hill, B.K., and Bruininks, R.H. Environmental Characteristics of Residential Facilities for Mentally Retarded Persons in the United States. *American Journal of Mental Deficiency* 88:49–56, 1983.

Rubin, H.R. Can Patients Evaluate the Quality of Hospital Care? *Medical Care Review* 47(3):267–326, 1990.

Rudman, D., Slater, E.J., Richardson, T.J., and Mattson, D.E. The Occurrence of Pressure Ulcers in Three Nursing Homes. *Journal of General Internal Medicine* 8:653–658, 1993.

Runde, P., Giese, R., Kerschke-Risch, P., Scholz, U., and Wiegel, D. Einstellungen und Verhalten zur Pklegeversicherung und zur Haulichen Plege. Translated by Hopperger, J.P. Hamburg, Germany: University of Hamburg, 1996.

Ryan, J.A. *Statement. Testimony before the Senate Special Committee on Aging Forum on Nursing Home Staffing.* Presented to the U.S. Senate. Washington, DC: American Health Care Association, 1999.

Sabatino, C.P., and Litvak, S. Consumer-Directed Homecare: What Makes It Possible? *Generations* Winter:53–58, 1992.

Salomon, J., Polivka, L., and Weber, S. *Quality of Life in Long-Term Care: The Role of Control.* Aging Research and Policy Report, Florida Exchange Center on Aging. Tampa, FL: University of South Florida, 1998.

Sano, M., Albert, S.M., Tractenberg, R., and Shittini, M. Developing Utilities: Quantifying Quality of Life for Stages of Alzheimer's Disease as Measured by the Clinical Dementia Rating. *Journal of Mental Health and Aging* 5(1):59–68, 1999.

Savashitsky, J. *The Ends of Time: Life and Work in a Nursing Home.* New York: Bergin and Garvey, 1991.

Scala, M.A., and Mayberry, P.S. *Consumer-Directed Home Services: Issues and Models.* Oxford, OH: Ohio Long-Term Care Research Project, Miami University, 1997.

Scanlon, W.J. A Theory of the Nursing Home Market. *Inquiry* 17(Spring):25–41, 1980.

Schlenker, R.E., Shaughnessy, P.W., and Crisler, K.S. Outcome-Based Continuous Quality Improvement as a Financial Strategy for Home Health Care Agencies. *Journal of Home Health Care Practice* 7(4):1–15, 1995.

Schmidt, M.G. *Negotiating a Good Old Age: Challenges of Residential Living in Late Life.* San Francisco: Jossey-Bass, 1990.

Schmitz, R., Chatterji, P., Murphy, M., and Feuerberg, M. Changes in Resident Status Pre and Post. In *A Report to Congress: Study of Private Accreditation (Deeming) of Nursing Homes, Regulatory Incentives and Non-Regulatory Incentives, and Effectiveness of the Survey and Certification System.* Washington, DC: HCFA, 1998.

Schnelle, J. Treatment of Urinary Incontinence in Nursing Home Patients by Prompted Voiding. *Journal of the American Geriatrics Society* 38:356–360, 1990.

Schnelle, J.F., Sowell, V.A., Hu, T.W., and Traughbur, B.T. A Behavioral Analysis of the Labor Cost of Managing Continence and Incontinence. *Journal of Organizational Behavior Management* 9(2):137–153, 1988a.

Schnelle, J.F., Sowell, V.A., Hu, T.W., and Traughber, B.T. Reduction of Urinary Incontinence in Nursing Home: Does It Reduce or Increase Cost? *Journal of the American Geriatrics Society* 36:34–39, 1988b.

Schnelle, J.F., Newman, D.R., and Fogarty, T. Management of Patient Continence in Long Term Care Nursing Facilities. *The Gerontologist* 30:373–376, 1990.

Schnelle, J.F., Newman, D.R., White, M., Volner, T.R., Burnett, J., and Cronqvist, A. Reducing and Managing Restraints in Long-Term Care. *Journal of the American Geriatrics Society* 40:381–385, 1992a.

Schnelle, J.F., Simmons, S.F., and Ory, M.G. Risk Factors That Predict Staff Failure to Release Nursing Home Residents from Restraints. *The Gerontologist* 32(6):767–770, 1992b.

Schnelle, J.F., Newman, D.R., White, M., Abbey, J., Wallston, K.A., Fogarty, T., and Ory, M.G. Maintaining Continence in Nursing Home Residents Through the Application of Industrial Quality Control. *The Gerontologist* 33(1):114–121, 1993.

Schnelle, J.F., Keeler, E., Hays, R.D., Simmons, S.F., Ouslander, J.G., and Siu, A.L. A Cost Utility Analysis of Two Interventions with Incontinent Nursing Home Residents. *Journal of the American Geriatrics Society* 43(10):1112–1117, 1995a.

Schnelle, J.F., MacRae, P.G., Ouslander, J.G., Simmons, S.F., and Nitta, M. Functional Incidental Training, Mobility Performance, and Incontinence Care with Nursing Home Residents. *Journal of American Geriatrics Society* 43(12):1356–1362, 1995b.

Schnelle, J.F., Ouslander, J.G., and Cruise, P.A. Policy Without Technology: A Barrier to Changing Nursing Home Care. *The Gerontologist* 37(4):527–532, 1997.

Schnelle, J.F., Cruise, P.A., Rahman, A., and Ouslander, J.G. Developing Rehabilitative Behavioral Interventions for Long-Term Care: Technology Transfer, Acceptance, and Maintenance Issues. *Journal of the American Geriatrics Society* 46:771–777, 1998.

Schug, S.A., Zech, D., and Dorr, U. Cancer Pain Management According to WHO Analgesic Guidelines. *Journal on Pain and Symptom Management* 5:27–32, 1990.

Shapiro, J.P. *No Pity: People with Disabilities Forging a New Civil Rights Movement.* New York: Times Books, 1993.

Shaughnessy, P.W., and Kramer, A.M. The Increased Needs of Patients in Nursing Homes and Patients Receiving Home Health Care. *New England Journal of Medicine* 322(1):21–27, 1990.

Shaughnessy, P.W., and Kurowski, P.W. Quality Assurance Through Reimbursement. *Health Services Research* 17(2):157–183, 1982.

Shaughnessy, P.W., Crisler, K.S., Schlenker, R.E., Arnold, A.G., Kramer, A.M., Powell, M.C., and Hittle, D.F. Measuring and Assuring the Quality of Home Health Care. *Health Care Financing Review* 16(1):35–67, 1994a.

Shaughnessy, P.W., Schlenker, R.E., Crisler, K.S., Powell, M.C., Hittle, D.F., Kramer, A.M., Spencer, M.J., Beale, S.K., Bostrom, S.G., Beaudry, J.M., DeVore, P.A., Chandramouli, V., Grant, W.V., Arnold, A.G., Bauman, M.K., and Jenkins, J. *A Study to Develop Outcome-Based Quality Measures for Home Health Services, Vol. 1. Final Report: Measuring Outcomes of Home Health Care.* Denver, CO: Center for Health Services and Policy Research, University of Colorado Health Sciences Center, 1994b.

Shaughnessy, P.W., Crisler, K.S., and Schlenker, R.E. *Medicare's OASIS: Standardized Outcome and Assessment Information Set for Home Health Care, OASIS-B.* Denver, CO: Center for Health Services and Policy Research, University of Colorado Health Sciences Center, 1997a.

Shaughnessy, P.W., Crisler, K.S., Schlenker, R.E., and Arnold, A.G. Outcomes Across the Care Continuum: Home Health Care. *Medical Care* 35(11):NS115–NS123, and 35(12):1225–1226 (Addendum), 1997b.

Shaughnessy, P.W., Crisler, K.S., and Schlenker, R.E. Outcome-Based Quality Improvement in the Information Age. *Home Health Care Management and Practice*, 19(2):11–19, 1998a.

Shaughnessy, P.W., Crisler, K.S., Schlenker, R.E., and Hittle, D.F. OASIS: The Next Ten Years. *Caring* 17(6):32–42, 1998b.

Shavelle, R. M., and Strauss, D.J. Mortality of Persons with Developmental Disabilities After Transfer into Community Care: A 1996 Update. *American Journal of Mental Retardation* 104(2):143–147, 1999.

Shield, R.R. *Uneasy Endings.* Ithaca, NY: Cornell University Press, 1988.

Shorr, R.I., Fought, R.L., and Ray, W.A. Changes in Antipsychotic Drug Use in Nursing Homes During Implementation of the OBRA-87 Regulations. *Journal of the American Medical Association* 271(5):358–362, 1994.

Shortell, S.M., Bennett, C.L., and Byck, G.R. Assessing the Impact of Continuous Quality Improvement on Clinical Practice: What It Will Take to Accelerate Progress. *Milbank Quarterly* 76(4):593–624, 1998.

Siegler, E.L., Capezuti, E., Maislin, G., Baumgarten, M., Evans, L., and Strumpf, N. Effects of a Restraint Reduction Intervention and OBRA '87 Regulations on Psychoactive Drug Use in Nursing Homes. *Journal of the American Geriatrics Society* 45:791–796, 1997.

Simmons, S.F., and Reuben, D. Nutritional Intake Monitoring for Nursing Home Residents: A Comparison of Staff Documentation, Direct Observation, and Photography Methods. *Journal of the American Geriatrics Society* 48(2):209–213, 2000.

Simmons, S.F., and Schnelle, J.F. Strategies to Measure Nursing Home Residents' Satisfaction and Preference Related to Incontinence and Mobility Care: Implications for Continuous Quality Improvement. *The Gerontologist* 39(3):345–355, 1999.

Simmons, S.F., Schnelle, J.F., Uman, G., Kulvicki, A., Lee, K., and Ouslander, J.G. Selecting Nursing Home Residents for Satisfaction Surveys. *The Gerontologist* 37(4):543–550, 1997.

Simon, M., and Martin, F. *La Prestation Dependance: Rapport Final du Programme d'Evaluation de l'Expetrimentation d'une Prestation Dependance.* Translated by Tilly, J. Paris, France: Centre de Recherche pour l'Etude et l'Observation des Conditions de Vie, 1995.

Simon-Rusinowitz, L., Mahoney, K., Desmond, S., Shoop, D., Squillace, M., and Fay, B. Determining Consumer Preferences for a Cash Option: Arkansas Survey Results. *Health Care Financing Review* 19(2):73–96, 1997.

Singer, B.H., and Manton, K.G. The Effects of Health Changes on Projections of Health Service Needs for the Elderly Population of the United States. *Proceedings of the National Academy of Sciences* 95(26):15618–15622, 1998.

Singer, G.H.S., Irvin, L.K., Irvine, B., Hawkins, N.J., and Cooley, E. Evaluation of Communities-Based Support Services for Families of Persons with Developmental Disabilities. *Journal of the Association for the Severely Handicapped* 14(4):312–323, 1989.

Singh, D.A. *Nursing Home Administrators: Their Influence on Quality of Care.* New York: Garland Publishing, 1997.

Singh, D.A. and Schwab, R.C. Retention of Administrators in Nursing Homes: What Can Management Do? *The Gerontologist* 38(3):361–369, 1998.

Slack, W.V. The Patient's Right to Decide. *Lancet* 2:240, 1977.

Smith, D.M. Pressure Ulcers in the Nursing Home. *Annals of Internal Medicine* 123:433–442, 1995.

Spector, W.D., and Takada, H.A. Characteristics of Nursing Homes That Affect Resident Outcomes. *Journal of Aging and Health* 3(4):427–454, 1991.

Spector, W.D., Fleishman, J.A., Pezzin, L.E., and Spillman, B.C. *The Characteristics of Long-Term Care Users.* Paper prepared for the Institute of Medicine Committee on Improving Quality in Long-Term Care, Washington, DC, 1998.

Spore, D., Mor, V., Larrat, E.P., Hiris, J. and Hawes, C. Regulatory Environment and Psychotropic Use in Board and Care Facilities: Results of a 10 State Study. *Journal of Gerontology, Medical Sciences* 51(3):M131–M141, 1996.

SSA (Social Security Administration). *Annual Statistical Supplement, 1999 to the Social Security Bulletin.* Washington, DC: SSA, 1999.

SSA (Social Security Administration). *Children Receiving SSI: June 2000.* Washington, DC: SSA, 2000.

Stancliffe, R.J. Community Living-Unit Size, Staff Presence, and Residents' Choice-Making. *Mental Retardation* 35(1):1–9, 1997.

Stancliffe, R.J., and Abery, B.H. Longitudinal Study of Deinstitutionalization and the Exercise of Choice. *Mental Retardation* 35(3):159–169, 1997.

Starfield, B., Bergner, M., Ensminger, M., Riley, A., Ryan, S., Green, B., McGauhey, P., Skinner, A., and Kim, S. Adolescent Health Status Measurement. *Pediatrics* 91:430–435, 1993.

Stark, A., Kane, R.L., Kane, R.A., and Finch, M.D. Effect on Physical Functioning of Adult Foster Care Homes and Nursing Homes. *The Gerontologist* 35(5):648–655, 1995.

Steele, C.M., Greenwood, C., Ens, I., Robertson, C., and Seidman-Carlson, R. Mealtime Difficulties in a Home for the Aged: Not Just Dysphagia. *Dysphagia* 12(1):43–50, 1997.

Stein, R.E. *Issues in the Quality of Long Term Care for Children*. Paper prepared for the Institute of Medicine Committee on Improving Quality in Long-Term Care, Washington, DC, 1998.

Stein, R.E., and Jessop, D.J. Does Pediatric Home Care Make a Difference for Children with Chronic Illness? Findings from the Pediatric Ambulatory Care Treatment Study. *Pediatrics* 73:845–853, 1984.

Stein, R.E., and Jessop, D.J. Functional Status II(R). *Medical Care* 28:1041–1055, 1990.

Stein, R.E., and Jessop, D.J. Long-Term Mental Health Effects of a Pediatric Home Care Program. *Pediatrics* 88:490–496, 1991.

Strauss, D.J., Kastner, T.A., and Shavelle, R.M. Mortality in Persons with Developmental Disabilities Living in California Institutions and Community Care, 1985–1994. *Mental Retardation* 36:360–371, 1998.

Strumpf, N.E., and Tomes, N. Restraining the Troublesome Patient: A Historical Perspective on a Contemporary Debate. *Nursing History Review* 1:3–24, 1993.

Sundel, M.R., Garrett, R.M., and Horn, R.D. Restraint Reduction in a Nursing Home and Its Impact on Employee Attitudes. *Journal of the American Geriatrics Society* 42(4):381–387, 1994.

SUPPORT Principal Investigators. A Controlled Trial to Improve Care for Seriously Ill Hospitalized Patients: The Study to Understand Prognoses and Preferences for Outcomes and Risks of Treatments (SUPPORT). *Journal of the American Medical Association* 274(20):1591–1598, 1995.

Tangalos, E. The Future Practice of Long-Term Care. *Journal of the American Geriatrics Society* 41(4):459–463, 1993.

Tangalos, E., and Stone, D. The Medicine Fee Schedule in Long-Term Care. *Journal of the American Geriatrics Society* 41(5):574–575, 1993.

Tellis-Nayak, V., and Tellis-Nayak, M. Quality of Care and the Burden of Two Cultures: When the World of the Nurse's Aide Enters the World of the Nursing Home. *The Gerontologist* 29:307–313, 1989.

Teno, J.M. *Putting Patient and Family Voice Back into Measuring Quality of Care in Long Term Care Services*. Paper prepared for the Institute of Medicine Committee on Quality in Long-Term Care, Washington, DC, June 11–12, 1998.

Teno, J.M., Hakim, R.B., Knaus, W.A., Wenger, N.S., Phillips, R.S., Wu, A.W., Layde, P., Connors, Jr., A.F., Dawson, N.V., and Lynn, J. Preferences for Cardiopulmonary Resuscitation: Physician–Patient Agreement and Hospital Resource Use. *Journal of General Internal Medicine* 10:179–186, 1995.

Teno, J., Bird, C., and Mor, V. *The Prevalence and Treatment of Pain in U.S. Nursing Homes*. Providence, RI: Brown University's Center for Gerontology and Health Care Research, 2000.

Teresi, J.A., Holmes, D., and Monaco, C. An Evaluation of the Effects of Co-Mingling Cognitively and Non-Cognitively Impaired Individuals in Long-Term Care Facilities. *The Gerontologist* 33:350–358, 1993.

Thomas, W.H. *The Eden Alternative: Nature, Hope, and Nursing Homes*. Sherburne, NY: Eden Alternative Foundation, 1994.

Thyen, U., Terres, N.M., Yazdgerdi, S.R., and Perrin, J.M. Impact of Long-Term Care of Children Assisted by Technology on Maternal Health. *Journal of Developmental and Behavioral Pediatrics* 19(4):273–283, 1998.

Thyen, U., Kuhlthau, K., and Perrin, J.M. Employment, Child Care, and Mental Health of Mothers Caring for Children Assisted by Technology. *Pediatrics* 103:1235–1242, 1999.

Tilly, J., and Bectel, R. *Consumer-Directed Long-Term Care: Participants' Experiences in Five Countries*. Washington, DC: American Association of Retired Persons, 1999.

Tisdale, S. *Harvest Moon: Portrait of a Nursing Home*. New York: H. Holt Publishers, 1987.

Tobin, S.S., *Personhood in Advanced Old Age: Implications for Practices*. New York: Springer Publishing, 1991.

Tossebro, J. Impact of Size Revisited: Relation of Number of Residents to Self-Determination and Deprivatization. *American Journal of Mental Retardation* 100:59–67, 1996.

Tractenberg S., and Batshaw, M. Caring and Coping: The Family of Children with Disabilities. In Batshaw, M., and Perret, Y., eds. *Children with Disabilities: A Medical Primer*, 4th Edition. Baltimore: Paul H. Brookes, 1997

Trupin L., and Rice, D.P. Health Status, Medical Care Use, and the Number of Disability Conditions in the United States. *Disability Statistics Abstracts* No. 9. Washington, DC: National Institute for Disability and Rehabilitation Research, 1995.

Tulloch, J. *A Home is Not a Home*. New York: Seabury, 1975.

Ullman, S.G. Ownership, Regulation, Quality Assessment, and Performance in the Long-Term Health Care Industry. *The Gerontologist* 27(2):233–239, 1987.

United Hospital Fund. *Better Jobs, Better Care: Building the Home Care Work Force*. New York: United Hospital Fund of New York, 1994.

U.S. Senate Special Committee on Aging. *Betrayal: The Quality of Care In California Nursing Homes*. Washington, DC: U.S. Senate, July 28, 1998.

U.S. Senate Special Committee on Aging. *The Nursing Home Initiative: Results at Year One*. Washington, DC: U.S. Senate, June 30, 1999.

VA (Department of Veteran Affairs). *Future Directions in Long-Term Care: Veterans and Caregiver Perspectives*. Washington, DC: VA, 1994.

Van Ort, S., and Phillips, L.R. Nursing Interventions to Promote Functional Feeding. *Journal of Gerontological Nursing* 21(10):6–14, 1995.

Vickery, K. HIS Chapter 11 Filing Latest in Bankruptcy Trend. *Provider* 26(4):17, 2000.

Vital Research. REAL Overview [WWW document]. URL: www.vitalresearch.com/pages/ (accessed August 1, 2000), 2000.

Vladeck, B., and Miller, N.A. The Medicare Home Health Initiative. *Health Care Financing Review* 16(1):7–16, 1994.

Vouri, H. Patient Satisfaction: An Attribute or Indicator of the Quality of Care? *Quality Review Bulletin* 13:106–108, 1987.

Vourlekis, E., and Green, R.R., eds. *Social Work Case Management*. New York: Aldine de Gruyter, 1991.

Wagner, A.M., Goodwin, M. Campbell, B., Eulero, S., Frank, S.A., Shephard, P.A., and Wade, M. Pain Prevalence and Pain Treatments for Residents in Oregon Nursing Homes. *Geriatric Nursing* 18(6):268–272, 1997.

Walker, D.K., and Jacobs, F.H. Public School Programs for Chronically Ill Children. Pp. 615–655 in Hobbs, N., and Perrin, J.M. eds. *Issues in the Care of Children with Chronic Conditions*. San Francisco: Jossey-Bass, 1985.

Walker, L., Porter, M., Gruman, C., and Michalski, M. Developing Individualized Care in Nursing Homes: Integrating the Views of Nurses and Certified Nurses Aides. *Journal of Gerontological Nursing* 25(3):30–35, 1999.

Ware, J.E., and Hays, R.D. Methods for Measuring Patient Satisfaction with Specific Medical Encounters. *Medical Care* 26(4):393–402, 1988.

Weissert, W.G., and Musliner, M.C. Case-Mix Adjusted Nursing Home Reimbursement: A Critical Review of the Evidence. *Milbank Quarterly* 70(3):455–490, 1992.

Weissert, W., and Scanlon, W.J. Determinants of Nursing Home Discharge Status. *Medical Care* 23(4):333–343, 1985.

Weissert, W.G., Elston, J.M., Bolda, E.J., Zelman, W.N., Mutran, E., and Mangnum, A.B. *Adult Day Care: Findings from a National Survey*. Baltimore, MD: Johns Hopkins University Press, 1990.

Weissert, W.G. Home-Care Dollars and Sense. Pp. 121–134 in Fox, D.M., and Raphael, C., eds. *Home-Based Care for a New Century*. Malden, MA: Blackwell Publishers, 1997.

White House. Clinton–Gore Administration Announces Multi-Million Dollar Investment to Assure Quality Care in Nursing Homes. Washington, DC: January 14, 2000.

Wiener, J.M., Illston, L.H., and Hanley, R. *Sharing the Burden: Strategies for Public and Private Long-Term Care Providers in Thirteen States*. Washington, DC: Brookings Institution, 1994.

Wiener, J.M., and Stevenson, D.G. Long Term Care for the Elderly and State Health Policy. *Assessing the New Federalism: Issues and Options for States*. Number A-17. Washington, DC: Urban Institute, 1997.

Wiener, J.M., and Stevenson, D.G. *Long-Term Care Financing and Quality of Care*. Paper prepared for the Institute of Medicine Committee on Improving Quality in Long-Term Care, Washington, DC, 1998.

Wiener, J.M., Stevenson, D.G., and Goldenson, S.M. Controlling the Supply of Long-Term Care Providers in Thirteen States. *Journal of Aging and Social Policy* 10(4):51–72, 1999.

Williams, S.J., and Calnan, M. Convergence and Divergence: Assessing Criteria of Consumer Satisfaction Across General Practice, Dental and Hospital Care Settings. *Social Science and Medicine* 33:707–716, 1991.

Wilner, M.A. Recruiting Qualified Home Care Aides: New Candidate Pools. *Caring* 18(4):44–45, 1999.

Wilson, L., Huffman, C., and Conroy, J. *Evaluation of Supported Placements in Integrated Community Environments Project*. Springfield, IL: Illinois Planning Council on Developmental Disabilities, 1991.

Wolfe, W. Nursing Homes Shake Off Old Role as Place Only for Death. *Minneapolis Star Tribune*, April 11, 1999.

Wolinsky, F.D., and Johnson, R.J. The Use of Health Services by Older Adults. *Journal of Gerontology* 46(6):S345–S357, 1991.

Yee, D.L., Capitman, J.A., Leutz, W.N., and Sceigaj, M. Resident-Centered Care in Assisted Living. *Journal of Aging and Social Policy* 10(3):7–26, 1999.

Yoon, R., McKenzie, D.K., Bauman, A., and Miles, D.A. Controlled Trial Evaluation of an Asthma Education Programme for Adults. *Thorax* 48(11):1110–1116, 1993.

Zech, D.F., Grond, S., Lynch, J., Hertel, D., and Lehmann, K.A. Validation of World Health Organization Guidelines for Cancer Pain Relief: A 10-year Prospective Study. *Pain* 63:65–76, 1995.

Zimmer, J.G., Watson, N.M., and Levenson, S.A. Nursing Home Medical Directors: Ideals and Realities. *Journal of the American Geriatrics Society* 41(2):127–130, 1993.

Zimmerman, D.R. Testimony before the U.S. Senate Special Committee on Aging. The Nursing Home Initiative: Results at Year One. Washington, DC, June 30, 1999.

Zimmerman, D.R., Karon, S.L., Arling, G., Clark, B.R., Collins, T., Ross, R., and Sainfort, F. Development and Testing of Nursing Home Quality Indicators. *Health Care Financing Review* 16(4):107–127, 1995.

Zimmerman, S. The Mental Retardation Family Subsidy Program: Its Effects on Families with a Mentally Handicapped Child. *Family Relations* 33:105–118, 1984.

Zinn, J.S. Inter-SMSA Variation on Nursing Home Staffing and Management Practices. *Journal of Applied Gerontology* 12(2):206–224, 1993a.

Zinn, J.S. The Influence of Nurse Wage Differentials on Nursing Home Staffing and Resident Care Decisions. *The Gerontologist* 33(6):721–729, 1993b.

Zinn, J.S. Market Competition and the Quality of Nursing Home Care. *Journal of Health Politics, Policy, and the Law* 19(3):555–582, 1994.

Zinn, J.S., Aaronson, W.E., and Rosko, M.D. Variations in the Outcomes of Care Provided in Pennsylvania Nursing Homes. Facility and Environmental Correlates. *Medical Care* 31:475–487, 1993.

Appendix A

Committee Meetings and Presenters of Testimony

The Committee on Improving Long-Term Care held a total of eight meetings starting in 1997. These meetings involved segments open to the public, as well as closed sessions for committee deliberation. The dates of these eight meetings are listed below:

November 13–15, 1997, Washington, D.C.
March 12–14, 1998, Washington D.C.
June 11–12, 1998, Washington, D.C.
August 27–28, 1998, Woods Hole, MA
October 1, 1998, Irvine, CA
January 14–17, 1999, Washington, D.C.
April 9–10, 1999, Washington, D.C.
April 27–28, 2000, Washington, D.C.

The second meeting of the Committee, in March 1998, also comprised a public hearing. The committee heard testimony from various constituencies and interested parties at this hearing. The following people testified during this meeting:

Sally White and Sue Whitman, IONA Senior Services
Marsha Greenfield, Consumers United for Assisted Living (CUAL)
Elma Holder, National Citizens' Coalition for Nursing Home Reform
William Lasky, Assisted Living Federation of America

Cynthia Dunn, American Association of Homes and Services for the Aging

Reverend Monsignor Charles Fahey, National Center for Assisted Living

Joanne Schwartzberg, M.D., American Medical Association

Larry Lawhorne, M.D., American Medical Directors Association

Laurie Kennedy-Malone, Ph.D., R.N., National Conference of Geriatric Nurse Practitioners

Peter Rabins, M.D., American Psychiatric Association and the American Association for Geriatric Psychiatry

Linda Mondoux, M.S., R.N., C.S., American Nurses Association

Mary Ann Wilner, Paraprofessional Health Care Institute

Ingrid McDonald, Service Employees International Union

Toby Edelman, National Senior Citizens' Law Center

Nancy Coleman, J.D., American Bar Association

Faith Mullen, American Association of Retired Persons (AARP)

Pamela Nadash, National Council on Aging

Marianna Grachek, Joint Commission on Accreditation of Healthcare Organizations

William Keane, Alzheimer's Association

Karen Pace, National Association for Home Care

Paul Willging, American Health Care Association

Karen Tucker, American College of Health Care Administrators

Douglas Andrews, National Association of Boards of Examiners of Long Term Care Administrators

Bob Kafka, American Disabled for Attendant Programs Today (ADAPT)

Richard Bringewatt, National Chronic Care Consortium

Heather Bennet McCabe, Family Voices

The Committee also heard from numerous experts at two workshops. Presenters including the following:

Ruth Stein, M.D., Albert Einstein College of Medicine

Joshua Wiener, Ph.D., Urban Institute

David Stevenson, M.S., Urban Institute

Penny Feldman, Ph.D., Visiting Nurse Service of New York

Jeanette Price, Solomon Smith Barney

Jack Payne, U.S. Department of Housing and Urban Development

Gordon Beckwith, U.S. Department of Housing and Urban Development

Rosalie Kane, D.S.W., University of Minnesota Long-Term Care Resource Center

John Durso, J.D., Katten, Muchin, and Zavis
Andrew Kramer, M.D., University of Colorado Center on Aging
Marvin Feuerberg, Ph.D., Health Care Financing Administration
Robert Kane, Ph.D., University of Minnesota
Catherine Hawes, Ph.D., Myers Research Institute
Ted Benjamin, Ph.D., University of California in Los Angeles
Brenda Klutz, Deputy Director, California Department of Health
    Licensing and Certification
Patricia McGinnis, California Advocates for Nursing Home Reform
Melvin Matsumoto, Administrator, The Redwoods
Sara Sinclair, CEO, Sunshine Terrace Foundation
David Banks, CEO, Beverly Enterprises

APPENDIX B

Separate Dissenting Opinions

Seven members of the Committee have provided dissenting opinions regarding specific aspects of the final report.

DISSENT REGARDING RECOMMENDATION 3.1 AND RELATED ISSUES THAT SHOULD HAVE GREATER EMPHASIS

Rosalie A. Kane, Joshua Wiener, Janet E. George, Laurie E. Powers, Arthur Y. Webb, Penny H. Feldman, and Keren Brown Wilson disagreed with the wording of Recommendation 3.1, and offered the following explanation of their differences with the recommendation and the supporting text:

The recommendations and the content of the Report reflect a serious effort to grapple with the complex issues in defining and assuring quality of long-term care across a variety of service sites and target populations. We endorse all of the report's recommendations, but think that Recommendation 3.1 does not go far enough. Further, the report as a whole, fails to convey a coherent strategy and sense of direction justified by review of all the evidence presented to the committee.

Several important points were minimized or omitted from the Report. These points are briefly stated below to provide a backdrop for our concerns about Recommendation 3.1, in particular and also our discussion of regulations. References supporting these views are included:

1. Quality of life, as perceived by the long-term-care consumer (or, when

appropriate his or her agent) is an essential part of the quality of long-term care. Quality of life includes outcomes such as consumer choice and autonomy, dignity, individuality, comfort, meaningful activity, meaningful relationships, sense of security, and spiritual well-being (Noelker and Harel, 2000). As the report indicates, Health Care Financing Administration is currently funding a major effort to develop and test measures and indicators of such quality of life outcomes. Other researchers have also had considerable success in developing consumer self-report measures of quality of life, including persons with considerable cognitive impairment (Brod et al., 1999; Logsdon et al., 1999; Uman, 1995). Although long-term-care providers cannot be fully responsible for quality of life outcomes (which are also a function of health and disability status, family composition, and personality), long-term-care programs and settings can act to enhance or to retard these quality of life outcomes. The current regulatory system was not designed with quality of life issues as the focus.

2. If quality of life is seen as a legitimate goal of long-term care, the consumer's view of quality may sometimes involve conditions and circumstances that professionals view as a threat to health or safety. This tradeoff and the possibility that consumers might knowingly assume risks in order to maximize other benefits were not expressed in the final version of the report, yet it is an important reality (Kapp 1999; Kapp and Wilson, 1995; Kane and Caplan, 1993; Clemens et al., 1994). Even though there have been relatively few discussions or studies of how consumers and providers relate to these tradeoffs, the tradeoffs are widely recognized to occur routinely across all settings (Degenholtz et al., 1997).

3. Consumer-centered care (including consumer-directed care) is extensively discussed in the report. Consumer-centered care calls for the consumer (or his or her agent) to be involved to the extent desired and practical in all goal-setting and planning for care and to have direct input into the evaluation of his or her care. Consumer-directed care is a term sometimes reserved for situations where consumers are completely responsible for hiring, training, supervising, and evaluating the care that they receive. The report mistakenly described consumer-centered care as largely applicable to personal assistant services received by people under age 65. In fact, such principles are widely applicable to and have increasingly been applied to older people receiving care in a variety of settings.

The report marginalizes "consumer-centered care," stating that it is not for all people. This, we believe, is a misunderstanding of the concept. The principle of consulting consumer preferences directly or through their agents has widespread applicability to people of all ages, and in all settings including nursing homes. It has been applied to people with cognitive impairment including Alzheimer's disease and developmental disability. The emergence of new models of care, including client-directed home care and assisted living, is a direct result of consumer choice about how they want to live while needing care. The version of consumer-directed care that entails cash payments to consumers who are then responsible for purchasing and monitoring their own care, is merely one manifestation of consumer-centered and consumer-directed care. This level of consumer direction is inapplicable to some consumers because of their preferences, capabilities or level of social support. Consumer-centered care can be seen on a continuum, with consumer direction of various kinds at one end of the continuum. Throughout the long-term-care system in all types of settings, consumer-centered and consumer-directed care is insufficiently available. Although the lack of a consumer-centered focus in long-term care is mentioned in the report, it is under-stated and plays out in the recommendations as a concept that needs study before implementation rather than implementation with accompanying research. In our view, the evidence gathered for this Report already supports the value of and need for consumer centered care.

Recommendation 3.1

Recommendation 3.1 states: *The Committee recommends that the Department of Health and Human Services, with input from state and private organizations, develop and fund a research agenda to investigate the potential quality impact associated with access to, and limitations of, different models of consumer-centered long-term-care services, including consumer directed services.*

A research agenda is certainly appropriate and welcome but in our view insufficient to address the lack of consumer-centered approaches in the current long-term-care system. The need for greater access to a broader array of services and reconfiguration of long-term-care services so they better address consumer preferences is well-established. Research is not needed to establish the desirability of that goal, one that is already the focus of much state policy. Research is needed to examine barriers to access and barriers to consumer-centered care.

We, therefore, endorse language that calls for *state governments to work with providers and consumers to design and make available in each state an array of community-based long-term-care options for individuals of all ages with long-term-care needs* and *for individual consumers to be afforded the opportunity to specify the degree of control and influence that they are able to or wish to assume over the direction of their care.*

We dissent from the narrow research-only nature of recommendation 3.1, and maintain that the recommendation should also have included an action step because the evidence presented in the report and other evidence presented to the Committee, clearly shows that long-term-care consumers today do not have appropriate choices. Many receive care in forms and circumstances that do not comport with their preferences. Chapter 2 presents extensive information about the lack of access to an array of services. A research agenda about whether it is appropriate to center long-term care on consumer preferences is a pale response to an obvious goal. A research focused recommendation conveys a view that consumer-centered care might be unsafe or imprudent care that would not meet quality standards. In our view, the care cannot by definition meet quality standards if it is inconsistent with or interferes with what makes life worthwhile to the consumer.

Those who object to implementing an array of options and endorsing consumer-centered care as a policy raise the point that many older people who need care have cognitive impairment and may not even have an agent willing or able to be a proxy decision-maker. We concur that people with substantial cognitive impairment who also have no family agent acting on their behalf cannot direct their care in the sense of hiring, training, supervising, and firing staff. But not all consumer-centered care is consumer-directed care—that is, care where the consumer or his or her agent, directly control all care details. The general concept of determining and to the extent possible enabling consumer preferences is applicable, even for people with cognitive impairment. Moreover, consumer-centered care, in the sense of care that conforms as much as possible to consumer's preferences, is also possible and desirable in nursing homes and a wide variety of residential settings (Gamroth et al., 1995). Both consumer-centered care and the consumer-directed variant have been applied to and on behalf of people with severe developmental disabilities accompanied by cognitive impairment with good results and cost savings (Nerney and Shumway, 1996). Work is already underway to determine the extent to which the concept can be applied for community-dwelling persons with Alzheimer's disease (Robert Wood Johnson Foundation, 1995). There is nothing in the concept of consumer-centered care that is antithetical to care of high technical quality, nor anything that would impose the burden of organizing their own care on people without the capability or desire to do so.

We endorse the research aspect of Recommendation 3.1. However, such research should be oriented towards demonstrating and overcoming obstacles to consumer-centered care and demonstrating models by which consumer preferences and feedback can be elicited and applied in a variety of settings. Research is also needed to test approaches that enable consumers to live at home or in settings with little nursing oversight while still receiving help with medications and other services that in many states require a registered nurse. For example, a recent study done by the University of Washington School of Nursing, under a mandate from the state legislature, examined the effect of permitting registered nurses to delegate nursing functions to nonlicensed and noncertified workers. The study documented excellent outcomes; lower costs, more leadership of nurses in community long-term-care settings and no untoward events (Young and Sikma, 1998). Research of this nature advances consumer-centered care and is necessary to identify the best approaches to deliver such care.

In addition, research, evaluation and demonstration efforts are needed to provide practical information to consumers and decision-makers and to broaden the understanding of what consumer-centered care entails. Consumer-centered and consumer-directed care encourages consumers to make choices among types of care settings and on details of care within a particular setting. Adequate information is necessary to make such choices. Such information must be available to consumers in easily understood terms.

Consumer-centered care means also that providers cede some decision-making to consumers and that consumers be permitted to make tradeoffs that they consider important in choosing a care setting or provider and the details of a care plan. The idea that a single "appropriate" setting exists for each consumer based on disability level must give way to an understanding that more than one choice can work for many consumers. This requires a philosophical change for providers, care managers, regulators, and consumer advocates, such as nursing home ombudsmen, all of whom should receive training in the philosophy of consumer-centered care. Provider-centered care is so ingrained in long-term-care programs that a concerted effort is needed to identify and explore the biases that many professionals bring to planning and allocating long-term-care services.

In conclusion, we reiterate that we respect the deep deliberation conducted by the Committee and agree with the intentions of the report and its recommendations. We also reiterate that we are not dissenting from the report itself except for the formulation of Recommendation 3.1. Otherwise, the main point of this separate opinion is to highlight some issues and give greater emphasis to the salience of consumer-centered approaches. We are grateful for that opportunity.

Concerns Regarding Regulatory Issues

Rosalie A. Kane, Janet E. George, Laurie E. Powers, Arthur Y. Webb, and Keren Brown Wilson additionally expressed dissatisfaction with the report's discussion of regulatory issues. Their viewpoint on these issues is expressed below.

Recommendation 5.2 *"recommends that state agencies along with the private sector develop programs to disseminate information to consumers (a) on the various types of long-term-care settings available to them, and (b) where applicable information on the compliance with relevant state standards of individual long-term-care providers."*

Recommendation 5.3 states: . . . *"all states have appropriate standard-setting and oversight mechanisms for all settings where people receive personal care and nursing services. The committee recognizes that before this recommendation can be implemented, research examining the effectiveness of the state survey and enforcement activities for residential care be undertaken."*

Taken together, these recommendations contain many important concepts with which we agree. However, the report gives insufficient recognition to the complexity of standard-setting and monitoring of alternative settings, given the diversity of models within and across states. Further, standards are in flux, and new methods of regulatory oversight are under development. Therefore, while supporting the recommendations, we offer several observations about their relationship to consumer-centered care.

Consumer understanding of the options available to them is a critical requirement in the implementation of consumer-centered care. Especially in residential care, terminology tends to be confusing and states have many different licensed entities with a variety of regulatory mandates and prohibitions. At a minimum, state bodies should make these definitions transparent to the public and publicize them widely. Recommendation 5.2 supports this point. In addition, we urge states to reexamine the standards. Some standards serve merely to delimit the amount of care that may be given or the disability levels of people that may be served in a particular setting. Standard-setting should include review of standards that pertain to building and equipment, to staff and program, and to consumers who may be admitted or retained. The point is to ensure an appropriate standard setting process and effective oversight mechanisms. The recommendation and the discussion supporting it, however, do not discuss the complexities, difficulties, and tradeoffs in standard setting for home and community-based services, or suggest that consumers be part of the standard setting and oversight processes.

The quality of residential care, including assisted living, is uneven. Some residential care settings offer neither homelike settings with a likelihood of a better quality of life nor a service capacity to meet the needs of people with higher levels of frailty. Further, we recognize the scandals that have occasionally erupted over problems in assisted living, and endorse strong state enforcement to curb such abuses. Beyond identifying indisputably poor care, however, little agreement has been reached on desired standards for various types of residential care. Assisted Living providers have combined with advocacy organizations including the American Association of retired Persons and the Alzheimer's Association to discuss draft standards for assisted living (ALQC, 1998). Great diversity exists among states in the current regulatory expectations, and many experts believe that some states have standards that are too minimal in terms of expectations for aging in place and for private accommodations. Some states use regulations more to limit the kind of care that may be offered and the people who may be admitted or retained rather than to specify care outcome expectations.

Recommendation 5.3 recognizes these issues and responds by calling for research on the effectiveness of state survey and enforcement activities. We would have preferred that the recommendation specify who should undertake the activity. Further, some prior effort to develop a national classification system and typology including considerable conceptual work on what effectiveness means in this context is necessary before a survey could yield useful information. Without clarity on a number of definitions, studies could do more harm than good by adding to confusion, and perhaps cutting off meaningful options to consumers.

Despite the uncertainties of assisted living and the diversity across states, significant numbers of consumers who are functionally eligible for nursing homes are selecting assisted living. Medicare and/or Medicaid waiver coverage for assisted living is now available in at least 30 states. Washington, New Jersey, Texas, and Oregon have shown that apartment style assisted living can be provided for moderate-income people with heavy long-term-care needs. It is therefore important that efforts be undertaken to develop and implement appropriate classifications and standards for enforcement.

In conclusion, we reiterate that we respect the Committee's deliberations and agree with the intentions of the report and the majority of its recommendations. Our dissent is limited to Recommendation 3.1. Otherwise, this separate opinion highlights some issues and gives greater emphasis to the salience of consumer-centered approaches than is reflected in the report. We are grateful for that opportunity.

REFERENCES

ALQC, Assisted Living Quality Coalition Report. Washington, D.C.: National Association for Retired Persons, 1998.

Albert, S, Catillo-Castaneda, C., Sano, M., Jacobs, D, Marder, K. Bell, K, Blysma, F., Lafleche, G, Brandt, J., Albert, M., and Stern, Y. Quality of Life in Patient's With Alzheimer's Disease as Reported by Patient Proxies. *Journal of the American Geriatrics Society,* 44:1342–1347.

Brod, M., Stewart, A.L., Sands, L. and Walton, P. Conceptualization and measurement of quality of life in dementia: The Dementia Quality of Life Instrument (DqoL). *The Gerontologist,* 39 (1), 25–35.

Clemens, E., Wetle, T., Feltes, M., Crabtree, B., and Dubitzky, D. Contradictions in case management: Client-centered theory and directive practice with frail elderly. *Journal of Aging and Health,* 6:70–88, 1994.

Degenholtz, H.D., Kane, R.A. and Kivnick, H.Q. Care-Related Preferences and Values of Elderly Community Based Long-Term-Care Consumers: Can Case Managers Learn What's Important to Clients? *The Gerontologist,* 37:767–776, 1997.

Gamroth, L.M., Semradek, J., and Tornquist, E.M. (eds). *Enhancing Autonomy in Long-Term Care: Concepts and Strategies.* New York: Springer Publishing Company, 1995.

Kane R.A. and Caplan, A.L. *Ethical Conflict in the Management of Home Care: The Case Manager's Dilemma,* New York: Springer Publishing Company, 1993.

Kapp, M.B. Quality of Care and Quality of Life in Nursing Facilities: What's Regulation Got to Do with It? *McGeorge Law Review,* 31(3):707–731.

Kapp, M.B. Who Is Responsible for This? Assigning Rights and Consequences in Elder Care. *Journal of Aging and Social Policy,* 9(2):51–65, 1997.

Kapp, M.B. and Wilson, K.B. Assisted Living and Negotiated Risk: Reconciling Protection and Autonomy. *Journal of Ethics, Law and Aging,* 1 (1):5–13, 1995.

Lawton, M.P., Van Haitsma, K., and Klapper J. Observed Affect in Nursing Home Residents with Alzheimer's disease. *Journal of Gerontology,* 51B:3–14, 1996.

Logsdon, R., Gibbons, L., McCurry, S. and Teri, L. Quality of Life in Alzheimer's Disease: Patient and Caregiver Reports. *Journal of Mental Health and Aging.* 5 (1):21–32,1999.

Mattimore, T.J., Wenger, N.S., Desbiens, N.A., Teno, J.M., Hamel, M.B., Lit, H., Califf, R., Connors, A.F., Lynn, J., and Oye, R.K. Surrogate and Physician's Understanding of Patient's Preferences for Living Permanently in a Nursing Home. *Journal of the American Geriatrics Society,* 45 (7):818–824, 1997.

Nerney, T. and Shumway, D. *Beyond Managed Care: Self-Determination for People With Disabilities,* Concord, NH: University of New Hampshire Institute on Disabilities, 1996.

Noelker L.S. and Harel, Z. (eds). *Quality of Life and Quality of Care in Long-Term Care.* New York: Springer Publishing Company, 2000.

Rabins, P., Kasper, J., Kleinman, L., Black, B. and Patrick, D. Concepts and Methods in the Development of the ADRLQ: An Instrument for Assessing Health-Related Quality of Life with Alzheimer's Disease. *Journal of Mental Health and Aging,* 5(1):33–49.

Robert Wood Johnson Foundation. *Independent Choices: Enhancing Consume-Direction for People With Disabilities*: Washington, D.C., The Brookings Institute.

Uman, G (1995). *Measuring Consumer Satisfaction in Nursing Homes: A Small Business Innovation Research (SBIR) Grant Study,* Paper presented at the Annual Meeting of the Gerontological Society of America, November 4, 1995. Available from Gwen Uman, Vital Research, 8380 Melrose Avenue, # 309, Los Angeles, CA.)

Young, H.M. and Sikma, S.K. *The Evaluation of the Implementation of Nurse Delegation in Washington State: Final Report.* Prepared by University of Washington School of Nursing for the Aging and Adult Services Administration, Washington State Department of Social and Health Services, November 1998.

Wilson, K.B. *Assisted Living: Reconceptualizing Regulation to Meet Consumers' Needs and Preferences.* Washington, D.C.: American Association of Retired Persons, 1996.

Acronyms

AAHSA	American Association of Homes and Services for the Aging
AARP	American Association of Retired Persons
ACHCA	American College of Healthcare Administrators
ADA	Americans with Disabilities Act
ADAPT	American Disabled for Attendant Programs Today
ADL	activity of daily living
AGS	American Geriatrics Society
AHCA	American Healthcare Association
AHCPR	Agency for Health Care Policy and Research
AHRQ	Agency for Healthcare Research and Quality
AIDS	acquired immune deficiency syndrome
ALF	assisted living facility
ALQC	Assisted Living Quality Coalition
AMDA	American Medical Directors Association
AoA	Administration on Aging
BBA 97	Balanced Budget Act of 1997
BLS	Bureau of Labor Statistics
CBO	U.S. Congressional Budget Office
CCAL	Consumer Consortium for Assisted Living
CHSPRA	Center for Health System Policy Research and Analysis
CHSRA	Center for Health Systems Research and Analysis

CMP	civil monetary penalty
CNA	Certified Nursing Assistant
CUAL	Consumers United for Assisted Living
DHHS	U.S. Department of Health and Human Services
DRG	Diagnosis Related Groups
FFS	fee for service
GAO	General Accounting Office
GNP	geriatric nurse practitioner
GNS	gerontological nurse specialist
HCBS	home- and community-based services
HCFA	Health Care Financing Administration
HEDIS	Health Plan Employer Data and Information Set
HHA	home health agency
HMO	health maintenance organization
IADL	instrumental activity of daily living
IDEA	Individuals with Disabilities Education Act
IOM	Institute of Medicine
JCAHO	Joint Commission on Accreditation of Healthcare Organizations
LPN	licensed practical nurse
LTC	long-term care
MDS	Minimum Data Set
MedPAC	Medicare Payment Advisory Commission
MEPS	Medical Expenditure Panel Survey
MMACS	Medicare and Medicaid Automated Certification System
MR/DD	mental retardation/developmental disability
NA	nursing assistant or nursing aide
NAHC	National Association for Home Care
NCCNHR	National Citizens' Coalition for Nursing Home Reform
NCHS	National Center for Health Statistics
NCPSSM	National Committee to Preserve Social Security and Medicare
NHCMQ	Nursing Home Casemix and Quality Demonstration Resident Status Measurement

NHIS	National Health Interview Survey
NHIS-D	National Health Interview Survey—Disability Supplement
NIC	National Investment Conference for the Senior Living and Long-Term Care Industries
NMES	National Medical Expenditure Survey
OASIS	Outcome and Assessment Information Set
OBQI	outcome-based quality improvement
OBRA 87	Omnibus Budget Reconciliation Act of 1987
OIG	Office of the Inspector General
OSCAR	On-Line Survey and Certification Assessment Reporting System
PACE	Program of All-Encompassing Care for the Elderly
PCS	personal care services
PPRC	Physician Payment Review Commission
PPS	prospective payment system
ProPAC	Prospective Payment Assessment Commission
PSDA	Patient Self-Determination Act
PSSRR	Preadmission Assessment Screening and Annual Resident Review
QI	quality indicator
RAI	Resident Assessment Instrument
RAI-RCF	Resident Assessment Instrument for Residential Care Facilities
RAP	resident assessment protocol
RCF	residential care facility
REAL	real experiences and assessment of life
RN	registered nurse
RUG	Resource Utilization Group
RUG-III	Resource Utilization Group—Version III
SCHIP	State Children's Health Insurance Program
S.D.	standard deviation
SNF	skilled nursing facility
SSA	Social Security Administration
SSI	Supplemental Security Income
SSP	State Supplemental Payments
VA	Department of Veterans Affairs or Veterans Administration

Biographical Sketches of
Committee Members

Peter O. Kohler, M.D. (*Chair*), is president of Oregon Health Sciences University. Prior to coming to Oregon, he was dean of the School of Medicine at the University of Texas Health Sciences Center in San Antonio and was previously interim dean and chairman of the Department of Medicine at the University of Arkansas. He served as chair of the Oregon Health Council, a statewide group advising the governor on health policy issues. Of special interest to him is the Area Health Education Center program. Dr. Kohler is immediate past chair of the Association of Academic Health Centers. He previously served on the Committee on Evaluating Telemedicine of the Institute of Medicine.

Richard D. Della Penna, M.D., holds several concurrent positions: assistant clinical Professor of medicine, University of California (San Diego) School of Medicine; physician-in-charge of continuing care services, home health, and hospice with the San Diego Kaiser Permanente Medical Program; and regional elder care coordinator for the Southern California Permanente Medical Program and national clinical lead of Kaiser Permanente's Care Management Institute's Elder Care Initiative. He serves on the Interregional Committee on Aging for the Kaiser Permanente National Program and is a member of the Regional Home Health Committee for the Southern California region. Additionally, he is the principal investigator, Implementing Geriatric Interdisciplinary Team Training for Practicing Professionals in association with the John A. Hartford Foundation and the Garfield Foundation; as well as a planning group and faculty member for the Institute for Healthcare Improvement, End of Life Collaborative. He received his M.D. from Tufts University School of Medicine in 1969, completing his internship and residency with Harvard Medical Service, Boston City Hospital. Dr. Della Penna is currently licensed to practice medicine in the State of California. He is American board certified in family practice with added qualifications in geriatrics.

Penny Hollander Feldman, Ph.D., is vice president for research and evaluation and director of the Center for Home Care Policy and Research at the Visiting Nurse Service of New York (VNSNY). Prior to joining VNSNY, Dr. Feldman served on the faculties of the Kennedy School of Government and the Department of Health Policy and Management at the Harvard School of Public Health, where she continues as visiting lecturer. At VNSNY, she directs research projects focused on improving the quality, outcomes, and cost-effectiveness of home-based care; supporting informed policy making by federal, state, and local decision makers; promoting equitable access and outcomes for older persons, especially those who are disadvantaged; and strengthening methods for home care research. Dr. Feldman is the program director of the Home Care Research Initiative, a national research program established by the Robert Wood Johnson Foundation in 1995. She has served as the chair of the Strategic Planning Committee and on the Board of Directors of the Visiting Nurse Affiliates of Cambridge as well as on the Board of Directors of the Health Action Forum of Boston and the Policy Advisory Committee of Health Care for All of Boston. She earned her Ph.D. in political science from Harvard University.

Janet E. George, R.N., M.A., is recently retired from the positions of assistant vice president, director of clinical systems, with HCR ManorCare and was previously vice president of quality improvement with ManorCare, Inc. In these capacities, Ms. George developed and directed quality improvement programs and supervised quality improvement specialists who facilitated and trained facility staff in the integration of the quality process into management and delivery of care. Until her retirement after 22 years of long-term care experience, Ms. George contributed to the development of practice standards within HCR ManorCare and to clinical practice guidelines in the long-term care industry. Ms. George is a past member of American Healthcare Association's Ethics Subcommittee and of its Professional Development Work Group and Clinical Practice Guidelines Subcommittee. Ms. George is a registered nurse with a bachelor's degree in nursing and a master of arts degree in human resource development.

Charlene Harrington, Ph.D., R.N. (who earned her Ph.D. at the University of California, Berkeley), is professor of sociology and nursing and immediate past chair of the Department of Social and Behavioral Sciences, School of Nursing, University of California, San Francisco. She is a fellow in the American Academy of Nursing and a member of the Institute of Medicine (IOM). She is the principal investigator of several research studies on state long-term care policies and program characteristics (since 1980), a study to design and develop a nursing home consumer information system about quality (Agency for Healthcare Policy and Research 1995–1999), and a study of Medicare consumer quality-of-care complaints. She evaluated the Social Health Maintenance Organizations demonstration (1985-1990) and is a member of the team developing second-generation projects. She served on the IOM Committee to Study Nursing Home Regulation (1983–1985), the Committee to Study Hospital and Nursing Home Staffing (1995-1996), and the current Committee on Improving Quality in Long-Term Care. In her 20 years of research experience at the University of California, San Francisco, she has completed numerous research studies and articles on long-term care and managed care.

Rosalie A. Kane, D.S.W., is a professor of public health at the University of Minnesota, where she is also on the faculty of the Center for Biomedical Ethics and the School of Social Work. Since 1989, she has directed a Long-Term Care Resource Center, providing technical assistance, research and development, and information dissemination to advance state efforts in home and community-based care. Previously, she was a social scientist at the Rand Corporation in Santa Monica, California, and a faculty member at the University of California at Los Angeles and, before that, at the University of Utah, from which she also received a doctoral degree in social work. Her research emphases focus on long-term care for disabled older persons and other dependent groups, including quality of care, assessment, case management, home care, nursing home care, and more recently, the study of values and ethics. Between 1988 and 1992, she was editor-in-chief of *The Gerontologist*. Presently, she leads a national study on "Measurement, Indicators, and Improvement of the Quality of Life in Nursing Homes" and a national study on the "Home Care/Assisted Living Connection."

    Dr. Kane has served on the IOM Committee on Nursing Home Regulation, 1983–1985, its Committee to Evaluate the LTC Ombudsman Programs (1993–1994), the National Advisory Council on Geriatrics and Gerontology for the Veterans Administration, and the 1997–1998 Veteran Administration's Committee on the Future of Aging Programs. She is a senior fellow of the Brookdale Foundation and has served on numerous task forces and committees, including the Scientific and Medical Advisory

Board of the Alzheimer's Association. Publications include *The Heart of Long-Term Care* (1988), coauthored with Robert L. Kane and Richard C. Ladd; (with Robert Kane) *Long-Term Care: Principles, Programs and Policies* (1987), *Assessing the Elderly: A Practical Guide to Measurement* (1981); *Long-Term Care in Six Countries: Implications for the United States* (1976); (with Arthur Caplan) *Everyday Ethics: Resolving Dilemmas in Nursing Home Life* (1990); *Ethical Conflict in the Management of Home Care: Case Manager's Dilemma* (1993), and (with Joan D. Penrod) *Family Caregiving in an Aging Society: Policy Perspectives* (1995).

Vincent Mor, Ph.D., is director of the Center for Gerontology and Health Care Research at Brown University. Dr. Mor has been the principal investigator of more than 12 National Institutes of Health grants and contracts to conduct program evaluations in aging and long-term care. He was one of the authors of the congressionally mandated Minimum Data Set for nursing home resident assessment and has published widely on a range of topics in gerontology including hospice, physical functioning, long-term care, cancer treatment patterns, patient outcomes, and residential care facilities.

Vivian Omagbemi, M.S., R.N., is the long-term care ombudsman for the Montgomery County Aging and Disability Services in Rockville, Maryland, a position she has held since 1983. Prior to this appointment, she was a community health nurse for the Montgomery County Health Department in Rockville, Maryland, and a nurse practitioner in occupational health at Howard University in Washington, D.C. She holds a B.S. in nursing from Adelphi University in New York and an M.S. in nursing from Catholic University in Washington, D.C. She is also a registered nurse in the State of Maryland.

James M. Perrin, M.D., is associate professor of pediatrics at Harvard Medical School, director of the Division of General Pediatrics at the Massachusetts General Hospital (MGH) for Children, and director of the MGH Center for Child and Adolescent Health Policy. He formerly chaired the American Academy of Pediatrics Committee on Children with Disabilities and was president of the Ambulatory Pediatric Association, whose journal, *Ambulatory Pediatrics,* he currently edits. For the American Academy of Pediatrics, he also co-chairs a committee to develop a practice guideline for attention deficit hyperactivity disorder. A graduate of Harvard College and Case Western Reserve University School of Medicine, he had his training in pediatrics at the University of Rochester and has been on the pediatric faculties of the University of Rochester and Vanderbilt University, with an additional appointment at the Institute for

Public Policy Studies at Vanderbilt University. His research has examined asthma, middle-ear disease, children's hospitalization, and chronic childhood illnesses and disabilities, with a recent emphasis on studies of the Supplemental Security Income Program for children and adolescents. He coauthored *Chronically Ill Children and Their Families* and *Home and Community Care for Chronically Ill Children*. He is a member of the National Advisory Council of the Agency for Healthcare Research and Quality. He served on the Institute of Medicine's Committees on Maternal and Child Health Under Health Care Reform and on Home-Based and Long-Term Care and Quality, the National Commission on Childhood Disability, and the Disability Policy Panel of the National Academy of Social Insurance.

Laurie E. Powers, Ph.D., is associate professor of pediatrics, psychiatry, and public health, co-director of the Center on Self-Determination, and director of research for the Rehabilitation Research and Training Center on Health and Wellness for Persons with Long-Term Disabilities at Oregon Health Sciences University. She specializes in issues related to disability, self-determination, and health through research, policy analysis, and model development activities.

At Dartmouth Medical School, Dr. Powers was an assistant professor and the associate director of the Hood Center on Family Support. Dr. Powers serves as a member of many professional committees and has served as a reviewer for a number of different professional journals. She is editor of several books and author of numerous chapters, articles, videotapes, and lectures. She earned her Ph.D. in counseling psychology (American Psychiatric Association approved) at the University of Oregon.

Ellen T. Reap is vice president at Adventist HealthCare where she heads the Senior Living Services company, which operates nursing homes, assisted living facilities, adult day care programs, and a HUD senior housing facility. She formerly served as the State of Delaware's director of the Office of Health Facilities Licensing and Certification, where she was responsible for regulating all levels of health facilities and programs, as well as directing the State Survey Agency. She was twice president of the National Association of Health Facility Survey Agencies, the professional organization of the states' health inspection officials. She served as an impact assessment adviser to the Health Care Financing Administration administrator on the implementation of nursing home enforcement regulations and has testified on nursing home quality of care issues before the Senate Special Committee on Aging. She previously served with HCFA, where she was involved with the survey and certification programs for nursing homes, home health, and end-stage renal disease. Prior to entering government service, she served in a variety of leadership roles in home health, nursing homes, and hospitals. Ms. Reap received her B.S. in nursing from The Catholic University of America.

John F. Schnelle, Ph.D., is director of the UCLA–Jewish Home Borun Center, and research health scientist, Veterans Administration Medical Center—Sepulveda. His research has focused on ways to improve quality health care for nursing home residents. In addition, Dr. Schnelle has received various awards and honors including the Shannon Award from the National Institutes of Health and the Brookdale Award from the National Institute on Human Resources and Aging. Dr. Schnelle received his Ph.D. in psychology from the University of Tennessee.

Paul M. Schyve, M.D., is senior vice president of the Joint Commission on Accreditation of Healthcare Organizations (JCAHO). From 1989 until 1993, he was vice president for research and standards, and from 1986 until 1989, the Director of Standards at the Joint Commission. Prior to joining JCAHO, Dr. Schyve was the clinical director of the State of Illinois Department of Mental Health and Developmental Disabilities. He received an undergraduate degree from the University of Rochester. He completed his medical education and residency in psychiatry at the University of Rochester, and has subsequently held a variety of professional and academic appointments in the areas of mental health and hospital administration, including director of the Illinois State Psychiatric Institute and clinical associate professor of psychiatry at the University of Chicago. Dr. Schyve is certified in psychiatry by the American Board of Psychiatry and Neurology and is a fellow of the American Psychiatric Association. He has published in the areas of psychiatric treatment and research, quality assurance, continuous quality improvement, health care accreditation, and health care ethics.

Eric G. Tangalos, M.D., is professor of medicine at the Mayo Clinic School of Medicine and chair of the Division of Community Internal Medicine at Mayo Rochester. He is director of information transfer at the Mayo Alzheimer's Disease Center and an investigator in Mayo's Alzheimer's Disease Patient Registry. Dr. Tangalos has served as President of the Minnesota Medical Directors Association and is past president of the American Medical Directors Association. He is a governor of the American College of Physicians–American Society of Internal Medicine. He is also a member of the board of the National Alzheimer's Association and the board of Friends of the National Library of Medicine. He was one of only two physicians appointed by President Clinton to the Advisory Committee of the 1995 White House Conference on Aging.

Arthur Y. Webb has been president and CEO of Village Care of New York since 1993. Village Care of New York is a community-based health care organization providing services to geriatric persons and people with AIDS. Previously, Mr. Webb was a research professor and senior fellow at the Institute for Health Policy, the Heller School, Brandeis University, and commissioner of the New York State Office of Mental Retardation and Developmental Disabilities. He is a member of the Board of Directors and of the Executive Committee for the New York Association of Services and Homes for the Aging. Other associations of which he is a member include the Healthcare Association of New York State and the Greater New York Hospital Association. Arthur Webb received his education from New York University, completing comprehensive exams in health policy, American government, and comparative political systems.

Joshua M. Wiener, Ph.D., is a specialist in Medicaid, health care for the elderly, and long-term care and has worked more than 25 years as a health care researcher and government official. Dr. Wiener is the author or editor of seven books and more than 70 articles on long-term care, health reform, health care rationing, and maternal and child health. His books include *Caring for the Disabled Elderly: Who Will Pay?*, *Sharing the Burden: Strategies for Public and Private Long-Term Care Insurance;* and *Rationing America's Medical Care: The Oregon Plan and Beyond*. His most recent book is *Persons with Disabilities: Issues in Health Care Financing and Service Delivery*. Along with Lewin-VHI, Inc., he developed the Brookings-ICF Long-Term Care Financing Model, a microsimulation model that projects the use and cost for long-term care into the future.

Prior to coming to the Urban Institute in April 1996, Dr. Wiener was a senior fellow at the Brookings Institution for almost 12 years. Before that, he worked for the Health Care Financing Administration, the Massachusetts Department of Public Health, the Congressional Budget Office, the New York State Moreland Act Commission on Nursing Homes and Residential Facilities, and the New York City Department of Health. Dr. Wiener earned his Ph.D. in sociology from Harvard University.

Keren Brown Wilson, Ph.D.,* co-founded Assisted Living Concepts, Inc., and served as its president, CEO, vice chair, and a director of the com-

---

*In 1999, class action securities litigation (unrelated to assisted living quality of care issues) was filed against Assisted Living Concepts, Inc., several of its former and present officers and directors, including Dr. Wilson, its independent auditors and underwriters. In September, 2000, the Company, its underwriters, and the individuals, including Dr. Wilson, stipulated to settlement. The Company's auditors remain in the pending litigation.

pany until October 19, 2000. She currently serves as founder/advisor to the company and as president of the Jessie F. Richardson Foundation. Dr. Wilson has 25 years of experience in aging services delivery systems and has, for the past 20 years, focused primarily on assisted living. From 1988 to September 1994, she was president and sole director of CCL, a company specializing in the development and management of assisted living residences. From 1986 to 1988, she served as senior vice president at Milestone, Inc., an assisted living development and management company. She was responsible for designing, developing, and managing the State of Oregon's first assisted living residence along with the state's first Medicaid-eligible assisted living residence. She serves on the Board of the American Society on Aging, is chair of Assisted Living Federation of America, and is a member of the Portland State University Foundation Board.

Index

A

Accountability, general, 14, 33, 134, 138
   see also External oversight; Regulatory
     issues; Standards
Accreditation, 4, 135, 137, 178
   adult foster care and small group
     homes, 49, 94, 164
   assisted living, 47
   board and care homes, 45, 91-92
   home health care agencies, 171-172
   Medicaid, 178
   Medicare, 178
   nongovernmental, 122, 137, 171-172,
     178, 223
   residential care facilities, 45, 47
Acute care services, 28, 124, 129, 182
   see also Special care units; Subacute care
     units
Adult foster care homes, 45, 49-50, 94-95,
     164, 250
   see also Group homes
Adults, *see* Elderly persons; Nonelderly
     adults
Advocacy, 11, 19, 135, 140, 174-177, 250
   American Association of Retired
     Persons (AARP), 68, 164-165, 293
   care management, 58
   children, 174-175
   funding, 19, 175-176
   home and community-based services
     organizations, 55, 58, 67
   information systems, promotion of, 177
   Long-Term Care Ombudsman Program,
     11, 79, 175-176
   Medicaid, 67
   nursing homes, 148, 161, 162, 176-177, 191
   personal care services, 67, 177
   residential care, 168, 202-203, 293
African Americans, 39
Age factors, 23-24
   employment issues, 212
   number in long-term care, 1, 39
   population, aging of, 2, 22-23
   see also Children and young adults;
     Elderly persons; Nonelderly
     adults
Agency for Health Care Policy and
     Research, 114, 127
AIDS, *see* HIV/AIDS
Alabama, 101
Alcohol and drug abuse, 126, 164
Alzheimer's Association, 293
Alzheimer's disease, *see* Dementia
American Academy of Nursing, 196
American Association of Retired Persons
     (AARP), 68, 164-165, 293
American Board of Family Practice, 62

American Board of Medical Specialities, 62(n.9)
American Geriatrics Society, 222
American Health Care Association, 194, 216, 223
American Medical Directors Association, 199, 222
American Nursing Association, 196
American Society of Internal Medicine, 62
Americans with Disabilities Act, 29, 103
Archstone Foundation, 3, 25
Arizona, 101
Assessment instruments, 8-10, 18, 37, 40, 47, 109, 117-120, 121-122, 127-134, 150-152
Assets and Health Dynamics of the Elderly Survey, 37(n.1)
Assisted living, 6, 8, 10, 42, 45, 47-49, 92-94, 109
    administrators, 47-48
    defined, 47, 50, 168-169
    elderly persons, 48(n.6), 92-94
    financing, general, 64
    functional status, 47, 49
    General Accounting Office studies, 93, 94, 202, 249
    licensure, 47
    Medicare/Medicaid, 293
    medication, 93, 166
    number of facilities, beds, and residents, 47, 48
    personal care services, 47, 48(n.6)
    personnel and personnel standards, 202, 203-204
    privacy and dignity, 47, 49, 92-93
    regulatory issues, 38, 93, 94, 166
    state standards, 10, 47, 93, 164, 166, 168-169. 292-293
Assisted Living Quality Coalition, 169, 203, 216
Auditory impairments, 116
Australia, 107

B

Balanced Budget Act, 16, 51, 193, 235, 236, 241-244
Bathroom facilities
    assisted living, 49
    home health care, 207
    nursing homes, 88, 229-230

Bed sores, *see* Pressure sores
Board and care homes, 10, 45-47, 64, 68, 91-92, 124, 163-169, 202-203, 250
    developmental disabilities, 46, 71
    medication, 46, 91-92, 202, 203
    regulatory issues, 45, 46, 91, 92, 163-169
    safety, 92, 163
    Supplemental Security Income, 47, 64, 68, 163
Bureau of Census, 250
Bureau of Labor Statistics, 13, 212

C

California
    assisted living, 93
    consumer-centered programs, 106-107
    developmentally disabled persons, residential care, 96
    home health care, 209
    nursing homes, 78, 145, 153, 158, 197
    personal care services, 55, 68, 209-210
Cardiovascular disease, 40
Care management, 3, 9, 15, 22, 69-70, 127, 135
    children, 58, 71-72
    consumer-centered services, 29, 71-72
    developmentally disabled persons, 96
    home and community-based services organizations, 54, 55, 58-59
    individualization of care, 6, 28, 29, 127-128, 189, 229
    restorative care, 8, 116
    state government, 58, 68
    see also Managed care
Casemix, 242
    nursing homes, 19, 74, 88, 90, 114, 117, 118, 123-124, 182, 188-195 (passim)
    residential care settings, 202
    see also Resource Utilization Groups
Casemix reimbursement, 19, 240-241
Centers for Advancement of Quality in Long-Term Care, 20, 234
Certification, 4, 8, 9, 10, 18, 135, 136-137, 172
    home health care agencies, 7, 8, 43, 51, 52, 97, 171-172, 173-174, 206, 207, 208
    Medicaid, 7, 8, 10, 17, 44, 47, 49, 51, 52, 174, 178, 207
    Medicare, 7, 8, 10, 44, 47, 49, 51, 52, 174, 178, 207

nongovernmental, 122, 137
nursing homes, 7, 8, 18, 42, 43, 44, 76,
    77, 137, 140-141, 143-163, 182
state survey activities, 18, 137, 142-163
voluntary, 122, 137, 171-172, 178, 223
Chains, *see* Multi-facility organizations
Chemical restraints, *see* Physical and
    chemical restraints
Children and young adults, 30, 40, 201
advocacy, 174-175
assessment design, 132-134
care management, 58, 71-72
cognitive factors, 40, 133, 217
consumer-centered care, 71-72
coordination of services, 70-71
diseases/conditions of children in care,
    40
family issues, 104, 105
functional status, 133
home and community-based services
    organizations, 58, 104-105, 210
home care, 210
home health care agencies, 104-105, 207-
    208
informal care for, 217
informal caregivers for elderly, 59-60, 217
long-term care defined, 28
number in care, 2, 23-24
nursing home visits by, 88
physician skills, 61
professional education for, 61, 104-105
Supplemental Security Income
    program, 68
Children with Special Health Care Needs,
    58
Clinical practice guidelines, 14, 15, 221-222,
    224, 226-228, 232, 234
cost factors, 15, 221, 232
Clinton, William, 113
Cognitive factors, 24, 288, 289, 290
assessment instruments, 7, 8, 116, 127, 132
assisted living facilities, 49
board and care homes, 46-47
care management, 70
children, 40, 133, 217
elderly persons, 2, 38, 290
nursing home patients, 7, 43, 84, 85, 86,
    116
residential care, 46-47, 166, 203-204
see also Dementia; Developmental
    disabilities; Mental retardation

Community-based services, 3, 6-7, 8, 16, 27,
    100-108
adult foster care homes, 45, 49-50, 94-95,
    164, 250
advocacy, 174
assisted living facilities
board and care homes, 10, 45-47, 64, 68,
    91-92, 124, 163-169, 202-203
consumer-centered services, 29, 105-108,
    131, 209
defined, 9, 41-42, 45, 91
demographics of users, 39
developmentally disabled persons, 24,
    54, 95-96
elderly persons, 37, 48(n.6), 52, 54, 55,
    92-94, 126-127, 131
functional status, 91
group homes, 41, 45, 49-50, 71, 94, 250
licensure, 45
Medicaid, 16, 22, 55, 66-67, 70, 101-103,
    106, 125-127, 164, 235-236
personal attendant services, 29
residential care, 22, 41, 45-50, 91-96
state government role, 8, 45, 91, 289-290
see also Assisted living; Home and
    community-based services
    organizations
Community Health Accreditation Program,
    171
Complaints and complaint resolution, 19,
    136, 138
advocacy, promotion of, 177
home health care, 170
Long-Term Care Ombudsman Program,
    11, 79, 175-176
nursing homes, 79, 115, 144, 153, 162
Confidence Satisfaction Survey, 85
Connecticut, 244
Consumer Assessment of Health Plans, 134
Consumer attitudes, 5, 6, 22, 29-30, 31, 89,
    94, 107, 108, 109, 127-131, 136,
    174, 249
Consumer-centered care, 7, 28, 29, 31-34,
    71-72, 75-76, 106-107, 138, 214,
    249-250, 288-293
assessment instrument design, 127-132
care management, 29, 71-72
children, 71-72
decision making, general, 7, 28, 88-
    89(n.3), 166
defined, 29, 288, 289

Department of Health and Human
Services role, 18, 108, 289
elderly persons, 29
financial issues, general, 29, 33
home and community-based health
care, 29, 105-108, 109, 131
home care, 29, 71, 128, 131
home health care agencies, 128, 209
informal care, 29, 71, 128, 131
information systems, 8, 32, 110
nursing homes, 31, 32, 71, 88-89(n.3),
131, 148, 222, 289
personal care services, 29, 250
professional education, 29, 71
providers, general, 29, 33-34, 214
quality of life, 29, 32-33
regulatory issues, 33, 136, 138, 148, 165-
166, 170
research funding, 18, 108, 289-290
state government role, 18, 108, 289
see also Advocacy; Complaints and
complaint resolution
Consumer Consortium on Assisted Living,
202, 204-205
Continence care, *see* Incontinence
Continuing Care Retirement Communities,
42
Contracting practices, 9, 25, 33, 136, 165-
166, 170, 249
home health care fraud, 96-97
Contractures, 78
Cost and cost-effectiveness, 15, 16-17, 22,
63-64, 223, 227, 236-239, 242
assessment instrument categories for,
115, 127
assisted living, 93, 94
board and care homes, 46
clinical practice guidelines, 15, 221, 232
home health care, 63-64, 97-98, 205, 242
nursing homes, 1, 63-64, 89, 90, 115, 162,
194-195, 221-224 (passim), 227,
229-230, 232, 236-238, 242-243
personnel standards and oversight, 13,
194-195, 205, 219
private health insurance, 69
process monitoring technology, 232
regulation, general, 139, 140
standards, 13, 15, 194-195, 219, 205,
221, 232
residential care, 166
see also Funding

Criminal behavior
abuse and neglect, 1, 13, 24, 78, 79, 138,
189, 192, 215-217
legislation, 13, 19, 216-217

D

Day care, 43, 59
Decision making, consumer, general, 7, 28,
291
nursing home residents, 88-89(n.3)
residential care, 166
see also Consumer-centered care
Decubitus ulcers, *see* Pressure sores
Dehydration, 82, 150, 192
Dementia, 40, 43, 49, 83, 86, 113, 204-205,
209, 211, 289
Demographic factors, 39
Baby Boom, 2, 23
educational attainment of care users, 39,
187
marital status, 39
number in long-term care, 1, 2, 22-23, 38
nursing home residents, 39, 43-44
race/ethnicity
see also Age factors; Gender factors
Dental health and care, 113, 116, 143, 182,
184, 189, 191
Department of Health and Human Services
access to care, 18, 20
Agency for Health Care Policy and
Research, 114, 127
assessment instrument development,
127
assisted living, 48(n.6)
board and care homes, 46
Centers for Advancement of Quality in
Long-Term Care, 20, 234
consumer-centered care research, 18,
108, 289
home and community-based services,
103
Medicaid/Medicare reimbursement
research, 20, 238
National Center for Health Statistics, 37
nursing home staff study, 192
organizational capacity research, 20,
233-234
see also Health Care Financing
Administration
Department of Justice, 103

Department of Veterans Affairs, 3, 25, 81
    see also Veterans Administration
Depression, 116, 133
Developmental disabilities, 24, 40, 41, 71,
        95-96, 201, 211, 290
    board and care homes, 46, 71
    community-based services, 24, 54, 95-96
    defined, 24(n.2)
    home and community-based services
        organizations, 54
    state government role, 24, 96
    see also Mental retardation
Diet, *see* Nutrition
Dignity, *see* Privacy and dignity
Dispute resolution, *see* Complaints and
        dispute resolution
District of Columbia, 101
Drug abuse, *see* Alcohol and drug abuse
Drugs, *see* Medication

E

Economic factors, *see* Cost and cost-
        effectiveness; Employment issues;
        Financial issues; Funding; Health
        insurance; Ownership of facilities;
        Poverty; Wages and salaries
Eden Alternative, 88
Education, *see* Patient education;
        Professional education and
        training; Public education
Educational attainment of care users, 39, 187
Education for All Handicapped Children
        Act, 71
Elderly persons, 2, 23, 40, 164
    abuse and neglect of, 215
    assisted living, 48(n.6), 92-94
    board and care homes, 46, 91, 202-203
    care management, 70
    cognitive impairments, 2, 38, 290
    community-based services, 37, 48(n.6),
        52, 54, 55, 92-94, 126-127, 131
    Continuing Care Retirement
        Communities, 42
    consumer-centered services, 29
    functional status, 2, 38, 59-60
    gender of care users, 2, 38, 43, 46, 51
    geriatric specialists, 12, 62
    home and community-based services
        organizations, 52, 54, 55, 126-127,
        131

home care, 210
home health care, 51, 97-98, 205
informal care, 59-60, 217
number in long-term care, 1, 2, 22-23,
        37, 38, 39, 59
physician training, 62
private insurance, 69
    see also Medicare
Emergency care, *see* Acute care services
Emotional well-being, *see* Mental health
        and illness
Employment issues, 13-14, 19, 60, 180-181,
        211-218
    assisted living, 94
    children in care, training of, 71-72
    criminal background checks, 1, 13, 24,
        78, 79, 138, 189, 192, 215-217
    home health care agencies, 207
    nonelderly adults with disabilities, 55
    number of long-term care workers, 60-
        61, 181
    nursing homes, 12-13, 89, 113, 187, 189,
        194-195, 199, 212, 213
    occupational therapy, 11, 71, 180, 182,
        190, 206, 207
    personal attendants, 55, 209-210
    see also Professional education and
        training; Providers and provider
        quality; Wages and salaries
Ethnicity, *see* Race/ethnicity of care users
External oversight, 9-11, 135-179
    committee recommendations, 18-19
    family members, 9, 11, 128, 135, 166, 174
    mass media, 1, 9, 21, 24, 61, 135, 213
    see also Accreditation; Advocacy;
        Certification; Licensure;
        Regulatory issues; Standards

F

Family members, 3, 7, 27, 36, 59, 60, 69, 95,
        128, 174, 217-218, 249, 250, 288
    child health care, 104, 105
    coordination of services, 70-72
    counseling of, 62
    dementia patients, 86
    external oversight and, 9, 11, 128, 135,
        166, 174
    of nursing home residents, 86, 87
    personal attendant programs, 55
    residential care, 166

social services defined, 27
see also Children and young adults;
  Informal care
Financial issues, 15-17, 20, 36, 62-69, 235-252
  adult foster care and small group
    homes, 49-50, 94
  assisted living, 94
  board and care homes, 46, 47
  casemix reimbursement, 19, 240-241
  consumer-centered care, 29, 33
  contracting practices, 9, 25, 33, 136, 165-
    166, 170, 249
  home care, 16, 62, 63-64, 247
  home health care, 63, 99, 100, 242, 243-244
  informal caregivers, 60, 63, 69
  information systems, 110
  nursing homes, 62, 63-64, 236-238, 242-
    243
  social services defined, 27
  see also Cost and cost-effectiveness;
    Funding; Health Care Financing
    Administration; Health insurance;
    Medicaid; Medicare; Regulatory
    issues; Wages and salaries
Fines and penalties, 10, 18, 137
  federal government, general, 10, 18, 137,
    141-142, 148, 153-156, 158, 159-161
  home health care agencies, 172-173
  nursing homes, 10, 18, 137, 141-142, 148,
    153-156, 158-162
  residential care facilities, 165
Florida, assisted living, 93
Food, *see* Nutrition
Foreign countries, *see* International
    perspectives; *specific countries*
Foundation for Accountability, 134
France, 107
Friends, 3, 27, 59, 60
  see also Informal care
Functional mobility
  board and care homes, 47
  defined, 27
  nursing home residents, 5, 7-8, 12, 76,
    229-230
  physical therapy, 11, 12, 51, 53, 54, 61,
    71, 182, 190
  residential care, 76, 125
Functional status, 36, 37, 39, 75, 127
  adult foster care homes, 94-95
  assisted living, 47, 49
  board and care homes, 46

children, 133
community-based residential care, 91
defined, 27
elderly persons, 2, 38, 59-60
home health care, 97, 98
informal care, 59-60
information systems on, 113
nursing home residents, 45, 79, 84, 94-
  95, 113, 116, 176, 189, 224
Resident Assessment Instrument (RAI),
  7-8, 116, 125
staffing and, 12, 189
see also Developmental disabilities;
  Incontinence; Personal care
  services
Funding, 64-69, 75, 233-234
  access to care, research, 18
  advocacy, 19, 175-176
  assessment instrument development/
    use, 119-120, 127, 152, 153
  consumer-centered care research, 18,
    108, 289-290
  home and community-based services
    organizations, 55, 120, 138
  Medicaid/Medicare reimbursement
    research, 20, 238
  nursing home assessment, 119-120, 152,
    153, 195-196
  organizational capacity, 20
  public education, 19
  regulatory accountability and, 18, 138
  residential facilities assessment, 127
  standards and, general, 136
  state survey regulations and
    certification, 18
  see also Financial issues; Medicaid;
    Medicare

G

Gender factors, 38, 39, 46
  consumer satisfaction, 129
  home care, 51
  informal caregivers, 59
General Accounting Office, 68
  assisted living, 93, 94, 202, 249
  home and community-based services,
    126-127
  home health care, 96-97, 99-100, 169,
    170-171, 172-173, 243

nursing homes, 68, 76, 77-78, 145, 148, 150-151, 152-153, 158, 160, 161
residential care, 93, 94, 163, 165-166, 202
Germany, 107
Government Accounting Office, 229
Government role, *see* Advocacy; Regulatory issues
Group homes, 41, 45, 49-50, 71, 250
licensure, 49, 94

H

HCBS, *see* Home and community-based services organizations
Health Care Financing Administration (HFCA), 3-4, 25, 137, 178, 182, 242, 244
certification requirements, 10, 18
developmentally disabled persons, 96
home and community-based care, 66
home health care, 7, 96-99, 169-173
nursing home care, 3-4, 7, 12, 18, 25, 42, 79, 86, 119, 142, 195
nursing home personnel, 12, 19, 184-187, 192, 193, 195-196, 201
On-line Survey Certification and Reporting (OSCAR) System, 7, 12, 76, 77, 81-82, 90, 112-115, 153, 183, 187, 236-237
personal care services, 101-103
Resident Assessment Instrument, 7-8, 111, 115-120, 124-125, 128
see also Minimum data set
see also Medicaid; Medicare
Health insurance, 4, 69
elderly persons, 69
external oversight, 9
home health care, 63
information systems, 110
nursing home care, 63, 64
see also Managed care
Health Insurance Portability and Accountability Act, 216
Health Plan Employer Data and Information Set, 133
Hearing impairments, *see* Auditory impairments
Historical perspectives, 21-22, 220-221, 250-251, 252
attitudes of caregivers, 228-229
care management, 58

consumer-centered care, 28
developmentally disabled persons, 95
home health care, 169
number in care, various settings, 2, 37, 38, 43, 169
nursing homes, 25, 42-43, 44, 110-111, 141-144, 150, 153-154, 235
professional licensure, 136
HIV/AIDS, 4, 34, 54, 102, 209, 211
Home and community-based services organizations, 3, 52, 54-59, 100-108, 109, 125-127, 179
advocacy, 55, 58, 67
children, 58, 104-105, 210
consumer-centered services, 29, 105-108, 109, 131
defined, 41-42
developmentally disabled persons, 24, 54, 95-96
elderly persons, 37, 48(n.6), 52, 54, 55, 92-94, 126-127, 131
employment issues, 60, 61
General Accounting Office studies, 126-127
Medicaid, 55, 66-67, 70, 101-103, 106, 125-127, 164, 235-236
Medicare, 55, 103
nonelderly adults, 55, 59
nursing home care, avoidance of, 100-101
regulatory issues, 102-103, 138
state government role, 54-58, 66-67, 68, 69, 101-103, 111, 125-127, 238, 246
see also Personal care services
Home care, 1, 3, 6, 16, 22, 25, 50-52, 53, 96-100, 109, 135-136, 138
attitudes toward, 31
casemix, 122
children, 210
consumer-centered services, 29, 71, 128, 131
elderly persons, 210
financing of, general, 16, 62, 63-64, 247
gender factors, 51
Medicaid, 7, 22, 51, 52, 55, 63, 64, 70
Medicare, 7, 16, 22, 50, 51, 52, 63, 64, 97-98, 99-100, 109
Resident Assessment Instrument, 111
number and number of residents, 43, 50-51, 169
On-line Survey Certification and Reporting (OSCAR) System, 7

Outcome and Assessment Information Set (OASIS), 8, 96, 97, 120-122, 128, 171
personnel, general, 13, 51, 53, 61, 180, 209-210, 214
personnel standards, 11, 96-97, 167
state government role, 96, 97, 173, 238
surveys, 37, 173
    see also "On-line..." and "Outcome..." supra
see also Assisted living; Informal care
Home health care agencies, 3, 50-52, 55, 70, 290-291
administrators, 96, 208
adolescents, 104-105
board and care homes, 10, 45-47, 64, 68, 71, 91-92, 124, 163-169, 202-203
children, 104-105, 207-208
certification, 7, 8, 43, 51, 52, 97, 171-172, 173-174, 206, 207, 208
consumer-centered care, 128, 209
cost factors, 63-64, 97-98, 205, 242
defined, 206
elderly persons, 51, 97-98, 205
employment issues, 207
financial issues, general, 63, 99, 100, 242, 243-244
functional status, 97, 98
General Accounting Office studies, 96-97, 99-100, 169, 170-171, 172-173, 243
Health Care Financing Administration, 7, 96-99, 169-173
hospitalization, 50
inspection of facilities, 170
licensed practical nurses, 51, 54, 61, 208
licensure, 7, 172, 173-174, 207
Medicaid, 43, 50, 170-171, 174, 207, 216
Medicare, 6, 8, 43, 50, 169-171, 172, 174, 206, 207, 208, 216, 236, 243
multi-facility organizations, 51
nurses, general, 51, 53, 54, 98-99, 100, 104, 206, 207, 208
nursing aides, 54
nutrition, 53, 54, 59, 68
outcomes, general, 8, 97-98
ownership of facilities, 51, 52, 53, 99
paraprofessional personnel, 51, 54, 181, 208-209, 291
patient education, 99
personnel and personnel standards, 181, 205-209, 212-213, 216

physical and chemical restraints, 206
physicians, 53, 54, 206
privacy and dignity, 207, 209
private insurance, 63
professional education, 206, 207-209
registered nurses, 51, 54, 61, 169-173, 206, 207, 208, 213, 291
regulation and standards, facilities, 167-168, 169-173, 206-209
state government role, 168, 170, 171, 173-174, 207, 208-209, 238
time factors, 50, 106, 121, 123, 208, 209
voluntary, 51, 52, 53, 54
see also Personal care services
Homeless persons, 46(n.4)
Hospice care, 37, 42, 50, 51, 52, 53, 54, 216
Hospitals and hospitalization
acute care services, 28, 124, 129, 182
financial issues, general, 63
home health care and, 50
labor force, 61
managed care, 45
Medicaid, 65
Medicare, 64
nursing home residents hospitalized, 84, 89, 188, 190, 195
nursing homes, hospital based, 44, 63, 82, 183, 185
nursing staff, 187, 192
Housebound and Aid and Attendance Allowance Programs, 29, 106
Housekeeping personnel, 11, 51, 60, 63, 77, 88, 95, 180, 183, 184

I

Illinois, 209, 244
Improving the Quality of Care in Nursing Homes, 3, 21
Incontinence
board and care homes, 47
nursing homes, 82-83, 108, 113, 188, 223, 228, 229-230
Individualization of care, 6, 28, 29, 127-128, 189, 229
Individuals with Disabilities Act, 71
Informal care, 3, 7, 11, 37, 41, 59-60, 217-218, 249
children, 217
consumer-centered care, 29, 71, 128, 131
defined, 27

demographics of caregivers, 59-60
elderly persons, 59-60, 217
financial issues, 60, 63, 69
functional status, 59-60
gender factors, 59
nonelderly adults, 60
number using, 1-2, 38
religious organizations, 3, 59
social services defined, 27
training, 218
see also Paraprofessionals; Volunteers
and voluntary organizations
Information systems, 7-9, 14, 31, 33, 110-
134, 224-227
advocacy, promotion of, 177
assessment instrument design/use
issues, 8-10, 18, 37, 40, 47, 109,
117-123 (passim), 127-134, 143-
144, 150-152
assisted living, 94, 109
community-based residential care, 45
consumer-centered, 8, 32, 110
education of caregivers, 218
financial issues, general, 110
managed care, 110, 111
mass media, 1, 9, 21, 24, 61, 135, 213
nursing home surveys of, 18, 37, 42,
142-153
Outcome and Assessment Information
Set (OASIS), 8, 96, 97, 120-122,
128, 171
quality of care, general, 3, 31, 33
Resident Assessment Instrument (RAI),
7-8, 111, 115-120, 124-125, 128
see also Minimum data set
see also Internet; Public education
In-Home Supportive Services Program, 55,
68
Injuries, *see* Safety issues
Inspection of facilities
home health care, 170
nursing homes, 18, 37, 42, 76, 81, 82, 84-
87, 90, 112, 113, 114-115, 137, 142-
158
residential care, 165, 166
Institutional care, 32
attitudes of professionals in, 28
children in, 40
defined, 3, 41
number in care, 2, 37, 38, 40
special care units, 22, 43, 65, 113, 241-244

see also Nursing homes
Institutional factors, *see* Organizational and
institutional factors
Insurance, *see* Health insurance; Managed
care; Medicaid; Medicare
Intermediate care, 4, 34, 37, 41, 42(n.2), 43,
216
International perspectives
home and community-based care, 107
see also specific countries
Internet
nursing homes, On-line Survey
Certification and Reporting
(OSCAR) System, 7, 12, 76, 77,
81-82, 90, 112-115, 153, 183, 187,
236-237
nursing homes, other, 161
Irvine Health Foundation, 3, 25

J

Joint Commission on Accreditation of
Healthcare Organizations, 171,
178, 223

K

Kansas, 209

L

Language therapy, *see* Speech and
language therapy
Legislation
Americans with Disabilities Act, 29, 103
Balanced Budget Act, 16, 51, 193, 235,
236, 241-244
criminal background, provider checks,
13, 19, 216-217
Education for All Handicapped
Children Act, 71
Health Insurance Portability and
Accountability Act, 216
home and community-based services,
102-103, 216
Individuals with Disabilities Act, 71
Medicare Catastrophic Coverage Act, 45
Nursing Home Reform Act, 25, 142-143,
174, 176, 250-251

Older Americans Act, 11, 54, 59, 68
  Long-Term Care Ombudsman
    Program, 11, 79, 175-176
Omnibus Budget Reconciliation Acts
    (OBRA), 3, 5-6, 7-8, 12, 14, 15, 16,
    21, 25, 45, 79, 80, 81, 83, 90, 95,
    108, 139-144 (passim), 150, 151,
    153-154, 161, 162, 170, 171, 179,
    182, 187, 190, 192-193, 206, 221,
    224, 233, 234, 247
  Patient Abuse Prevention Act
    (proposed), 216
  Patient Self-Determination Act, 29
  Rehabilitation Act, 55
  Resident Assessment Instrument (RAI),
    7-8, 111, 115-120, 124-125, 128
    see also Minimum data set
  Social Security Act, 66, 68, 163, 206, 207
    see also Supplemental Security
      Income program
  see also Regulatory issues
Licensed practical nurses (LPNs), 11, 60,
    180, 216
  board and care homes, 202
  care management, 70
  education, 196-197
  home health care, 51, 54, 61, 208
  number of, 61
  nursing homes, 89, 61, 113, 182, 183,
    187, 188-189, 196, 200, 201, 212,
    213
  wages, 194, 213
Licensure, 4, 9, 10, 135, 137, 172,
  board and care homes, 202, 203
  home health care agencies, 7, 172, 173-
    174, 207
  Medicaid, 7, 174, 207
  Medicare, 7, 174, 207
  nursing homes, 7, 89, 182
  personal care attendants, 210
  residential care facilities, 45, 47, 49, 92,
    94, 137, 163, 164, 165, 202
  state survey activities, 42, 137, 142-163,
    164
  see also Licensed practical nurses;
    Registered nurses
Local services, *see* Community-based
    services
Long-term care, defined, 1, 3, 27-28, 36
Long-Term Care Ombudsman Program, 11,
    79, 175-176

M

Maine, 101, 124
Managed care, 22, 69
  Medicaid, 22, 69, 70, 111
  Medicare, 22, 45, 50, 69
  nursing homes, 45, 200-201
  information systems, 110, 111
Marital status, 39
Massachusetts, 101, 226
Mass media, 1, 9, 21, 24, 61, 135, 213
Maternal and Child Health programs, 58
MDS, *see* Minimum data set
Medicaid, 4, 8, 15-17, 20, 136-137, 214, 235-
    247
  adult foster care and small group
    homes, 49-50, 94
  advocacy, 67
  assisted living, 293
  board and care homes, 163
  certification, 7, 8, 10, 17, 44, 47, 49, 51,
    174, 178, 207
  community-based services, 16, 22
    home and community-based care,
      55, 66-67, 70, 101-103, 106, 125-
      127, 164, 235-236
  home care, 7, 22, 51, 52, 55, 63, 64, 70
  home health care agencies, 43, 50, 170-
    171, 174, 207, 216
  hospitalization, 65
  incentives, 4, 244
  licensure, 7, 174, 207
  managed care, 22, 69, 70, 111
  nursing homes, 10, 15-17, 19, 20, 42(n.3),
    43, 44, 63, 64, 67, 70, 80, 142, 161,
    235, 239-240, 244-246
    external oversight, 9, 10, 18, 42, 137,
      142-153
    personnel, general, 183, 185-187,
      193-195, 237
    personnel standards, 182, 193, 198,
      201, 215, 216
    Resident Assessment Instrument
      (RAI), 7-8, 111, 115-120
    state survey and certification, 18, 42,
      137, 143-153
  On-line Survey Certification and
    Reporting (OSCAR) System, 7,
    12, 76, 77, 81-82, 90, 112-115, 153,
    183, 187, 236-237
  personal care services, 55, 56-57, 66, 67,
    101-103, 106

research funding, 20, 238
residential care, 70, 96, 202, 204, 293
state government, 10, 16, 17, 18, 19, 20,
   42, 55, 56-57, 65, 66-67, 68, 69, 80,
   101-103, 111, 125-127, 136, 137,
   142-153, 170, 174, 207, 236, 238-
   241, 246, 251
see also Home and community-based
   service organizations
Medical records, 153
Medicare, 4, 64-65, 69, 136-137, 214, 236,
   239-240, 251
assisted living, 293
certification, 7, 8, 10, 44, 47, 49, 51, 52,
   174, 178, 207
Department of Health and Human
   Services research, 20, 238
historical perspectives, 22
home and community-based services,
   55, 103
home care, 7, 16, 22, 50, 51, 52, 63, 64,
   97-98, 99-100, 109
home health care agencies, 6, 8, 43, 50,
   169-171, 172, 174, 206, 207, 208,
   216, 236, 243
hospitalization, 64
licensure, 7, 174, 207
managed care, 22, 45, 50, 69
nursing homes, 10, 16, 42(n.3), 43, 44-45,
   63, 64-65, 142, 161, 236, 240, 242-
   243
   certification, 42(n.3), 43-44
   external oversight, 9, 10, 18, 42, 137,
      142-153
   On-line Survey Certification and
      Reporting (OSCAR) System, 7,
      12, 76, 77, 81-82, 90, 112-115, 153,
      183, 187, 236-237
   personnel, general, 183-187, 195
   personnel standards, 182, 193, 197-
      198, 201, 216
   prospective payment system, 16, 20,
      22, 50, 63, 65, 96-99 (passim), 117,
      118, 122, 185, 186. 236, 238-244
      (passim)
research funding, 20, 238
residential care, 202, 204, 293
state government, 10, 16, 18, 42, 97, 136,
   142-153, 170, 174, 207, 240-241, 251
survey and certification, 18, 42, 137,
   143-153

Medicare Catastrophic Coverage Act, 45
Medicare Payment Advisory Commission
   (MedPAC), 241-242, 243
Medication, 10, 121, 291
assisted living, 93, 166
board and care homes, 46, 91-92, 202,
   203
nursing homes, 143, 182, 184, 191, 199,
   241
see also Physical and chemical restraints
Men, see Gender factors
Mental health and illness, 24, 40
adult foster care homes, 94
assessment instruments, 7-8, 9, 127, 133
assisted living facilities, 49
board and care homes, 46
children, 133
depression, 116, 133
family members, counseling, 62
home and community-based services
   organizations, 53-54
home health care, 53
nursing home care, 7-8, 43, 45, 113, 116,
   184, 199
residential care, 46, 164
see also Dementia; Physical and
   chemical restraints
Mental retardation, 4, 34, 37, 40, 41, 164,
   201, 216
advocacy, 177
developmental disability defined,
   34(n.7)
group homes, 45
special education for children, 71
Methodology, see Research methodology
Michigan, 101, 244
Minimum data set (MDS)
integrated assessment instruments, 126
nursing homes, 8, 14, 15, 76, 90, 116-120,
   149, 150, 221, 225-227
residential care, 124-125
Minnesota, nursing homes, 80, 189, 245,
   246
Minorities, see Race/ethnicity of care users
Missouri, 101
Mobility, see Functional mobility
Multi-facility organizations
home health care, 51
nursing homes, 10, 43, 44, 149-150, 243

N

National Center for Health Statistics, 37, 42, 123
National Citizens' Coalition for Nursing Home Reform, 191
National Council on Quality Assurance, 134
National Health Interview Survey, 37(n.1)
National Health Provider Inventory, 45
National Home Health Agency Prospective Payment Demonstration, 96
National Institutes of Health, 85
National League for Nursing, 171
National Long-Term Care Survey, 37(n.1), 59, 246
National Nursing Home Survey, 42
National Study of Assisted Living for the Frail Elderly, 48(n.6)
Netherlands, 107
New Hampshire, 209
New Jersey, 209, 293
New York State, 200, 241
Nonelderly adults, 2, 24, 38-40
    adult foster care homes, 45, 49-50, 94-95, 164, 250
    advocacy, 174-175
    care management, 59
    diseases requiring care, 40
    home and community-based services organizations, 55, 59
    informal care, 60
    number in long-term care, 1, 23, 39
North Carolina, 124, 125
North Dakota, 101, 245
Nurses and nursing, general, 12-13, 17, 18, 65, 70, 89, 212
    adult foster care homes, 95
    assisted living facilities, 49, 93
    board and care homes, 46, 202-203
    care management, 58
    education and training, 156, 196-198, 202-203
    home health care, 51, 53, 54, 98-99, 100, 104, 206, 207, 208
    hospitals, 187, 192
    nursing homes, 113, 142, 143, 183-195, 230, 237
    pressure sores, 80-81
    residents-to-nurses ratios, 12, 187, 190, 191, 192

    see also Licensed practical nurses; Nursing assistants; Registered nurses
Nursing assistants (NAs), 11, 12, 17, 60-61, 180, 212, 215-216
    board and care homes, 202-203
    education, 156, 197-198, 202-203
    home health care, 54
    nursing homes, 61, 88, 113, 143, 188, 189, 190, 191, 192, 212, 229, 232
    wages, 194, 213, 214
Nursing Home Casemix and Quality Demonstration project, 117, 118
Nursing Home Casemix and Quality Demonstration Resident Status Measurement, 118
Nursing Home Reform Act, 25, 142-143, 176, 250-251
Nursing homes, 1, 2, 5-6, 12-16 (passim), 20, 24, 41, 42-45, 76-90, 108, 244-246, 250-251
    accreditation, 7, 42, 43, 44, 76, 89, 140-141, 161-162, 182
    administrators and administration, 143, 161-162, 182, 184, 191, 196-197, 198-202, 212, 242-243
    advocacy, 148, 161, 162, 176-177, 191
    bathroom facilities, 88, 229-230
    care management, 70, 71
    casemix, 19, 74, 88, 90, 114, 117, 118, 123-124, 182, 188-195 (passim)
    casemix reimbursement, 19, 240-241
    certification, 7, 42, 43, 44, 76, 89, 140-141, 161-162, 182
    children, visits to homes, 88
    clinical practice guidelines, 14, 15, 221-222, 224, 226-228
    cognitive factors, 7, 43, 84, 85, 86, 116
    complaints and complaint resolution, 79, 115, 144, 153, 162
    consumer-centered care, 31, 32, 71, 88-89(n.3), 131, 148, 222, 289
    cost factors, 1, 63-64, 89, 90, 115, 162, 194-195, 221-224 (passim), 227, 229-230, 232, 236-238, 242-243
    definitional issues, 42(n.3), 221, 250
    dementia patients, 40, 43, 83, 86, 113, 204-205, 209, 211, 289
    demographics of users, 39, 43-44

Department of Health and Human Services study, 192
employment issues, 12-13, 89, 113, 187, 189, 194-195, 199, 212, 213
family members, 86, 87
financing of care, general, 62, 63-64, 236-238, 242-243
functional mobility, 5, 7-8, 12, 76, 229-230
functional status, general, 45, 79, 84, 94-95, 113, 116, 176, 189, 224
General Accounting Office studies, 68, 76, 77-78, 145, 148, 150-151, 152-153, 158, 160, 161
Health Care Financing Administration, 3-4, 7, 12, 18, 25, 42, 79, 86, 119, 142, 195
    personnel, 12, 19, 184-187, 192, 193, 195-196, 201
    state survey and certification, 18, 42, 137, 143-163
historical perspectives, 25, 42-43, 44, 110-111, 141-144, 150, 153-154, 235
home and community-based services and avoidance of, 100-101
hospital-based, 44, 63, 82, 183, 185
hospitalization of residents, 84, 89, 188, 190, 195
incontinence, 82-83, 108, 113, 188, 223, 228, 229-230
information systems, 110, 122-123, 223-227
inspection of facilities, 18, 37, 42, 78, 81, 82, 84-87, 90, 112, 113, 114-115, 137, 142-158
Internet, 161
licensure, 7, 89, 182
managed care, 45, 200-201
Medicaid, *see* Medicaid, nursing homes
Medicare, *see* Medicare, nursing homes
medication, 143, 182, 184, 191, 199, 241
mental health and illness, 7-8, 43, 45, 113, 116, 184, 199; *see also* *"dementia patients" supra*
multi-facility organizations, 10, 43, 44, 149-150, 243
number in care, 1, 2, 22-23, 37, 39, 42, 43
nutrition, 77, 78, 82, 85, 113, 116, 142, 143, 150, 153, 182, 184, 188, 191-192, 198, 229, 230

On-line Survey Certification and Reporting (OSCAR) System, 7, 12, 76, 77, 81-82, 90, 112-115, 153, 183, 187, 236-237
organizational factors, 14, 200, 221-234
outcomes of care, general, 4, 7-8, 14, 15, 17, 80-81, 223
ownership of facilities, 44, 47, 88, 113, 114, 149-150
pain and pain management, 77, 78, 80, 83-84, 150
personnel, 12, 15, 17, 19, 79, 89, 90, 114-115, 149, 180, 183-201, 212, 213, 223-224, 228-232, 237
    education and training, 156, 187, 196-201, 223
    licensed practical nurses, 61, 89, 113, 182, 183, 187, 188-189, 196, 200, 201, 212, 213
    nurses, general, 113, 142, 143, 183-195, 230, 237
    nursing aides, 61, 88, 113, 143, 188, 189, 190, 191, 192, 212, 229, 232
    paraprofessionals, general, 181
    physicians, 113, 143, 199-201
    registered nurses, 61, 113, 182, 183, 187, 188-190, 191, 192-194, 212, 237
    standards, 11, 12, 71, 74, 142, 181, 182-183, 191-198, 201, 215, 216
physical and chemical restraints, 77, 78, 79, 80, 89, 108, 153, 197, 184, 195, 199-202, 251
pressure sores, 77, 78, 79, 80-82, 84, 150, 188, 192, 199
privacy and dignity, 5, 77, 85, 88, 108, 110, 198, 229
private insurance, 63, 64
private sector, 43, 44, 243
quality management systems, 14, 15, 221, 222-223
quality of life, general, 5, 6, 12, 32, 84-90, 108, 142, 143, 155, 156, 192, 231
    pain and pain management, 77, 78, 80, 83-84, 150
race/ethnicity of residents, 39, 43
record keeping, 153, 195-196

regulatory issues, *see* Regulatory issues, nursing homes
research funding, 119-120, 152, 153, 195-196
research methodology, 84-87, 90, 143-144, 150-152, 153
resident councils, 176
Resident Assessment Instrument (RAI), 7-8, 111, 115-120
  minimum data set (MDS), 8, 14, 15, 76, 90, 110, 116-120
resident assessment protocols (RAPs), 8, 115, 225, 226, 227-228
Resource Utilization Groups (RUGs), 117, 118, 184-186, 193
safety issues, 5, 7, 10, 76, 77, 78-79, 85, 86, 142, 153, 155, 156-158, 198
social factors and services, 88, 94, 116, 182, 184, 191
special care units, 22, 43, 113, 241-244
standards, 114, 140-163, 176-177, 182, 191-195, 235
state government, 10, 16, 17, 18, 19, 42, 79, 80, 81, 118, 126, 137, 142-163, 197, 198, 236, 238, 241, 246
subacute care units, 22, 43, 65, 113, 241-244
surveys of, 18, 37, 42, 137, 142-158
time factors, 15, 89, 118, 123, 151, 153, 156, 159, 160, 182, 183-187, 188, 189, 194, 199-200, 226-227, 229-231, 237
volunteers, 44
Nutrition
  assisted living, 48(n.6)
  food handling, 10, 163
  home health care, 53, 54, 59, 68
  nursing homes, 77, 78, 82, 85, 113, 116, 142, 143, 150, 153, 182, 184, 188, 191-192, 198, 229, 230
  regulatory issues, 3, 10, 142, 143, 150, 153
  weight problems, 74, 78, 118, 150

O

OASIS, *see* Outcome and Assessment Information Set
Occupational therapy, 11, 71, 180, 182, 184, 190, 206, 207
Office of the Inspector General, 215-216

Ohio, assisted living, 93
Old age, *see* Elderly persons
Older Americans Act, 11, 54, 59, 68
  Long-Term Care Ombudsman Program, 11, 79, 175-176
Omnibus Budget Reconciliation Acts (OBRA), 3, 5-6, 7-8, 12, 14, 15, 16, 21, 25, 45, 79, 80, 81, 83, 90, 95, 108, 139-144 (passim), 150, 151, 153-154, 161, 162, 170, 171, 179, 182, 187, 190, 192-193, 206, 221, 224, 233, 234, 247
On-line Survey Certification and Reporting (OSCAR) System, 7, 12, 76, 77, 81-82, 90, 112-115, 153, 183, 187, 236-237
Oregon
  adult foster care homes, 94, 95
  assisted living, 93, 293
  board and care homes, 202-203
  nursing homes, 246
  personal attendant programs, 5
Organizational and institutional factors, 2-3, 14-15, 69-72, 180, 220-234
  child care, 70-72, 105
  clinical practice guidelines, 14, 15, 221-222
  coordination of services, 69-72, 105
  family issues, 70-72
  nursing homes, 14, 200, 221-234
  quality management systems, 14, 15, 221, 222-223
  see also Accreditation; Care management; Certification; Community-based services; External oversight; Information systems; Licensure; Managed care; Ownership of facilities; Regulatory issues; Residential care settings; Standards
OSCAR, *see* On-line Survey Certification and Reporting (OSCAR) System
Outcome and Assessment Information Set (OASIS), 8, 96, 97, 120-122, 128, 171
Outcomes of care, 4, 5, 7-9, 33, 74-75, 110-134, 233-234
  chronically poor providers, 18, 111, 141, 148-150, 158-161, 251
    see also Fines and penalties
  consumer-centered care, 74-75
  definitional issues, 8-9, 29-30, 31, 74

home health care, 8, 97-98
nursing homes, 4, 7-8, 14, 15, 17, 80-81,
    223
see also External oversight; Information
    systems
Ownership of facilities, 213
    adult foster homes, 50
    home health care agencies, 51, 52, 53, 99
    hospices, 51, 53
    nursing homes, 44, 47, 88, 113, 114, 149-
        150
    see also Multi-facility organizations

P

Pain and pain management, nursing
    homes, 77, 78, 80, 83-84, 150
Paraprofessionals, 3, 11, 59, 60-61, 180, 181,
    214, 215
    home health care, 51, 54, 181, 208-209, 291
    nursing homes, 181
    regulatory requirements, 9, 138-139
    residential care, 205
    see also Housekeeping personnel;
        Nursing assistants; Personal care
        services
Patient Abuse Prevention Act (proposed), 216
Patient education, 55, 71, 138
    home health care, 99
Penalties, *see* Fines and penalties
Personal care homes, 41, 164, 202
Personal care services, 1, 3, 4, 6, 13, 22, 60,
    101-103, 109
    adult foster care homes, 94, 95
    advocacy, 67, 177
    assisted living, 47, 48(n.6)
    community-based, 29, 54-55, 56-57, 66-
        67, 101
    consumer-centered, 29, 250
    defined, 27
    education of staff, 174
    employment issues, 55, 209-210
    family members, 55
    Health Care Financing Administration,
        101-103
    licensure, 210
    Medicaid, 55, 56-57, 66, 67, 101-103, 106
    personnel, 61, 174, 209-210, 212
    regulation and standards, 18, 102-103,
        173, 174

state government role, 54-55, 56-57, 66-
    67, 68, 101-103, 174, 209-210
Pharmaceuticals, *see* Medication
Physical and chemical restraints, 3
    board and care homes, 91-92
    community-based residential care, 91
    home health care agencies, 206
    nursing homes, 77, 78, 79-80, 89, 108,
        153, 182, 184, 195, 199-202, 251
    regulations, 3, 6, 139
Physical therapy, 11, 12, 51, 53, 54, 61, 71,
    182, 190
Physicians, 11, 51, 62, 125
    board and care homes, 203
    education and training, 61, 62, 199-201
    home health care, 53, 54, 206
    nursing homes, 113, 143, 199-201
Poverty, *see* Medicaid; Supplemental
    Security Income program
Practice guidelines, *see* Clinical practice
    guidelines
Pressure sores, 123
    nursing homes, 77, 78, 79, 80-82, 84, 150,
        188, 192, 199
Primary care, 28
Privacy and dignity, 5, 6, 10, 71, 76, 288
    assisted living, 47, 49, 92-93
    contracting practices, 9, 25, 33, 136, 165-
        166, 170, 249
    home health care agencies, 207, 209
    nursing homes, 5, 77, 85, 88, 108, 110,
        198, 229
    residential care, 164, 169
    see also Bathroom facilities; Physical and
        chemical restraints
Private sector, general, 22, 70
    adult foster care and small group
        homes, 50
    home health care, 51, 52, 53
    hospice care, 51, 53
    nursing homes, 43, 44, 243
    residential care, 108, 166-167
    state collaboration in information
        dissemination, 18
    see also Assisted living; Board and care
        homes; Health insurance;
        Managed care; Multi-facility
        organizations; Ownership of
        facilities

Professional education and training, 13, 19, 60, 74, 139, 180, 181, 210-211, 215, 234
  administrators, 196-197, 198-202, 208
  assessment instruments, surveyors, 8, 115, 117, 152-153
  assisted living, 93
  child care, 61, 104-105
  consumer-centered services, 29, 71
  home health care, 206, 207-209
  informal caregivers, 218
  nursing aides, 156, 197-198, 202-203
  nursing home personnel, 156, 187, 196-201, 223
  personal care, 174
  physicians, 62, 199-201
  registered and licensed practical nurses, 196-197
  residential care staff, 93, 166, 168, 202-203, 204-205
  standards, 19, 71, 181
Program of All-Inclusive Care for the Elderly, 70
Proprietary care facilities, see Private sector
Prospective payment system, 16, 20, 22, 50, 63, 65, 96-99 (passim), 117, 118, 122, 185-187, 236, 238-244 (passim)
Providers and provider quality, 1, 3, 4, 10, 11-14, 41-62, 180-219
  accountability, general, 33
  attitudes, 28, 187, 195, 228-229, 232
  chronically poor providers, 10, 18, 111, 137, 141-142, 148-150, 153-156, 158-162, 251
  criminal behavior by providers, 1, 13, 24, 78, 79, 138, 189, 192, 215-217
  day care, 43, 59
  personnel standards, 11, 12, 13, 19, 71, 74, 96-97, 142, 167, 180-219 (passim)
    assisted living, 202, 203-204
    cost factors, 13, 205, 194-195, 219
    federal government, general, 11, 181, 182-183, 191-194
    home health care agencies, 181, 205-209, 212-213, 216
    Medicaid, 182, 193, 198, 201, 215, 216
    Medicare, 182, 193, 197-198, 201, 216
    nursing homes, 11, 12, 71, 74, 142, 181, 182-183, 191-198, 201, 215, 216

    personal care services, 18, 102-103, 173, 174
    residential care, general, 202-203
    state, 11, 19, 181, 182-183, 202, 215-216
    personnel-to-residents ratios, 12, 187, 190, 191, 192, 202
    staffing issues, general, 11-14, 19, 32, 61, 109, 112, 113, 114-115, 134, 163
    standards, facilities, 11, 33-34, 135-179
Psychological factors, see Mental health and illness
Psychotropic medications, see Physical and chemical restraints
Public education, 3, 19, 249, 292
  advocacy and, 175, 177
  children, 133
  children, special education, 71
  mass media, 1, 9, 21, 24, 61, 135, 213
  social services defined, 27

Q

Quality management systems, 14, 15, 221, 222-223
Quality of life, general, 10, 12-13, 20, 23, 42, 74, 179, 234, 287-288
  adult foster care homes, 95
  advocacy, 176
  attitudes and, 29-30
  board and care homes, 46, 92
  consumer-centered care, 29, 32-33
  cultural attitudes, 22
  defined, 29-30, 84
  nursing homes, 5, 6, 12, 32, 84-90, 108, 142, 143, 155, 156, 192, 231
  pain and pain management, 77, 78, 80, 83-84, 150
  REAL (real experiences and assessment of life), 85, 86
  regulatory issues, 10, 77, 78, 80, 83-84, 139, 141, 142, 143, 150
  research methodology, 84-87, 90
  residential care, general, 10, 108, 292-293
  see also Functional status; Incontinence; Nutrition; Pressure sores; Privacy and dignity; Safety issues

R

Race/ethnicity of care users, 39
  board and care homes, 46
  consumer satisfaction, 129
  home health care, 51
  nursing homes, 39, 43
RAI, *see* Resident Assessment Instrument
REAL (real experiences and assessment of
    life), 85, 86
Recreational services, 46, 92, 95
Registered nurses (RNs), 11, 60, 180, 216
  board and care homes, 202
  education, 196-197
  home health care, 51, 54, 61, 169-173,
    206, 207, 208, 213, 291
  number of, 61
  nursing homes, 61, 113, 182, 183, 187,
    188-190, 191, 192-194, 212, 237
  wages, 194, 213
Regulatory issues, 3, 4, 5, 7, 9-10, 135, 136-
    140, 291-293
  advocacy and, 177
  arguments for and against regulation,
    138-140
  assisted living, 93, 94, 166
  attitudes of enforcement personnel, 141
  board and care homes, 45, 46, 91, 92,
    163-169
  consumer-centered care, 33, 136, 138,
    148, 165-166, 170
  cost factors, general, 117, 140
  dispute resolution, 144, 162
  funding and, 18, 138
  home and community-based services,
    102-103, 138
  home health care agencies, 167-168, 169-
    173, 206-209
  information systems, 7, 110
  nursing homes, 138, 140-153
    advocacy and, 176-177
    dispute resolution, 144, 162
    federal, 3, 5-6, 7-8, 9, 10-11, 12, 14,
      15, 16, 18, 21, 79, 80, 81, 83, 89,
      90, 136-137, 139-163
    inspection of facilities, 18, 37, 42, 76,
      81, 82, 112, 113, 114-115, 137, 142-
      158
    sanctions for noncompliance, 10, 18,
      137, 141-142, 148, 153-156, 158,
      158-162
    state, 9, 10-11, 18, 20, 89, 140-163

nutrition, 3, 10, 142, 143, 150, 153
On-line Survey Certification and
    Reporting (OSCAR) System, 7,
    12, 76, 77, 81-82, 90, 112-115, 153,
    183, 187, 236-237
  paraprofessionals, general, 9, 138-139
  personal care services, 18, 102-103, 173,
    174
  physical and chemical restraints, 3, 6, 139
  quality of life, 10, 77, 78, 80, 83-84, 139,
    141, 142, 143, 150
  Resident Assessment Instrument (RAI),
    7-8, 111, 115-120
    minimum data set (MDS), 8, 14, 15,
      76, 90, 116-120, 149, 150, 221, 225-
      227
  residential care, 8, 10, 45, 46, 91, 92, 163-
    169, 202-204, 292-293
  sanctions for noncompliance, 10, 18,
    137, 141-142, 148, 153-156, 158,
    159-160
  state survey regulations, 18, 42, 137,
    142-163, 164, 251
  see also Accreditation; Certification;
    Legislation; Licensure; Standards
Rehabilitation Act, 55
Rehabilitation services and facilities, 8, 12,
    22, 30, 41, 55, 64, 65, 77, 79, 89,
    98, 113, 116, 143, 182, 190
  see also Occupational therapy; Physical
    therapy; Speech and language
    therapy
Relatives, *see* Family members
Religious institutions, informal caregivers,
    3, 59
Research methodology, 37
  assessment instruments, 8-10, 18, 37, 40,
    47, 109, 117-123 (passim), 127-
    134, 143-144, 150-152
  nursing home research/inspection
    surveys, 84-87, 90, 143-144, 150-
    152, 153
  quality of life studies, 84-87, 90
  see also Information systems
Resident Assessment Instrument (RAI), 7-8,
    111, 115-120, 124-125, 128
  see also Minimum data set
Resident assessment protocols (RAPs), 8,
    115, 225, 226, 227-228

Residential care settings, 1, 3, 6, 22, 25, 108-
        109, 124-125, 127
    advocacy, 168, 202-203, 293
    casemix, 202
    cognitive factors, 46-47, 166, 203-204
    community-based services, 22, 41, 45-
        50, 91-96
    cost factors, 166
    developmentally disabled persons, 24,
        95-96
    employment, general, 13, 61, 181
    family members, 166
    functional mobility, 76, 125
    functional status, general, 91
    General Accounting Office studies, 93,
        94, 163, 165-166, 202
    group homes, 41, 45, 49-50, 71, 94, 250
    inspection of facilities, 165, 166
    licensure, 45, 47, 49, 91-92, 94, 137, 163,
        164, 165, 202
    Medicaid, 70, 96, 202, 204, 293
    Medicare, 202, 204, 293
    mental health and illness, 46, 164
    minimum data set, 124-125
    number of, 43
    number of residents in, 1-2, 22-23, 43
    paraprofessional personnel, 181
    personnel, 108-109, 181, 202-205
    personnel, education of, 93, 166, 168,
        202-203, 204-205
    personnel standards, 202-203
    privacy and dignity, 164, 169
    quality of life, 10, 108, 292-293
    regulatory issues, 8, 10, 45, 46, 91, 92,
        163-169, 202-204, 292-293
    research funding, 127
    safety, 5, 76, 205
    time factors, 204-205
    see also Adult foster care homes; Assisted
        living; Board and care homes;
        Hospice care; Institutional care
Resource Utilization Groups (RUGs), 117,
        118, 184-186, 193
Respiratory disease, 40
Restraints, see Physical and chemical
        restraints
Rhode Island, 101
Robert Woods Johnson Foundation, 3, 25,
        103, 120

S

Safety issues, 7, 10, 13, 31, 138, 139, 288
    abuse and neglect, 13, 78, 79, 138, 189,
        192, 215-217
    board and care homes, 92, 163
    community-based residential care, 91
    home health care agencies, 205
    nursing homes, 5, 7, 10, 76, 77, 78-79, 85,
        86, 142, 153, 155, 156-158, 198
    residential care, 5, 76, 205
    see also Physical and chemical restraints
Salaries, see Wages and salaries
Sanctions, regulatory, see Complaints and
        complaint resolution; Fines and
        penalties
Securities and Exchange Commission, 213
Social factors and services, 11, 75
    adult foster care homes, 94, 95
    assessment instrument design, 116, 131
    assisted living, 93
    attitudes about long-term care needs, 22
    board and care homes, 92
    care management, 58
    definition of social services, 27
    friends, 3, 27, 59, 60
    funding from 75
    home health care, 53, 54
    number of social workers, 61
    nursing homes, 88, 94, 116, 182, 184, 191
    recreational services, 46, 92, 95
    residential care, 203
    standards of care, 5, 10, 182, 184, 191, 203
    see also Family members; Informal care
Social Security Act, 66, 68, 163, 206, 207
    Social Services Block Grant, 68
    see also Supplemental Security Income
        program
Special care units, 22, 43, 113, 241-244
    Alzheimer's disease, 113
Specialists and specialization, 12, 62, 70,
        104, 124, 187, 189, 190-191, 196
    see also Occupational therapy; Physical
        therapy
Speech and language therapy, 11, 71, 121,
        180, 182, 184, 189, 206, 207
SSI, see Supplemental Security Income
        program

Standards, 3, 5, 9-10, 11, 18, 75, 76, 33-34,
    135-179
  advocacy and, 177
  assessment instruments and
      methodologies, 8-9, 14, 114, 115-
      116, 123
  assisted living, 10, 47, 93, 164, 166, 168-
      169, 202, 203-204, 292-293
  child care, 104-105
  clinical practice guidelines, 14, 15, 221-
      222, 224, 226-228, 232, 234
  cost factors, 13, 15, 194-195, 219, 205,
      221, 232
  definitional issues, substandard quality
      of care, 156, 158-159
  funding for, 136
  home care, 11, 96-97, 167
  home health care agencies, 169-173, 181,
      205-209, 212-213, 216
  inspection of facilities,
    home health care, 170
    nursing homes, 18, 37, 42, 76, 81, 82,
        84-87, 90, 112, 113, 114-115, 137,
        142-158
    residential care, 165, 166
  nursing home audit procedures, 114
  nursing homes, 140-163, 176-177, 182,
      191-195, 235
  personnel, 11, 12, 13, 19, 71, 74, 96-97,
      142, 167, 180-219 (passim)
    assisted living, 202, 203-204
    cost factors, 13, 194 195, 205, 219
    federal government, general, 11, 181,
        182-183, 191-194
    home health care agencies, 181, 205-
        209, 212-213, 216
    Medicaid, 182, 193, 198, 201, 215, 216
    Medicare, 182, 193, 197-198, 201, 216
    nursing homes, 11, 12, 71, 74, 142, 181,
        182-183, 191-198, 201, 215, 216
    personal care services, 18, 102-103,
        173, 174
    residential care, general, 202-203
    state, 11, 19, 181, 182-183, 202, 215-216
  professional education, 19, 71, 181
  purchaser of care, set by, 135
  residential care, 8, 10, 45, 46, 91, 92, 163-
      169, 202-204, 292-293

  sanctions for noncompliance, 10, 18,
      137, 141-142, 148, 153-156, 158,
      159-160
  social factors and services, 5, 10, 182,
      184, 191, 203
  state, 10, 11, 19, 181, 182-183, 202, 215-
      216, 292-293
  substandard facilities and programs, 10,
      18, 137, 141-142, 148-150, 153-156,
      158-162, 251
  voluntary, 137, 171-172, 178, 202-203,
      204-205
  see also Accreditation; Certification;
      Licensure; Outcomes of care;
      Regulatory issues
State Supplemental Payments, 47, 64, 68
Stroke, 40
Subacute care units, 22, 43, 65, 113, 241-244
Supplemental Security Income program, 68
  adult foster care and small group
      homes, 49
  board and care homes, 47, 64, 68, 163
  children, 68
  State Supplemental Payments, 47, 64, 68

T

Tennessee, nursing homes, 80
Texas, 209, 293
Toilet facilities, *see* Bathroom facilities;
      Incontinence
Training, *see* Patient education;
      Professional education and
      training; Public education
Transportation services, 46, 53, 59

U

United Hospital Fund, 213

V

Veterans Administration, 29, 106
  see also Department of Veterans Affairs
Visual impairments, 40, 116

Volunteers and voluntary organizations, 3, 59
    accreditation agencies, 122, 137, 171-172, 178, 223
    children, consumer-centered care, 72
    external oversight, 9
    home health care and hospice facilities, 51, 52, 53, 54
    nursing homes, 44
    religious organizations, 3, 59
    residential care, 168-169
    standards, voluntary, 137, 171-172, 178, 202-203, 204-205
    see also Advocacy; Informal care

W

Wages and salaries, 13-14, 19, 61, 180, 187, 194-195, 210, 211, 213-215, 242
    assisted living, 94
Washington, D.C., *see* District of Columbia
Washington State, 293
Weight problems, 74, 78, 118, 150
Welfare, *see* Medicaid; Supplemental Security Income program
Wisconsin, 245, 246
Women, *see* Gender factors
World Wide Web, *see* Internet